Y0-CCF-756

HANDBOOK OF PSYCHIATRY · 3
PSYCHOSES OF
UNCERTAIN AETIOLOGY

Bc

RC 512 .P745 1982

Psychoses of uncertain aetiology

HANDBOOK OF PSYCHIATRY

General Editor: Professor M. Shepherd

Edited by: Professor N. Garmezy, Dr. L. A. Hersov, Professor M. H. Lader, Professor P. R. McHugh, Professor G. F. M. Russell, Professor J. K. Wing, Professor O. L. Zangwill

Assisted by the Editorial Board and International Advisory Board of *Psychological Medicine*

Volume 1: General psychopathology
Edited by M. Shepherd and O. L. Zangwill

Volume 2: Mental disorders and somatic illness
Edited by M. H. Lader

Volume 3: Psychoses of uncertain aetiology
Edited by J. K. Wing and L. Wing

Volume 4: The neuroses and personality disorders
Edited by G. F. M. Russell and L. A. Hersov

Volume 5: The scientific foundations of psychiatry
Edited by M. Shepherd

Handbook of PSYCHIATRY Volume 3

PSYCHOSES OF UNCERTAIN AETIOLOGY

Parts I and II edited by J. K. Wing
Part III edited by Lorna Wing and
J. K. Wing

CAMBRIDGE UNIVERSITY PRESS
Cambridge
London New York New Rochelle
Melbourne Sydney

RC
512
.P745
1982

Published by the Press Syndicate of the University of Cambridge
The Pitt Building, Trumpington Street, Cambridge CB2 1RP
32 East 57th Street, New York, NY 10022, USA
296 Beaconsfield Parade, Middle Park, Melbourne 3206, Australia

© Cambridge University Press 1982

First published 1982

Printed in the United States of America by
Vail-Ballou Press, Inc., Binghamton, NY

Library of Congress catalogue card number: 81-17092

British Library cataloguing in publication data
Handbook of psychiatry.
Vol. 3: Psychoses of uncertain aetiology
1. Psychiatry
I. Wing, J. K.   II. Wing, Lorna
616.89   RC454
ISBN 0 521 24101 4 hard covers
ISBN 0 521 28438 4 paperback

v

CONTENTS

Contents

Contributors

George Ashcroft, MB, FRCPE, MRC Psych,
Professor of Mental Health,
University Medical Buildings,
Foresterhill, Aberdeen AB9 2ZD, UK

Paul E. Bebbington, MA, MB, MRCP, MRC Psych,
MRC Social Psychiatry Unit,
Institute of Psychiatry,
De Crespigny Park, London SE5 8AF, UK

D. H. Bennett, MD, FRC Psych,
Consultant Psychiatrist,
Bethlem Royal and Maudsley Hospital,
Denmark Hill, London SE5 8AZ, UK

Anthony W. Clare, MD, M.Phil, MRCP, MRC Psych,
Senior Lecturer,
Institute of Psychiatry,
De Crespigny Park, London SE5 8AF, UK

C. Robert Cloninger, MD,
Department of Psychiatry,
Washington University School of Medicine and
Jewish Hospital of St. Louis,
216 South Kingshighway,
St. Louis, Missouri 63110, USA

Donald J. Cohen, MD,
Professor of Pediatrics, Psychiatry and Psychology,
Child Study Center,
Yale University School of Medicine,
333 Cedar Street, New Haven, Connecticut 06510, USA

John A. Corbett, MB, FRC Psych, MRCP,
Consultant Psychiatrist,
Bethlem Royal and Maudsley Hospital,
Denmark Hill, London SE5 8AZ, UK

Uta Frith, PhD,
MRC Developmental Psychology Unit,
Drayton House,
Gordon Street, London WC1H OAN, UK

James L. Gibbons, MD, FRCP, FRC Psych,
Professor of Psychiatry,
Royal South Hants Hospital,
Southampton SO9 4PE, UK

I. I. Gottesman, PhD,
Professor of Psychiatric Genetics,
Departments of Psychiatry and Genetics,
Washington University School of Medicine,
Saint Louis, Missouri 63110, USA

Judith Gould, MPhil, PhD,
MRC Social Psychiatry Unit,
Institute of Psychiatry,
De Crespigny Park, London SE5 8AF, UK

Philip J. Graham, FRCP, FRC Psych,
Professor of Child Psychiatry,
Institute of Child Health,
Great Ormond Street, London WC1N 3JH, UK

D. R. Hanson, PhD,
Postdoctoral Fellow,
Dight Institute for Human Genetics,
University of Minnesota,
Minneapolis, Minnesota 55455, USA

Edward Hare, MD,
Consultant Psychiatrist,
Bethlem Royal and Maudsley Hospital,
Denmark Hill, London SE5 8AZ, UK

Steven R. Hirsch, MD, MPhil, MRCP, FRC Psych,
Professor of Psychiatry,
Charing Cross Hospital Medical School,
Fulham Palace Road, London W6 8RF, UK

Patricia Howlin, PhD,
Departments of Psychology and Child Psychiatry,
Institute of Psychiatry,
De Crespigny Park, London SE5 8AF, UK

I. Kolvin, MD, FRC Psych,
Professor of Child and Adolescent Psychiatry,
Nuffield Psychology and Psychiatry Unit,
Director, Human Development Unit,
Fleming Memorial Hospital, Great North Road,
Newcastle upon Tyne NE2 3AX, UK

Julian P. Leff, MD, MRCP, FRC Psych,
Assistant Director,
MRC Social Psychiatry Unit,
Institute of Psychiatry,
De Crespigny Park, London SE5 8AF, UK

John M. Neale, PhD,
Professor of Psychology,
State University of New York at Stony Brook,
Stony Brook, New York 11794, USA

Thomas F. Oltmanns, PhD,
Assistant Professor of Psychology, Indiana University,
Bloomington, Indiana 47405, USA

E. S. Paykel, MD, FRCP, FRCP Ed, FRC Psych,
Professor of Psychiatry,
St. George's Hospital Medical School,
Cranmer Terrace, London SW17 ORE, UK

Felix Post, MD, FRCP, FRC Psych,
Emeritus Physician,
Bethlem Royal and Maudsley Hospital,
Denmark Hill, London SE5 8AZ, UK

John D. Rainer, MD,
Chief of Psychiatric Research (Genetics),
New York State Psychiatric Institute and
Professor of Clinical Psychiatry,
Department of Psychiatry,
Columbia University,
722 West 168th Street, New York, NY 10032, USA

K. Rawnsley, MB, FRCP, FRC Psych, DPM,
Professor of Psychological Medicine,
Welsh National School of Medicine,
Heath Park, Cardiff CF4 4XN, UK

Theodore Reich, MD,
Professor of Psychiatry and Genetics,
Department of Psychiatry,
Washington University School of Medicine and
Jewish Hospital of St. Louis,
216 South Kingshighway,
St. Louis, Missouri 63110, USA

John Rice, PhD,
Department of Psychiatry,
Washington University School of Medicine and
Jewish Hospital of St. Louis,
216 South Kingshighway, St. Louis, Missouri 63110, USA

D. M. Ricks, MD, MRC Psych,
Children's Department,
Harperbury Hospital,
Harper Lane,
Shenley, Radlett, Herts WD7 9HQ, UK

Richard Rodnight, D Sc,
Professor of Neurochemistry,

Institute of Psychiatry,
De Crespigny Park, London SE5 8AF, UK

Peter Sainsbury, MD, FRCP, FRC Psych,
Director,
MRC Clinical Psychiatry Unit,
Graylingwell Hospital,
Chichester, Sussex PO19 4PQ, UK

Bennett A. Shaywitz, MD,
Associate Professor of Pediatrics and Neurology,
Child Study Center,
Yale University School of Medicine,
333 Cedar Street,
New Haven, Connecticut 06510, USA

Erik Strömgren, MD,
Formerly Professor of Psychiatry,
University of Aarhus,
Psychiatric Hospital, Risskov DK 8240, Denmark

Brian Suarez, PhD,
Department of Psychiatry,
Washington University School of Medicine and
Jewish Hospital of St. Louis,
216 South Kingshighway,
St. Louis, Missouri 63110, USA

J. K. Wing, MD, PhD, FRC Psych, DPM,
Professor of Social Psychiatry and
Director, MRC Social Psychiatry Unit,
Institute of Psychiatry,
De Crespigny Park, London SE5 8AF, UK

Lorna Wing, MD, FRC Psych, DPM,
MRC Social Psychiatry Unit,
Institute of Psychiatry,
De Crespigny Park, London SE5 8AF, UK

J. Gerald Young, MD,
Associate Professor of Pediatrics and Psychiatry,
Child Study Center,
Yale University School of Medicine,
333 Cedar Street,
New Haven, Connecticut 06510, USA

Foreword

The idea of this handbook originated from a survey of the available British books on psychiatry in the late 1960s (1). It became apparent then that the post-war development of the subject as a major, independent branch of medicine had been accompanied by a spate of textbooks and specialized monographs from the rapidly increasing number of academic and clinical departments. The time seemed ripe 'to compile the comprehensive authoritative multi-authored handbook which has yet to appear in this country' (2).

In the event almost another decade was to pass before the enterprise was to be realized. During this time the climate of opinion has come to favour the appearance of a representative statement of what has been termed the 'Maudsley' approach to psychological medicine. Modern British psychiatry, as Lord Taylor has pointed out, is 'largely the product of the Maudsley Hospital' (3). It embodies not so much a national school of opinion as a continuation of the broad, central tradition of psychiatric theory and practice which originated on the European mainland, was transported through the psychobiology of Adolf Meyer to North America and returned to Europe via the United Kingdom, where its pre-eminent representative has been Sir Aubrey Lewis (4). At its core is an adherence to the principles of scientific enquiry in clinical and basic research, with due acknowledgement of the role played by social and psychological investigation as well as by the natural sciences.

The prospects for the production of a handbook were further improved by the creation in 1969 of *Psychological Medicine*, a journal devoted to research in the field of psychiatry and the allied sciences, which brought together an editorial board which has played an important part in this undertaking. The participation of the journal's international advisory board also helped to ensure a wide base for the work which, from its inception, has received sympathetic encouragement from Cambridge University Press.

Why call a handbook what is clearly so much more than a manual or guide which can be held in the hand? If the term is a misnomer it is one which has been blessed by tradition and usage. In the German-speaking countries, where so many of the roots of modern psychiatry are embedded, a *Handbuch* is much weightier than a *Lehrbuch* and the massive volumes associated with the names of Aschaffenburg and Bumke exemplify the fruits of German scholarship at its most diligent. The format has, of course, been applied to other medical disciplines in other languages, largely to meet a need which has been clearly expressed in the preface to the *Handbook of Clinical Neurology*, now comprising some forty volumes: 'only a Handbook designed on the principle of exhaustive, critical, balanced and comprehensive reviews written by acknowledged experts, is in the position of reflecting the state of neurology in the second half of the twentieth century' (5).

While the *Handbook of Psychiatry* has a similar objective, it is less expansive in content and more ambitious in form. An encyclopaedic compilation of all the theories and speculations which impinge on contemporary psychiatry would call for more than forty volumes, but would become outdated very soon. Here we have preferred to concentrate on the fabric of psychological medicine and the loom of observations and concepts on which it has been woven. Accordingly, volumes 2–4 contain the clinical substratum of the subject, flanked by one volume devoted to general psychopathology and another to the various scientific modes of enquiry on which the discipline is founded.

A full list of contents, with titles of chapters and names of authors, is provided in each volume. An outline of the material contained in all five volumes is as follows:

All the volumes are self-contained and edited separately, but they are intended to reinforce one another. Every effort has been made to avoid overlap and duplication of material and the inclusion of cross-references, some in the text and others at the back of each volume, should facilitate the process of integration. The whole is designed to be more than the sum of its parts.

Michael Shepherd
Institute of Psychiatry
October 1980

References

(1) Shepherd, M. (1969) British books on psychiatry, I & II. *British Book News*, Feb/Mar., pp. 85–8 and 167–70

(2) (1980) Psychiatry: personal book list. *Lancet*, i, 937

(3) Taylor, Lord (1962) The public, parliament and mental health. In *Aspects of Psychiatric Research*, ed. Richter, D., Tanner, J. M., Taylor, Lord & Zangwill, O.L., p. 13. London: Oxford University Press.

(4) Shepherd, M. (1977) *The Career and Contributions of Sir Aubrey Lewis*. Bethlem Royal & Maudsley Hospitals

(5) Vinken, P. J. & Bruyn, G. W. (1969) Preface to *Handbook of Clinical Neurology*, vol. I, p. v. Amsterdam: North Holland

Preface

A word of explanation may be necessary concerning the title of this third volume of the *Handbook of Psychiatry*. In conventional usage schizophrenic, paranoid and manic-depressive disorders are grouped under the heading of 'functional psychoses'. Conditions such as early childhood autism and Asperger's syndrome have often been included as well, perhaps because of an assumption that they were related in some way to schizophrenia. Jaspers pointed out that 'we give the term "functional" to those psychic changes for which no physical cause can be found and where at present there is in the somatic sphere no real ground for supposing that such causes exist, and where such a supposition can only rest on the postulate that there must be physical causes for all psychic changes'. Since we do, in fact, now have some useful clues to somatic causes or good grounds for supposing that such causes exist, for most of the so-called 'functional psychoses', the latter term seems inappropriate. On the other hand, to group them under the heading of 'other psychoses', as is done in the ninth revision of the *International Classification of Diseases,* does not solve the problem of a title for this volume.

The term 'psychosis' also needs comment. It has a certain descriptive and clinical utility, but is by no means unambiguous. It is retained in the *International Classification of Diseases* as a generic label and it is used clinically to describe mental states characterized by gross distortions of thought, perception, or affect. But someone with a mild schizophrenic condition may have considerable insight and be well able to function socially, while someone with a 'neurosis' may occasionally act in a blind panic and may become severely socially disabled. Moreover, terms like 'psychosis' and 'neurosis' often carry theoretical connotations since there is a range of holistic theories, both psycho-dynamic and organic, purporting to explain their nature and origins.

These matters are discussed in more detail in volume 1 of this Handbook. The title chosen for volume 3 is descriptive rather than theoretical. The conditions dealt with are the 'psychoses' covered by categories 295–299 of the *International Classification*, ninth revision (schizophrenias, affective psychoses, paranoid states and psychoses with origin specific to childhood). Their causes are indeed still uncertain but the title is intended to indicate that we are not entirely ignorant of aetiology and can with confidence expect further advances in knowledge.

It is a pleasure to acknowledge the contribution made by Miss Christine Durston, Mrs Joan Head, Miss Florence Suggars and Mrs Yvonne Walters during the long process of editing this multi-author volume.

J. K. Wing
June 1981

PART I

Schizophrenia and paranoid psychoses

Section 1

Clinical

1
Development of concepts of schizophrenia

ERIK STRÖMGREN

The term schizophrenia is used to cover a number of different concepts, some of which are strikingly different from the others. Not all of these concepts can be equally useful. There is a set of characteristics which nearly all psychiatrists will recognize as 'schizophrenic', and which they can be confident their colleagues will label in the same way. Beyond this there are other sets of characteristics which some psychiatrists will call 'schizophrenic' while others will not. It is not, however, possible to give a strict *theoretical* definition of a central concept of schizophrenia which the majority of psychiatrists all over the world would agree upon. The International Pilot Study on Schizophrenia, organized by the World Health Organization (1973), did show that it was possible to create an *operational* definition of such a core group. By means of a standard technique for interviewing patients (Wing, Cooper & Sartorius, 1974), groups of psychiatrists in nine countries in different parts of the world identified similar groups of patients among which the large majority had also received a diagnosis of schizophrenia on ordinary clinical examination by local psychiatrists.

This was an important practical achievement but nobody would expect the group of conditions identified in this way to conform to a single disease entity. The advantage of a central operational definition is that it provides a sound basis for comparing groups of patients and therefore for testing hypotheses about causation, pathology, treatment, or prognosis. In this way, the value of the various concepts will gradually be clarified and the many contradictions which characterize the results of research within the field of schizophrenia eventually resolved.

Schizophrenia has probably existed as long as mankind but attempts to conceptualize it began only about a hundred years ago. When, during the nineteenth century, advances in pathology and later in bacteriology made it possible to single out those cases of mental disorder which were based on verified somatic disorder the majority of patients in mental hospitals could still not be characterized in this way; many psychiatrists, however, tended to believe that, in these cases too, the underlying disorder was of a physical nature. Among this very large group, some subgroups with characteristic symptomatology were singled out. French clinicians described the *'folie circulaire'* which corresponds closely to the manic-depressive disorder of our time (Falret, 1854). Kahlbaum (1874) described patients with catatonia, and Hecker patients with hebephrenia (1871). In the first editions of Kraepelin's psychiatric textbook (1883 to 1893) the same descriptive approach predominated. During the 1890s, however, Kraepelin's follow-up studies convinced him that there were important correlations between symptomatology and course, with the consequence that he tried to delimit 'disease entities' characterized by unity of cause, course, and outcome. It was clear to him that according to these principles the manic-depressive cases could be distinguished from a number of other groups. In the 1893 edition of his textbook he had already used the term dementia praecox (introduced by Morel in 1860), but at that time it covered a narrow concept, excluding catatonia and dementia paranoides. In the 1896 edition these three forms were grouped together under the subheading 'deterioration processes' within the main group of 'metabolic disorders'. In the 1899 (sixth) edition Kraepelin presented his views on dementia praecox and manic-depressive psychosis in the form in which they have been known since then, the main point being the correlation between symptomatology and prognosis. He stressed, however, that there were exceptions to this correlation, some of the dementia praecox cases seeming to recover, although some minor traces of disease might still be left.

At this point, Kraepelin's dementia praecox included the three subgroups hebephrenia, catatonia, and paranoid deterioration. Following a suggestion by Diem (1903) he added the group of dementia simplex. Kraepelin regarded the following symptoms as

characteristic of dementia praecox: hallucinations, usually of an auditory or tactile nature; decrease of attention towards the outer world; lack of curiosity; disorders of thought especially of the *'Zerfahrenheit'*-type, with unusual and partly incomprehensible associations and, as a consequence, incoherence of speech; lack of insight and judgment; delusions; emotional blunting; negativism; stereotypies. Kraepelin stressed that many of these symptoms could occasionally appear in other patients and that what was characteristic of patients with dementia praecox was that such symptoms appeared in clear consciousness and with unimpaired perception and memory. The fact that many intellectual functions were completely unimpaired made it necessary to distinguish these patients terminologically from patients with 'deterioration' (*'Verblödung'*) similar to that in general paralysis or senile disorders. Kraepelin used the term 'dementia' in order to make this distinction. However, 'dementia' has remained in common use for organic deteriorations as well and this has led to a great deal of confusion about Kraepelin's terminology.

In spite of the fact that no somatic disorder could be found as the basis for dementia praecox Kraepelin was inclined to believe that such a condition would eventually be discovered. The same view was held by Eugen Bleuler who gave a more comprehensive description of dementia praecox than Kraepelin had until then done. In his historic paper (1908) in which he introduced the term 'schizophrenia' and in his classic monograph *Dementia praecox oder Gruppe der Schizophrenien* (1911) he stressed that the term dementia praecox was not appropriate: first, the disorder need not always start 'precociter', at an early age; second, the mental changes were not of the same nature as those characterizing the organic 'dementias' – there was no real deterioration of intellectual faculties. Since one basic feature of the symptomatology of these patients was a 'mental splitting' he found the term 'schizophrenia' more adequate. By 'splitting', Bleuler meant two things. First, a changed pattern of associations, as if ordinary connections had lost their meaning and unusual associations could occur, under the influence of accidental and, above all, emotional stimuli, thus losing logical continuity and creating the typical schizophrenic 'thought disorder'. Second, 'splitting' was a useful term to describe the common incongruity between ideas and emotions.

Bleuler's monograph contained two basic and very important innovations. First he distinguished between 'Grundymptome' and *'akzessorische Symptome'*, primary and secondary symptoms, or essential and accessory symptoms, the primary symptoms being caused directly by the aetiological agent, whereas the secondary symptoms represented the psychological reactions of the personality to the primary disorders. He emphasized that, although in many patients the secondary symptoms dominated the clinical picture, they were in principle reversible. Being pure psychological reactions, he thought they could often be understood and interpreted only on psycho-analytic lines. This introduction of psycho-analytic theory and technique into the study of schizophrenia was Bleuler's second major innovation.

Bleuler regarded the following symptoms as being of primary nature: disturbance of associations, thought disorder, changes in emotional reactions, tendency to prefer phantasy to reality and to seclude oneself from reality, being autistic. (The term 'autistic' has since been used in a different sense; see chapter 29.) As secondary symptoms he regarded hallucinations, delusions, catatonic symptoms, and all kinds of behavioural anomalies.

Although Bleuler regarded the primary process as being physical in nature, he admitted that nothing could be said about the exact nature of the aetiological agents. He regarded it as very likely that there was no uniform causation, and for this reason he preferred the term 'group of schizophrenias' instead of simple schizophrenia.

Since the days of Kraepelin and Bleuler the search for aetiological agents responsible for the origin of schizophrenia has continued with great intensity and diversity. On many occasions claims have been made for specific biochemical or physiological abnormalities but other research workers have rarely been able to reproduce the findings. It can safely be stated that no such abnormality is yet of value in making a clinical diagnosis, although some theoretical progress has been made (see chapter 12). Of greater importance are the results of genetic studies. Twin studies and adoption studies show clearly that genetic factors play a part in the causation of schizophrenia. Studies of monozygotic twins seem, however, to demonstrate that genetic factors are responsible for less than 50 per cent of the causation. In addition, twin and family studies have shown that there is no genetic distinction between the different subgroups of schizophrenia. There is some correlation in the sense that different cases of schizophrenia in one family have some tendency to be of the same clinical type, but there are many exceptions to this rule. Progress in genetic studies is reviewed in chapter 11.

With regard to the environmental factors which must necessarily be responsible for a great part of the aetiology there are very few illuminating facts. It is true, however, that some drugs can produce clinical syndromes which cannot be distinguished from schizophrenia; in particular, amphetamine and related drugs, marihuana, and occasionally LSD. In principle, therefore, it is possible that hitherto unrecognized toxic agents might be responsible for a part of the schizophrenias. It is a matter of convention whether such cases should be regarded as subgroups of schizophrenia or be discarded from that concept.

With regard to psychological factors which could be of primary aetiological importance very little is known. Manfred Bleuler has undertaken the most intensive studies concerning such factors and their interaction with genetics. On the basis of follow-up studies of a large number of schizophrenic patients and their relatives over a period of more than 30 years Bleuler (1972) has formulated definite views concerning the delimitation and causation of schizophrenia. He says that there is no impairment of memory and no deterioration of intellect; neither is consciousness disturbed. It is characteristic of schizophrenics that seriously abnormal mental processes can coexist with normal processes within the same personality. As primary symptoms he is nowadays inclined to regard 'autism' and 'splitting' as by far the most important symptoms, present in all schizophrenics.

With regard to the aetiology Bleuler feels that it is heterogeneous, being partly genetic, partly environmental. He regards it as very likely that there are no specific genes responsible for the development of schizophrenia. Instead, the genetic basis could consist in an unfavourable combination of genes that in other combinations do not result in abnormality. This disharmonious grouping could make the individual especially vulnerable to certain kinds of mental traumata. These traumata seem also to be of very different kinds. Even the intensive investigations which Bleuler has made of the environments of schizophrenics have not disclosed any specific noxious factors which appear in the majority of the life histories of schizophrenics. It seems, however, that emotional conflicts of an ambivalent nature with close relatives, originating in childhood, have harmful effects in some cases. These issues are further discussed in chapter 9.

Thus the results of studies of aetiological factors

do not provide us with a natural delimitation of the concept of schizophrenia. In this respect we are, in spite of a large accumulation of disconnected fragments of knowledge, in practically the same position as Kraepelin and Eugen Bleuler at the beginning of the century. Nevertheless, it is a fact that many experienced psychiatrists have a certain, rather indefinable, feeling that the patients whom they agree to call schizophrenic have something in common, in spite of the diversity of symptomatology. On the occasion of the International Congress of Psychiatry meeting in Zürich in 1957, Rümke (1958) gave expression to this widely experienced feeling by saying that when the diagnosis of schizophrenia is made it is often because in the presence of the patient the psychiatrist experiences a certain 'praecox-feeling'. This expression has been quoted so many times that it is likely to be the expression of some fact but as a scientific basis for delimitation of the concept of schizophrenia it is not very useful.

For the moment, therefore, the main basis for delimiting the group of schizophrenias must remain operational: the use of various techniques for recognizing patterns of symptoms. Even so there are difficulties enough. In all such techniques there will be a component of subjective interpretation of what the patient is saying or doing. In recent years much attention has been paid to some of the symptomatological criteria described by Kurt Schneider (1976) as essential for the diagnosis of schizophrenia. Among symptoms which appear in schizophrenia he suggests that some are of the 'first rank'. These symptoms are not like Bleuler's 'primary symptoms' which are supposed to be direct expressions of a basic schizophrenic disorder. Schneider does not feel that first-rank symptoms are of any theoretical value. He regards them simply as symptoms which empirically have turned out to be of great importance when psychiatrists make a diagnosis. First-rank symptoms are the following: patient hearing his own thoughts spoken aloud; hearing voices talking to each other about the patient; hearing voices which comment on the patient's behaviour; feelings of patient's body being influenced by outside forces; feelings of thoughts being removed or foreign thoughts being inserted into the mind; feeling that thoughts are broadcast to other people; feeling that emotions, drives, and intentions are dictated by external forces. Schneider concludes: 'When it is stated that the patient has such experiences and there is no evidence of physical disorder we, in all modesty, are talking about schizo-

phrenia.' Because of their operational importance, it is particularly necessary to adopt common definitions of these symptoms.

All schizophrenics are paranoid, more or less. In some schizophrenics the delusions are the dominant feature, such cases usually being labelled dementia paranoides or schizophrenia paranoides. In others, impairment of contact makes it difficult to ascertain the presence of delusions, and some intelligent schizophrenics find it useful to conceal their paranoid ideas as far as possible. But not all paranoid persons are schizophrenic. Whereas Eugen Bleuler was inclined to incorporate all paranoid psychoses of long duration in schizophrenia, Kraepelin kept his concept of '*paranoia*' separate. In the paranoia group he included patients characterized by incurable systematic delusions, very often concentrated on a certain topic. These patients did not deteriorate in any way, were not obviously 'autistic', and very seldom suffered from hallucinations. This disorder usually started in middle age and never receded. Kraepelin distinguished this group from the '*paraphrenias*', which he regarded as a subgroup of schizophrenia. These patients had florid delusions spreading unsystematically over a number of topics, sometimes accompanied by hallucinations. After having fallen into disuse in most countries this concept has made a reappearance in recent decades. The nosological place of the group is still under debate.

The same is true of Kretschmer's '*sensitiver Beziehungswahn*' or 'sensitive delusion of reference'. When Kretschmer (1918) (see 1966) published his classic monograph on this group most German psychiatrists were inclined to regard these cases simply as a variation of paranoid schizophrenia. Several decades of follow-up showed however that they did not necessarily develop into a typical schizophrenic condition. Kretschmer regarded them as psychogenic reactions, starting on the basis of a sensitive personality and precipitated by a specific key event of a very personal character representing an unbearable blow to the patient's self-esteem.

The fact that these psychoses can go on for several months or even years has contributed to the tendency to regard them as variants of schizophrenia. There are other psychoses of a paranoid character which do not seem to belong to the group of schizophrenias although they sometimes become chronic. First, there are the psychoses caused by difficulties in communication: for example paranoid psychoses in the deaf; Allers' '*Psychosen in sprachfremder*

Umgebung' arising in prisoners of war (Allers, 1920), refugees, and other persons who are suddenly placed in surroundings where nobody can understand their language; psychoses arising in persons who suffer from various kinds of organic loss – Anton's symptom, denial of the person's own blindness (Anton, 1899) and other forms of anosagnosia, for instance in hemiplegics. In these latter cases an emotional component causing the delusions is obvious; a simple desire for denial of the defect. On the other hand there is a definite organic component since anosagnosia only arises when the lesion is in the non-dominant hemisphere. These different kinds of disorders are mentioned in order to show that chronic paranoid psychoses need not be schizophrenic in nature. In general it can be said that these 'mono-symptomatic' delusions are devoid of any 'first rank' character. In French psychiatry (Magnan, 1893; Ey *et al.*, 1974) the *'bouffées délirantes'* play an important role: acute paranoid psychoses of short duration.* In Scandinavian psychiatry these psychoses would usually be thought of as 'psychogenic' or 'reactive' psychoses, in an aetiological sense, and labelled 'schizophreniform' from a symptomatological viewpoint (Strömgren, 1965, 1974).

---

* Acute delusional or hallucinatory states of brief duration, with no subsequent development of schizophrenic symptoms were classified by French psychiatrists as *bouffées délirantes*. There were two subdivisions. The first – *bouffées délirantes vraies, type Magnan* – is not a reactive psychosis. The other – *bouffées délirantes réactionelles* – is. Both, however, are classified in the ICD as 298.3, *Acute Paranoid Reaction*. These terms are not, however, much used in current practice.

Delusions in manic-depressives are usually easily distinguishable from schizophrenic delusions: they are 'holothymic', formed and nourished by the underlying mood, with which they are obviously compatible, and accessible to empathic understanding, in contrast to schizophrenic delusions, which are, at first sight, 'primary', originating from deeply hidden, uniquely personal, sources that may never be understood.

In conclusion it should be stressed that no theoretical aetiological definition of schizophrenia seems possible at present. The International Classification of Diseases (ICD) of the World Health Organization is intended only as a classification, but in an indirect way it does give a hint about aetiology: Schizophrenia (295), Affective Psychoses (296) and Paranoid States (297) are placed immediately before 'Other Non-Organic Psychoses' (298), suggesting that schizophrenia should be regarded as a non-organic psychosis. The introductory definition of group 295 does not actually say anything about aetiology. 'Schizophrenic psychoses' are supposed to be 'a group of psychoses in which there is a fundamental disturbance of personality, a characteristic distortion of thinking, often a sense of being controlled by alien forces, delusions which may be bizarre, disturbed perception, abnormal affect out of keeping with the real situation, and autism. Nevertheless, clear consciousness and intellectual capacity are usually maintained. The disturbance of personality involves its most basic functions which give the normal person his feeling of individuality, uniqueness and self-direction.'

2

Acute syndromes of schizophrenia

JULIAN P. LEFF

Harbingers

Careful descriptions of the modes of onset of illnesses have always been considered of the utmost importance in any account of their natural history. The early recognition of the presence of a particular disease gains enormously in significance when, as is the case with schizophrenia, a useful treatment is available. The problem with schizophrenia is that the earliest features that can be linked with the appearance of the disease are by no means characteristic. Thus certain parental attitudes, maternal over-involvement and parental conflict present during the patient's childhood, occur more commonly in the families of schizophrenics than in the families of patients with other psychiatric illnesses. However the overlap is large enough to render these features diagnostically useless (Hirsch & Leff, 1975). The same is true of minor developmental abnormalities in childhood (O'Neal & Robins, 1958), certain behaviours noted in the classroom (Lewine et al., 1978), and unexplained deterioration in academic performance or work record occurring before the appearance of any observable symptoms (Goldberg & Morrison, 1963). Each of these features increases our understanding of the early development of schizophrenia, but in the individual case their significance is understood only in retrospect.

Occasionally the development of behaviour in childhood and early adolescence is so unlike the known patterns of neurotic and antisocial behaviour as to raise a strong suspicion that it foreshadows the development of schizophrenia.

A boy of 12 years attended his brother's birthday party. They were entertained by a magician who made a rabbit disappear. The boy became intensely anxious about the disappearance of the rabbit, relating it to fears about his own disappearance. He could not be reassured by his parents and was referred to a child guidance clinic. He attended for a few months, during which time his anxiety subsided. Four years later he developed a florid schizophrenic illness.

Modes of onset

The characteristic symptoms of schizophrenia can develop in a few hours in a person who has previously been perfectly well, or may take years to attain a recognizable form. This chapter is concerned with the more acute forms of onset. Chapter 4 deals with the more chronic forms and with the chronic states that may supervene upon an acute onset.

Acute schizophrenia may appear abruptly, out of the blue, may develop out of an amorphous state known as delusional mood, or may be preceded by a prodromal period of neurotic symptoms.

Abrupt onset

This is characterized by the sudden appearance of abnormal behaviour, usually in response to the development of delusions and/or hallucinations. The rapid onset of such strange experiences without any warning is understandably very alarming to the sufferer, who often exhibits marked fear. This is commonly expressed in motor behaviour, the patient pacing up and down, sometimes running about in an apparently purposeless way, or attacking himself, other people, or inanimate objects in an attempt to put an end to his terrifying experiences. In this phase of the illness, the patient may be so restless, agitated, and preoccupied with inner experiences as to be inaccessible to examination. Such states of acute excitement tend to subside rapidly and pose difficult diagnostic problems, since by the time the patient can be communicated with, any psychopathology has disappeared and is frequently forgotten. Consequently their relationship to more classical schizophrenia remains conjectural. They have been termed *bouffées délirantes* (Collomb, 1957; Ey *et al.*, 1974) or schizophreniform psychoses (Strömgren, 1965, 1974; Tewfik, 1958) and are seen more commonly in developing countries than in the west (WHO, 1973). However, in developed countries immigrants, such as Africans and West Indians (Littlewood & Lipsedge, 1978), tend to present with states of excitement which are dominated by behavioural rather than psychological symptoms. Some states of undifferentiated excitement, without more specific schizophrenic or manic or organic features, may constitute a separate nosological entity.

Syndromes

Catatonia

Another predominantly behavioural form in which acute schizophrenia may present is *catatonia*. This has also become exceedingly rare in the West although it remains an occasional form of presentation in developing countries (see chapter 6 for its value in differential diagnosis). Speech in catatonia is characteristically scanty or absent, so that one relies on the behavioural manifestations to recognize the condition. There are a variety of these including:

Waxy flexibility. The patient's head, trunk, and limbs can be manipulated into unnatural postures which the patient will maintain for long periods of time, in a way which would be impossible for a normal person. Sometimes the patient will adopt such postures spontaneously, for example lying down but keeping his head raised a few inches above the bed for hours at a time, the so-called 'psychic pillow'. The cervical vertebrae may actually become ankylosed in this position.

Echopraxia. The patient spontaneously imitates movements made by other people. Chapman (1966) has recorded an illuminating subjective account of this;

> I get shaky in the knees and my chest is like a mountain in front of me, and my body actions are different. The arms and legs are apart and away from me and they go on their own. That's when I feel I am the other person and copy their movements.

Mitgehen. When given a slight push in one direction the patient will continue the movement initiated to its conclusion.

Negativism. The patient will do the exact opposite of what is asked; for example, will stand up when asked to sit down.

Ambitendence. The patient is caught between two opposing movements, for example, wavers backwards and forwards in a doorway.

Stupor. The patient remains completely motionless and may be incontinent of urine and faeces. Consciousness is not clouded or impaired, as may be discovered when the patient recovers. Periods of stupor may alternate with episodes of overactivity and excitement.

Delusional perception

Another rare presenting symptom of acute schizophrenia is *delusional perception*, one of Schneider's (1959, 1971) first-rank symptoms. The patient, who has been well up to that moment, is suddenly struck with the immense personal significance of a particular perception. The same perception is available to any observer, but the interpretation put on it by the patient is totally idiosyncratic.

> A man was standing on a station platform when his eye was caught by the British Rail insignia of two arrows pointing in opposite directions. He instantly knew that this meant he had to go to hospital.

Delusional mood

This is another kind of onset characterized by a mood of puzzlement and bewilderment. The patient feels that something out of the ordinary is going on around him and that it is centered on himself. He may be toying with various possible explanations but has not settled on any one of them. The essence of this symptom is the patient's certainty that some unusual activity is being directed at him, coexisting with puzzlement as to its nature.

> A patient complained that he felt as though he was on stage acting in some play, but that he didn't know which part he was playing or what the play was.

Delusional mood is usually a transient stage in the development of a full-blown psychosis, often but not always schizophrenia. Once the patient has decided on a definite delusional explanation for his experiences, delusional mood has passed and the nature of the psychosis can be determined. However, occasionally delusional mood subsides without the development of delusions, in which case the nature of the psychosis must remain in doubt.

Prodromal neurotic symptoms

The onset of florid schizophrenic symptoms is quite frequently preceded by a period lasting from a few days to several months, during which the patient exhibits neurotic symptoms. Every kind of neurotic symptom may be encountered (Chapman, 1966) so that there is nothing specific to enable one to anticipate the eventual appearance of schizophrenia. Hoch and Polatin (1949) have suggested that certain constellations of neurotic symptoms represent a form of schizophrenia, so-called 'pseudoneurotic schizophrenia', but the evidence for this is by no means conclusive.

First-rank symptoms

Delusional perception has already been described. A number of other first-rank symptoms can be grouped together as varieties of thought disturbance.

Thought insertion. Thoughts coming in to the patient's mind are not recognized as originating from his own mental activity, but are ascribed to an outside source. This may be unspecified or the patient may be convinced that these alien thoughts come from other people's minds. The essence of the symptom is the belief that alien thoughts are inserted into the mind from outside.

> Thoughts are put into my mind like 'Kill God'. It's just like my mind working, but it isn't. They come from this chap, Chris. They're his thoughts.
> Thoughts come into my mind from outer space.

Thought broadcast. The patient experiences his thoughts leaving his mind and travelling over a distance to other people's minds. The recipients may be a few people well-known to the patient or a multitude of strangers. In either case the process is a passive one over which he has no control, and which makes him feel that his most intimate thoughts are no longer private to himself.

> My thoughts go into other people's minds. It's telecommunication between people.
> My thoughts go out to all my close relatives and to psychiatrists.

Thoughts spoken aloud. The patient hears his thoughts spoken as if by a voice inside his own head. They may be experienced as so loud that he may wonder whether they are audible to other people.

> It was like my ears being blocked up and my thoughts shouted out.

Thought echo. The patient experiences his thoughts being repeated immediately after he thinks them. This is an involuntary repetition, just like an echo except that it is not audible.

> My thoughts come back again like a playback.

Thought withdrawal. The train of thought is abruptly terminated, leaving the patient's mind empty of all thoughts. This is the experience of thought block, which the patient may ascribe to his thoughts actually being removed from his head, the delusion of thought withdrawal.

> My thoughts are removed from my mind while I'm asleep so that when I wake up in the morning I can hardly think.

Third-person auditory hallucinations. Apart from these varieties of thought disturbance, one kind of auditory hallucination is included by Schneider as a first-rank symptom. The patient hears a voice or several voices discussing him in the third person. It is like eavesdropping on a conversation of which the patient is the subject. The tenor of the remarks may be neutral, pleasant, or hostile, the latter being commonest. A rarer variant of this symptom is hearing a voice or voices conducting a running commentary on the patient's thoughts or actions.

> He is an astronomy fanatic. Here's a taste of his own medicine. He's getting up now. He's going to wash. It's about time.

Delusions of control. This is one of the commonest first-rank symptoms, the patient's experience being that he is no longer exercising his own will in respect of his bodily actions, his speech, or his desires. The patient may explain this in terms of being taken over by an outside force or being possessed by a spirit or some other person. As in all such cases the explanation chosen by the patient directly reflects the beliefs extant in his culture about control by spiritual or physical forces.

> My grandfather hypnotized me and now he moves my foot up and down.
> They inserted a computer into my brain. It makes me turn to the left or right.

> I have been mesmerized by psychiatrists. A voice comes out of my mouth. It sounds like my voice but it's not.

Somatic passivity experiences. The patient experiences sensations on the surface of his body or internally, which he attributes to forces acting over a distance. The symptom is rare.

> I have tingling feelings in my legs caused by electric currents from an alternator.

These are the main types of Schneiderian first-rank symptoms. Gradations between some of them may be observed; in particular, thoughts spoken aloud and auditory hallucinations appear to lie on a continuum of experience, which can be traversed by an individual patient over a matter of days. As with any continuum more minute subdivisions can be made. Koehler (1979) has given detailed phenomenological analysis of first-rank symptoms.

These first-rank symptoms are very similar to the 'syndrome of mental automatisms' described by de Clérambault (1942), who also pointed out the tendency of patients to develop secondary delusional explanations for their experiences.

Disturbances of affect

In the absence of first-rank symptoms, acute schizophrenia can present with paranoid delusions, delusions of reference and misinterpretation, religious delusions, grandiose delusions, and hallucinations in any modality. These schizophrenic states are distinguishable from manic and depressive psychoses partly by the absence of the appropriate affect, either elation or depression. However a more positive identification of schizophrenia can be made from the quality of the affect, which may be blunted or incongruous.

Blunted affect. This is more commonly associated with chronic schizophrenia, but may be a prominent and transient feature of the acute state. In severe cases the patient's face is devoid of all expression; there are no expression marks on the forehead or around the eyes and the face looks as though it had been ironed smooth. The mouth only moves for the purpose of speech, and social smiling – an integral part of social intercourse – is absent. An expressionless face of this description may also be the result of drug-induced Parkinsonism, but there are other tell-tale signs of this to be observed in the limbs. Blunting of affect also registers in the voice, which lacks the usual rise and fall in tonality. This is particularly noticeable when the patient recounts dramatic and frightening experiences in a flat tone of voice. There is often an absence of gesture, of appropriate eye-contact, and of other essentials of non-verbal communication.

Incongruity of affect. This is occasionally shown by sudden weeping or wailing when the patient is talking about neutral or pleasant topics. The tears rapidly dry up and do not convey an associated depression of mood. Much more commonly incongruity is manifested by inexplicable smiling, giggling, or laughing. These may occur in the course of a conversation or when the patient is sitting on his own. In the latter instance they may be part of a 'conversation' the patient is conducting with his 'voices'. Whatever the context, the causeless mirth gives the impression of a private joke which is not shared with the onlooker, and may even be at his expense. The usual warmth of humour is not communicated to the observer, who is left with a chill feeling of estrangement. In some cases of schizophrenia the clinical picture is dominated by a shallow incongruous affect, leading to the subclassification of hebephrenia (see chapter 4).

Blunting and incongruity of affect can occur in organic disorders and it is unwise to make a diagnosis of schizophrenia on this basis alone.

Disturbances of speech

Full-fledged schizophrenic speech disturbances are rare but minor abnormalities are common. Schizophrenic patients may coin new words, *neologisms*, to convey their experiences to others, for example, 'computator' for a machine that sends out thought waves. They may also use recognizable English words in odd combinations or contexts, for example, 'people are the abomination of desolation'; 'my sister trades on my brain'. The more severe disturbances of speech take two main forms, *incoherence* and *poverty of content*.

Incoherence. This is produced by the patient answering a question with a completely irrelevant reply, or by suddenly shifting the topic either between sentences or within a sentence; so-called 'knight's move' or 'derailment of the train of thought'. If this occurs frequently, the listener's ability to follow the patient's speech is severely impaired. In very advanced cases, speech production is no longer constrained by grammatical rules and a 'word salad' or 'verbigeration' results, the so-called 'schizophasia'. Schizophrenic speech may also be interlaced with puns, rhymes, clang associations, and word associations, which further impair comprehension and make the differentiation from acute mania difficult. If the clinical picture of an acute psychosis is dominated by incoherence of speech it will be difficult to elicit any other symptoms. In such cases it is advisable to tape-record a sample of speech and transcribe it, as this procedure may enable a firm diagnosis to be made. In less severe cases, if incoherence of speech is suspected, the patient should be encouraged to speak spontaneously for several minutes without interruption. The longer the patient goes on speaking, the more likely incoherence is to emerge.

As I am as God made me and understand my position and you'll listen with intelligence your intelligence works lit again and is recorded in my head and gradually with the be telling the truth to wisdom that went to the top and worked down to my system even to my head blood pressure true expression of red this is what I thought confession and it is telling the truth.

Poverty of content. The patient speaks quite freely, but gives very little or no information. After listening for a few minutes, it is impossible to summarize what has been said because the patient is vague and repetitive, and fails to give any closure, or even to come to grips with any topic.

Interviewer: What are your plans for the future?

Patient: It would be a case then of which choice I'd have to take but you take the choice of going to the local record shop where they know me very well and taking charge of well going backwards and forwards up and down the street for a bit you know maybe like I could hint to them perhaps they could or perhaps a friend of mine next door might give me a lift if he thought he could help the situation help bring the lot of us but I feel a bit embarrassed about him we can have him in the car it's not far but it's a long way sometimes.

3
Chronic syndromes of schizophrenia

JULIAN P. LEFF

Schizophrenia may develop insidiously over a number of years; the acute florid state may persist unchanged for many years, or it may subside leaving a chronic defect state. Each of these different courses is subsumed under the general term chronic schizophrenia, but as they have different manifestations they will be dealt with separately here.

Insidious onset schizophrenia

This is usually assigned to the subclassification of simple schizophrenia (see chapter 4) and is a rare variety. Delusions and hallucinations may never appear in acute and dramatic form but only as minor and fragmented manifestations. The effects of the illness are mainly evident in the patient's social life, working ability, and emotional relationships. The process usually begins during adolescence or in early adulthood, but may not be recognized as an illness for some years. There is a gradual attrition of interest in social relationships, the patient becoming increasingly solitary and uncommunicative. Whatever interest the patient showed in hobbies or sports dwindles until he spends his leisure time completely unoccupied. Work also suffers. If the patient is carrying out a demanding job, he is soon found to be incapable of continuing with it. He tends to arrive late, is slowed down mentally and physically, and is unable to take responsibility. A more automatic job may be carried on for some time after other aspects of the patient's life have been severely affected but eventually patients with this condition lose their employment. The patient's emotional life also becomes progressively restricted; he ceases to show affection to his close relatives and no longer responds to pleasurable or unpleasant happenings with the expected ups and downs of mood. As the illness progresses habits that are the product of early socialization are affected; he may cease to dress and groom himself to an acceptable standard and neglect to wash himself as much as is necessary. The end result of this progressive deterioration is indistinguishable from the chronic state that sometimes follows an acute florid schizophrenia. Another link with the more usual schizophrenic picture is provided by the fact that patients with simple schizophrenia occasionally complain of paranoid or other delusions. However, it is difficult to elicit much psychopathology as they are often markedly uncommunicative by the time they are brought to a psychiatrist, restricting their answers to monosyllables.

Persistent florid states

About 5 to 7 per cent of schizophrenic patients presenting acutely with delusions and hallucinations show no response to antipsychotic drugs (Leff & Wing, 1971). It was at first thought that the introduction of parenteral long-acting fluphenazine would make substantial inroads into this drug-resistant population, since it bypasses problems involved in absorption from the gut. Unfortunately these hopes have been disappointed and it is the exceptional patient who shows a good response to long-acting injections after failing to improve on oral medication. In the current absence of any other effective form of treatment these patients are destined to a chronic course from the start of their illness. Although proportionately a small group, their accumulation over the years represents a serious therapeutic problem (see chapter 14). In such cases, the psychopathology is usually remarkably stable, the same delusions and hallucinations persisting unchanged over decades. Any emotional reactions shown by the patients to these experiences at the beginning of their illness soon subside as they come to accept them as an integral part of their everyday life. Indeed some patients come to regard their auditory hallucinations as regular companions and prefer to converse with them than with actual people, whose attempts to communicate are resented as unwarranted intrusions.

M. Bleuler (1972) followed up an unselected group of 208 schizophrenic patients over several decades. He found that a surprisingly high proportion, about two-thirds to three-quarters, showed an amelioration of their symptoms over long periods of time. It is arguable that the force of the abnormal experiences did not really abate, but that the patients learned to conceal them from others. Many patients learn that to discuss their experiences, particularly with professional people, can lead to disadvantages such as increased medication or cancelled leave. It is not surprising therefore that some patients become very guarded about revealing their delusions and hallucinations or deny them altogether. However, such patients may reveal the presence of active auditory hallucinations by their non-verbal behaviour; stopping in the middle of a conversation and glancing upwards and to one side.

Another persistent psychotic state, seemingly related to schizophrenia, that is sometimes encountered is the *monosymptomatic delusion*. Patients with this condition have a single abiding belief, for example, that they give off a bad smell noticeable to others, or that their nose is excessively large, which is demonstrably untrue but which they hold with unshakeable conviction. These beliefs have all the characteristics of delusions, but may be unaccompanied by any other psychotic symptoms and generally fail to respond to antipsychotic medication.

Chronic defect states

These may become apparent when the acute symptoms subside or they may accompany persistent florid states. Very occasionally they follow a protracted first attack of schizophrenia, but more usually they develop in the course of recurrent illnesses after some years of repeated episodes. They differ from the florid symptoms, which are readily identifiable abnormal behaviour, in that they are the *absence* of normal behaviour. Hence they are sometimes referred to as *negative symptoms*. They have already been mentioned in the description of simple schizophrenia above, but will be dealt with in more detail here. There is good evidence that the negative symptoms can be augmented by the socially deprived environment of a 'back ward' (Wing & Brown, 1970). However, with the increasing emphasis on community care it has become evident that such states can develop just as readily in sheltered settings outside hospital and in the patient's home. Furthermore, careful observation of long-term in-patients suggests that those with schizophrenia are much more liable to develop these defect states than are patients with other psychiatric conditions (Morgan, 1979). Hence a vulnerability to socially unstimulating environments appears to be an integral feature of schizophrenia. There are several types of defect which in general occur together but some may be more pronounced in individual patients than others.

Lack of initiative

Patients appear to lose the ability to initiate action. Whether this is due to a reduction in motivation or an inability to translate drives into action is unknown, but there is some evidence favouring the former explanation. Wing and Freudenberg (1961) conducted an experiment in which they examined the effects of active supervision and encouragement versus passive supervision on the productivity of chronic schizophrenics in a sheltered workshop. They found that these chronic patients did respond to praise and encouragement by a significant increase in production, but that this improvement was totally lost as soon as active supervision was replaced with passive supervision. Furthermore any improvement occurring in the workshop setting did not generalize to other situations. The fleeting nature of such improvements wrought by behavioural means and the lack of generalization appear to be specific to schizophrenia (Falloon *et al.*, 1977), and may indicate a basic psychological deficit (see chapter 10). As the defect state worsens, patients become progressively more inert until spontaneous activity may virtually be extinguished. Even fundamental drives such as sex usually diminish in strength and often disappear entirely. By contrast the need for oral satisfaction remains strong and may even be intensified; patients sometimes eat voraciously and as a consequence may become very obese. Phenothiazines, in particular chlorpromazine, can add to this problem. Patients often smoke heavily within the limits they can afford, and abuse of alcohol in chronic defect states also occurs. In addition to the oral satisfaction it provides, alcohol also acts to diminish social unease. Furthermore, the pub is a neutral meeting place where it is possible to be with other people without being obliged to interact socially.

Lack of energy

Another related feature of chronic defect states is the slowness with which patients carry out movements. They may complain of feeling that everything is more of an effort than it used to be and react by increasing inertia. It is not uncommon for such patients to spend the whole day lying on their beds if left to their own devices. The retardation of physical movements is another disadvantage in the way of keeping these patients in employment.

Lack of alertness

Coupled with the physical slowness is a retardation of mental activity. This feature is evident on cognitive testing. Here again phenothiazine drugs accentuate the problem because of their sedative properties. A further hindrance in the way of normal cognitive functioning is lack of concentration. The span of attention is greatly reduced in chronic schizophrenia and causes problems in gaining the patient's co-operation even in relatively simple tasks. There is evidence that this non-specific defect is responsible for the poor performance of schizophrenic patients on tests claimed to tap specific malfunctioning, such as the Repertory Grid Test of thought disorder (Frith & Lillie, 1972) and the pendulum tracking task (Brezinova & Kendell, 1977). As noted above, although patients may deny harbouring delusions and hallucinations they may be considerably preoccupied with abnormal experiences. This absorption in their inner mental activity renders it difficult to capture the patients' attention in conversation or during an interview, and questions often have to be repeated several times.

Lack of interest

A prominent feature of chronic defect states is a progressive restriction of the patient's erstwhile interests. Activities such as hobbies and sports are dropped early on in the condition, although patients may continue for much longer with less demanding interests such as reading and knitting. Occasionally patients may keep up an activity which is spurred on by a delusional motivation, such as collecting optical instruments in order to discover the secret of the universe, or writing a 'best-selling' novel. However, with these exceptions, most interests wither away, until the only 'activity' remaining is to sit passively in front of the omnipresent television set. Morgan (1979) carefully recorded the conversations he had had with a group of chronically handicapped patients over a number of years. He found that none of them watched television selectively and few could give a coherent account of what they saw. Morgan writes, 'They welcomed a holiday from work but had no idea what to do with it; alternatively, if you like, they knew exactly what they wanted to do with it – nothing.

They resented my efforts to stimulate them into activity and usually reacted with mute hostility.'

In addition to being a feature of the chronic syndromes in its own right, lack of interest must also be contributed to by inability to concentrate, withdrawal into an inner mental world, and loss of contact with the world outside the hospital or home. Morgan's patients were still expressing prices in shillings and pence six years after decimalization.

Lack of emotional responsiveness

This is manifested both in the patient's close relationships and in his reaction to events. The range of his emotional responses becomes narrowed so that he no longer evinces the heights and depths of emotion normally elicited by fluctuations in life circumstances. Close relatives frequently complain about the patient's emotional aloofness (Creer & Wing, 1975; Leff & Vaughn, 1976), experiencing a loss of love and warmth. Ultimately the patient may reach a state of severe emotional blunting, where no emotional responses are shown at all. To the observer the patient presents a face devoid of emotional expression, a monotonous voice, and an absence of expressive gestures.

Social withdrawal

Avoidance of other people's company is seen at an early stage of the chronic defect states. At first this appears as a failure to initiate social contacts but it later develops into an active rejection of company. Patients living at home can spend the majority of the day in their own room, only emerging for meals. Even then they may prefer to avoid communal meals and choose times to eat when they will be on their own. When visitors call, the more actively rejecting patients will leave the sitting room for the privacy of their bedroom. Even if they stay, they cannot easily be ignored since they project an atmosphere of brooding hostility that positively discourages conversation between others.

The need for privacy is so compelling that in the vast psychiatric institutions in California, where privacy could not be found on the wards, patients built individual shelters for themselves out of debris they found in the grounds. Even when these were demolished by the staff in the interest of tidiness, they rose again (Sommer, 1969).

Another manifestation of social withdrawal is a progressive restriction of speech. Evident at first as a lack of spontaneous conversation, it can reach a stage of near muteness where the patient responds to questions with monosyllables only.

Although usually considered to be one of the symptoms of chronic defect states, social withdrawal may actually be a protective strategy that enables the patient to avoid the recurrence of florid symptoms (Vaughn & Leff, 1976). Unfortunately it can lead to social isolation that exacerbates the other chronic defects.

Loss of social graces

At a later stage in the development of this syndrome patients lose patterns of social behaviour that are inculcated early in life. Table manners and the courtesies of greeting disappear, so that patients may eat greedily and wolfishly, scattering food debris around the table and over themselves. They may completely ignore visitors and fail to respond to the rituals of greeting. Their dress and grooming becomes careless if not perfunctory, so that they present a dishevelled and sometimes indecent appearance. They may pass loud flatus in public without seeming to notice, or make sexual overtures in inappropriate situations. Washing and bathing can be completely neglected, rendering the patient malodorous.

Disturbance of sleep patterns

Some patients seem to suffer a reversal of sleep rhythms, remaining awake throughout the night and sleeping during the day. However, this can also be a strategy to achieve social withdrawal rather than representing a disturbance in biological rhythms.

4
Subclassification of schizophrenia

ERIK STRÖMGREN

The symptomatology of the schizophrenias is so varied that it has taken time and experience to discern the similarities behind the differences. Until the end of the nineteenth century hebephrenia, catatonia and paranoid dementia were regarded as separate disease entities. In the 1899 edition of Kraepelin's textbook these three groups were finally combined as subgroups of dementia praecox. A few years later a fourth group, 'simple dementia', was added. This division of schizophrenia into four subgroups was accepted by Eugen Bleuler in his monograph of 1911.

Schizophrenia simplex is characterized by insidious fading of personality from an early age, without especially spectacular symptoms. Delusions and hallucinations are occasionally present but rarely predominant. There is increasing autism and social impoverishment.

In the *hebephrenic type* the affective changes are more conspicuous, emotions often seeming quite inadequate; behaviour becomes irresponsible and unpredictable, the patients are obviously deluded and hallucinated. Like schizophrenia simplex, this type usually starts before the age of 25.

In the *catatonic type* psychomotor disturbances are prominent, with symptoms such as hyperkinesia, stupor, stereotyped movements, and talk (see chapter 3). Hallucinations and delusions are usually conspicuous. This form also starts, often acutely, at a relatively young age. The *paranoid form,* by contrast, usually has a later age of onset and a more insidious onset. Delusions constitute the dominant symptoms. Appearance and behaviour may be normal and hallucinations absent.

There are no genetic distinctions between the four subgroups. In fact, they may all occur at different times in the same patient. Catatonic symptoms have been especially susceptible to the effect of somatic treatments. Until these treatments were introduced the catatonic types were dominant in the chronic wards of psychiatric hospitals. Nowadays they may be difficult to find even in a large hospital.

Kleist and his pupils (1928, 1953), particularly Leonhard (1979), attempted to isolate a number of schizophrenic subtypes which they regarded as separate disease entities. The genetic studies which they undertook gave little support to these theories (Schulz & Leonhard, 1940; Trostorff, 1968 a, b).

For a long time it was supposed that schizophrenia always began before the age of about 50 years. This is probably one of the reasons why Kraepelin kept *paraphrenia* apart as a separate condition. It is more likely however, that this group is a form of schizophrenia with somewhat atypical features because of the late age of onset. A psychosis which starts at an age when the personality has already become mature and fixed does not dissolve the personality in the same way as a psychosis which breaks into the development of personality at a young age.

During the 1930s two new terms came into widespread use: *schizo-affective psychosis* and *schizophreniform psychosis*. The first of these terms has had a curious fate. It was introduced by Kasanin (1933) who applied it to cases 'characterized by a very sudden onset in a setting of marked emotional turmoil with a distortion of the outside world. . . . The psychosis lasts a few weeks to a few months and is followed by a recovery'. Kasanin also emphasized that such psychoses usually started as a consequence of a severe mental stress. The term schizo-affective psychosis was soon introduced into the official *American Psychiatric Association Nomenclature* (1952) but was described there as a subgroup of schizophrenia characterized by a mixture of schizophrenic and affective symptoms, with the comment that 'on prolonged observation, such cases usually prove to be basically schizophrenic in nature'. The *International Classification of Diseases* (ICD) has the following definition of this type: 'A psychosis in which pronounced manic or depressive features are intermingled with schizophrenic features and which tends towards remission without permanent defect, but which is prone to recur'. Although many psychiatrists using the term have regarded this group as being a subgroup of schizophrenia the term has mainly served as a convenient buffer group between schizophrenia and affective disorder. Angst has shown that schizo-affective disorders, as diagnosed in Switzerland, have predominantly the same course as cases of manic-depressive disorder (Angst, 1980).

The other term which came into use during the 1930s was *schizophreniform psychosis*. It was introduced by Langfeldt (1937, 1939) who wished to distinguish between schizophrenic disorders that responded favourably to the newly introduced shock treatments and disorders that did not respond. The first group he labelled 'schizophreniform' in contrast to the 'true' or 'process' schizophrenias which in the long run, did not react satisfactorily to these treatments. He suggested that there were definite clinical differences between the two groups. The schizophreniform disorders usually had an acute onset, often in connection with severe mental stress; emotional contact with the patient was much better than with patients belonging to the true schizophrenic group. In addition, family studies showed that there was a difference between the two groups in the sense that some of the relatives of patients with schizophreniform disorders had mild and short-lived schizophrenia-like conditions, whereas the genetic loading in the schizophrenic families was much more uniformly schizophrenic. Unfortunately the term 'schizophreniform psychosis' has been used in many other ways. Etymologically, the term should only designate psychoses which show symptomatic similarities to schizophrenia although it is doubtful whether they belong to the group. Some schizophrenias, manic-depressive psychoses, reactive psychoses and toxic psychoses may thus be 'schizophreniform'. It should be kept in mind that the term does not imply any aetiological relationship to schizophrenia.

One further terminological innovation has come into use during the last decade: the *schizophrenia spectrum*. This term was introduced by Kety and his colleagues (1968) as an operational working tool to be applied in the Danish-American studies on adoptees and their relatives. When family studies of schizophrenics were started it was of interest not only to ascertain the cases of definite schizophrenia but also to register cases which might have some aetiological relationship to schizophrenia. It was impossible to know in advance where the borderline should be drawn, and it was found safe to include conditions which seemed to have only a faint relationship to schizophrenia. The spectrum was divided into two parts, the 'hard' and the 'soft'; the first comprising chronic (process) schizophrenia, doubtful chronic schizophrenia, acute schizophrenic episode, doubtful acute schizophrenic episode, borderline schizophrenia, and doubtful borderline schizophrenia, while the second contained paranoid states, paranoid personality, schizoid personality, and inadequate personality.

Although the idea of this schizophrenia spectrum was sound it may have given rise to some misunderstanding, since it implies that all the different states mentioned have now been proved to have a genetic relationship to schizophrenia. This is certainly not the case. On the contrary one important result of the studies was that the acute schizophrenic episodes seemed to have no genetic relationship to the 'true' schizophrenias (Kety *et al.*, 1971).

Two other groups seem to have considerably more aetiological relationship to schizophrenia: *pseudoneurotic schizophrenia* and *pseudopsychopathic schizophrenia*. The first of these groups was described by Hoch and Polatin (1949) and has since been studied by many other workers (Vanggaard, 1979). These individuals are said to be characterized by 'panneurosis' and chaotic sexuality. In the beginning they may be mistaken for neurotics, hypochondria and psychosomatic symptoms being in the foreground. However, in contrast to 'true' neurotics, the symptoms do not provide any secondary gain, while in contrast to most schizophrenics, it is possible to establish a reasonable psychotherapeutic relationship, and autism is not nearly as severe as in 'true' schizophrenia. Occasionally pseudoneurotic patients suffer from shortlasting 'micropsychotic' episodes with or without comprehensible psychological precipitation; such episodes have a definite schizophrenic symptomatology. There is rarely any serious schizophrenic deterioration. This is also characteristic of *pseudopsychopathic schizophrenia*, first described by Dunaif and Hoch (1955). There are many mechanisms in common with pseudoneurotic schizophrenia but behaviour is more disturbed. Most of the patients are described as having antisocial personalities and most are actually criminals. Such cases may be misdiagnosed sociopathy combined with addiction, and the 'micropsychoses' may be diagnosed as prison psychoses or toxic psychoses. The authors suggest that long observation in hospital is necessary in order to understand the true nature of the disorder.

Pseudoneurotic and pseudopsychopathic disorders are often included in the group of '*borderline states*', into which many otherwise unclassifiable conditions have been placed. According to the definition of Grinker and his colleagues (1968, 1977), young people suffering from 'borderline syndromes' only rarely develop true schizophrenic syndromes.

Finally one group should be mentioned which at the beginning of the century received much attention; the so-called *Urstein psychosis*. The Polish psychiatrist Urstein (1909) gave a penetrating and extensive description of a number of cases which started with typically manic-depressive attacks and later on developed into a state which could not be distinguished from catatonic schizophrenia. Although this was not a very common course, all experienced psychiatrists had seen cases of this kind. This was of great theoretical interest since it seemed to indicate a relationship between the two major psychoses, which at that time were regarded as being more or less mutually exclusive. When the shock treatments were introduced in the 1930s the Urstein riddle was solved. Many of these formerly chronic catatonic-like psychoses reacted favorably to the new treatments, leaving no trace of a schizophrenic personality change and, in some cases, unveiling a definite manic-depressive disorder.

The different forms and types described above are only a small selection from all those which, over the years, have been described as subgroups of schizophrenia or in some way aetiologically related to schizophrenia. Only one other concept will be mentioned, however, namely the so-called *psychogenic* or *reactive psychoses*. It should be emphasized that those who originated these terms did not regard the conditions as having any relationship to schizophrenia, but many American psychiatrists do so classify them. The term 'psychogenic psychosis' has been in current use in Scandinavian psychiatry since the beginning of the century. The group contains patients who develop an acute psychosis, usually of short duration and resulting in complete recovery, immediately following a severe mental trauma. Some of these cases show a confusional picture similar to the schizo-affective psychoses of Kasanin (1933), others are pure depressions, others again are predominantly paranoid in nature. Family studies have shown that the family background is widely different from that of schizophrenia.

To give a systematic view of all these different syndromes, forms and subtypes of schizophrenia is not easy. The problem has been one of the great headaches of those responsible for the creation of the *International Classification of Diseases* (ICD). Fortunately, such classifications do not aim to describe nosologically defined classes but to create classes which can be described in such a way that psychiatrists in all parts of the world will be able to place cases of the same nature in the same class, thus establishing the basis for comparable statistics.

The ninth edition (1975) of the ICD includes an important innovation, which unfortunately is only applied in the section on mental disorders. In this section each class is carefully defined. The basis for the definitions is the *Glossary of mental disorders and guide to their classification*, compiled by an international group of psychiatrists chaired by Sir Aubrey Lewis (1974). This was published in 1974 for use in conjunction with the 8th revision of the ICD. A new edition of the glossary (1978) provides similar definitions for the diagnoses contained in the ninth revision of the ICD.

In ICD 9 'schizophrenic psychosis' appears as group 295. There is an introductory comprehensive and lucid description which concludes as follows: 'The diagnosis "schizophrenia" should not be made unless there is, or has been evident during the same illness, characteristic disturbance of thought, perception, mood, conduct, or personality – preferably in at least two of these areas. The diagnosis should not be restricted to conditions running a protracted, deteriorating, or chronic course. In addition to making the diagnosis on the criteria just given, effort should be made to specify one of the following subdivisions of schizophrenia, according to the predominant symptoms'.

The subdivisions include first the four traditional types: Simple type (295.0), hebephrenic type (295.1), catatonic type (295.2), and paranoid type (295.3). The paranoid type contains 'paraphrenic schizophrenia', but excludes 'paraphrenia, involutional paranoid state' (297.2) and 'paranoia' (297.1). The paraphrenic types described within 295.3 and

297.2 do not, however, seem to be really different. Chapter 5 contains a more detailed discussion of the paranoid psychoses.

Next follows 'acute schizophrenic episode' (295.4). In these cases there is 'a dreamlike state with slight clouding of consciousness and perplexity' ('oneirophrenia') and 'there may be ideas of reference and emotional turmoil'. It is stated that remission may occur within a few weeks or months even without treatment. This description seems to come very close to Kasanin's description of schizo-affective psychoses and to differ essentially from the 'schizo-affective type' (295.7) described below.

Latent schizophrenia (295.5) contains such states as borderline, pre-psychotic, and prodromal schizophrenias and, in addition, pseudoneurotic and pseudopsychopathic schizophrenia.

Residual schizophrenia (295.6) is a form in which most of the symptoms have 'lost their sharpness' after a prolonged course.

Schizo-affective type (295.7) is described as 'a psychosis with manic or depressive features intermingled with schizophrenic features, tending towards remission without permanent defect but with proneness to recur'. This group contains cases with symptoms and course similar to that of manic-depressive disorder but where there are schizophrenic features in addition. The group is also supposed to contain such states as 'cyclic schizophrenia', 'mixed schizophrenic and affective psychosis', 'schizophreniform psychosis, affective type'.

There are two further subdivisions – 295.8 (other specified forms, including schizophrenia with an onset in late childhood) and 295.9, ('not otherwise specified'). The use of the latter is deprecated.

The chart at the end of this chapter (Fig. 4.1) illustrates the relations of the 'schizophrenic psychoses' to other ICD groups. The subgroups are likely to overlap, conceptually and diagnostically, across the borders, and the chart shows those where confusion is most likely to arise.

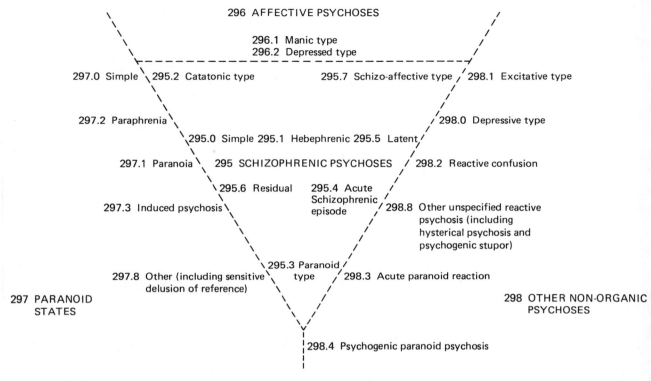

Fig. 4.1. Relation of 'schizophrenic psychoses' to other ICD groups.

5
Paranoid disorders
FELIX POST

Definitions

The history of the words 'paranoia' and 'paranoid' from the time of the Greeks to the present day has been reviewed by Lewis (1955, 1970) and the evolution of paranoia as a basic clinical concept is dealt with by Scharfetter in volume 1, chapter 2 of this Handbook. The relationship of the concepts 'paranoia' and 'paranoid' to schizophrenia has been discussed by Strömgren in chapter 1 of the present volume.

In the present chapter these concepts will be further examined in a wider context. It will be shown that the terms 'paranoiac' and 'paranoid' signify mental abnormalities which may be found in a considerable variety of psychiatric conditions. Leaving more remote history aside, Kraepelin's (1913) formulation of paranoia has come to be generally adopted: a condition which develops insidiously and is initiated by a single unshakeable delusion, not necessarily of persecutory content; secondary delusions usually arise later culminating in a complex delusional system. The other mental functions, both intellectual and emotional, remain unimpaired. More specifically, hallucinosis does not develop in 'paranoia' as it does in 'paraphrenia'.

The progress of the long and learned debate on the 'paranoia question' was reviewed by Kolle (1931a, 1957) who concluded that nearly all cases diagnosed as paranoia had turned out to have been schizophrenics. Considering the length of the debate the condition was extremely rare: among some 30 000 cases registered in Kraepelin's Clinic in Munich between 1904 and 1922, only 157 had diagnoses containing the word 'paranoid', and only 19 were classified as suffering from the narrowly defined condition described as 'paranoia' (Kolle, 1931b). A later enquiry found some 900 paranoid conditions, but only 11 were diagnosed as paranoia and even these included psychoses characterized principally by sensitive delusions of reference and delusions of jealousy (Kolle, 1957).

Confusion became worse confounded when Kolle (1931a) proposed to substitute the name 'paraphrenia' (a term which Kraepelin ultimately abandoned) for 'paranoia'. It is not surprising that Lewis (1970) wrote of paranoia: 'Its shadowy, fluttering existence qualified it for use in darkening counsel.'

As true paranoia is both an exceedingly rare condition and a dubious concept, the term 'paranoid' (i.e. like paranoia) has been found preferable. At the same time there has been a narrowing of its meaning. The main weight in paranoia was on the presence of a true central delusion regardless of content. The subject of the delusion could be divine identity, elevated parentage, scientific invention, being chosen for a mission, being loved and desired, being wronged by administrative or legal authorities, or being persecuted by other people out of envy or because of any of the minor interpersonal frictions that arise during social life.

In modern psychiatry the term 'paranoid' is used almost exclusively to describe any delusional form of self-reference concerned with persecution, litigation, jealousy, love, envy, hate, honour, or the supernatural. Underlying delusions of grandeur are often ill-concealed, but modern usage lays the main stress on hostility which the patient believes to be directed against him. However, the common practice of using the word 'paranoid' as though it were synonymous with 'hostile' or 'aggressive' is to be deprecated.

On first clinical contact with a person whose complaints or conduct disorder seem to be based on false beliefs of being slandered, disadvantaged, or persecuted, one may be justified in labelling the disorder as a *paranoid state*, in a preliminary fashion. The next task is to discover the nature of the disorder which has given rise to the paranoid symptomatology. For this purpose it might be useful to have in mind the following simple classificatory schema:

Acute and transient paranoid episodes

Persistent paranoid reactions
Paranoid symptoms in manic and depressive illnesses
Paranoia ('true' delusions without hallucinations or affective deterioration)
Paraphrenia (delusions and hallucinations without deterioration)
Paranoid schizophrenia (delusions and hallucinations with affective deterioration)
Paranoid symptoms in acute, subacute, and persistent brain syndromes

It is doubtful whether, in terms of their further course, paranoid schizophrenia and paraphrenia, and even perhaps paranoia, are separate conditions.

The paranoid spectrum

Paranoid clinical phenomena are present in so many different psychiatric conditions that their detailed discussion would lead to confusing overlap with other chapters in the present volume, and with several chapters in volumes 1 and 2. For this reason, paranoid symptomatology will in the present chapter be discussed from a bird's-eye view, and references to only a few particularly informative and important publications will be quoted.

The ubiquity of paranoid phenomena may be seen as related to a basic human tendency to anticipate hostility emanating from others. This tendency may have been of advantage during early human development (Monod, 1971). It is, however, of decided disadvantage in modern society, in which well-integrated people tend to adopt an attitude of trust towards those they know and to society more generally, though not always to members of other societies.

Both social and personality disintegrations may provoke the release of paranoid ways of experiencing, thinking, and behaving. Thus, paranoid symptomatology is rarely encountered in children, adolescents, or young people. Paranoid clinical phenomena become increasingly common from middle life onwards when, especially in the presence of unfavourable circumstances, an individual's bonds with significant others and with his group may become increasingly disrupted. Certain personality traits may sharpen and shape a personality type which has been found to pre-date the onset of many, though by no means all, mental illnesses with prominent paranoid symptomatology. Paranoid personalities have been described as violent, excitable, self-willed, and distrustful, but also as sensitive, shy, and tending to be preoccupied with what other people might be thinking about them; homosexual men have been held to be especially likely to develop these attitudes, although the evidence is not convincing. Homosexuality is also said by some to play a fundamental psycho-dynamic role in the origin of paranoid psychoses. (Henderson & Batchelor, 1962, pp. 290–95).

These personality developments may facilitate *acute paranoid reactions* lasting only for a few days or weeks, as in *bouffées délirantes* (see footnote on p. 7); or for longer periods under the impact of social isolation in prisoners or immigrants. Where sexual bonds have been unstable or have become fragile, conjugal paranoia (Revitch, 1954) or pathological jealousy with delusions of infidelity (Shepherd, 1961) may become established, and subside only when the precipitating relationship has been dissolved. On the other hand, deafness originating during early life may be an important factor in fostering paranoid personality deviations, which (possibly in relation to increasing social isolation) may develop into persistent paranoid psychoses in old age (Cooper, Garside & Kay, 1976).

In the case of all transient or persistent paranoid reactions, sudden or progressive social isolation acting on a vulnerable personality seems to have been at work. By contrast, transient or persistent disruption of personality functioning, as it occurs in major mental illnesses, may also lead to the release of paranoid phenomena.

This is seen most strikingly and most frequently in the case of the *schizophrenias*. Henderson and Batchelor (1962, pp. 261–2) were so impressed by the frequency of paranoid symptoms in all Kraepelinian types of schizophrenia that they proposed the abolition of 'paranoid schizophrenia' as a separate type, and suggested 'paranoid psychosis' as a substitute. They pointed out that paranoid psychoses develop later in life than does schizophrenia, e.g. at 35 or over; that paranoid psychoses are symptomatically more homogeneous and do not show the same mutual transitions and admixtures as the various types of schizophrenia; also that they have a stronger affective component, are often of a transitory or cyclical nature, and thus might be more responsive to treatment. Finally, Henderson and Batchelor were influenced by the often attested fact that patients with paranoid psychoses rarely exhibit the gross intellectual and emotional deterioration which is characteristic of many schizophrenics. Elsewhere (Post, 1966, 1978, 1980), a considerable volume of subsequent

experience has been summarized, showing that schizophrenic illnesses quite often arise for the first time after the age of 40 through to old age, that many of them bear the hallmark of Schneider's first-rank symptoms, and that resurrecting the term 'paraphrenia' for late onset schizophrenia is clinically unhelpful. Even those paranoid psychoses of late onset which do not exhibit Schneider's phenomena, but only a simple hallucinosis or paranoid delusional ideas without 'dissolution of ego boundaries', respond well to major tranquillizing drugs, and should therefore be classed among the schizophrenias, until these disorders come to be conceptualized in terms of basic pathology rather than of symptomatology or response to treatment.

Affective psychoses may also be complicated by paranoid symptoms. In *depression*, paranoid delusions can usually be derived from the patient's feelings of lowered self-esteem or from his delusional ideas of guilt, in that he regards pseudo-hallucinatory criticisms and derogatory remarks as well as imaginary persecutory experiences as deserved. In *mania*, paranoid beliefs often develop around the restraints that others attempt to place on the patient. *Mixed manic-depressive psychoses* are often associated with much perplexity and with paranoid symptoms not clearly derivable from any dominant affect: under these circumstances patients may be misdiagnosed as schizophrenics. A similar error can occur in elderly patients with so-called involutional and senile melancholias in which the depressive affect is often hostile in colouring and the paranoid content not clearly guilt-laden. At all ages, paranoid symptoms are likely to lead into the theoretical and therapeutic problems presented by the controversial concept of a schizo-affective type of illness (Procci, 1976).

Finally, paranoid phenomena may for a time be prominent when personality becomes disrupted by cerebral disease or deterioration. Paranoid symptomatology may lead to errors in diagnosis when associated with *acute* or *subacute brain syndromes*, in which diminished awareness, disorientation, and amnesia are not prominent. Delirium due to drugs like amphetamines, or related to alcohol abuse, presents the most striking example. *Chronic brain syndromes* may equally present with a largely paranoid symptomatology at a time when intellectual functioning is still relatively intact. Thus some persistent alcoholic psychoses may be descriptively indistinguishable from paranoid schizophrenia; the same problem used to arise frequently in the case of general paralysis of the insane, but is now more commonly encountered in long-standing temporal lobe epilepsy (Slater *et al.*, 1963). Many of the dementing illnesses of middle and late life, from Huntington's chorea to pre-senile, senile, and multi-infarct dementias, may exhibit, for a time at least, significant paranoid features (Davison & Bagley, 1969; see also chapter 6).

When paranoid reactions occur in relation to certain life-events or situations – for example, to litigation and claims for financial compensation, to imprisonment, to emigration, to long-standing deafness, or, in the case of *'folie à deux'*, to close contact with someone with a paranoid illness – the disorder almost always represents a disabling increase of personality traits which have been present for many years. Similarly, when one of the major functional psychoses is associated with paranoid symptoms, it can usually be demonstrated that this is due to a 'pathoplastic' influence of the previous personality. By contrast, paranoid symptoms in the course of cerebral disorders often arise in persons without conspicuous paranoid traits. Earlier suspiciousness, sensitivity, or schizoid traits are usually denied by friends and relatives. Also there is no evidence of hereditary predisposition to paranoid or schizophrenic illness. For example, paranoid psychotic patients with temporal lobe epilepsy did not have a higher incidence of schizophrenia in their families than was found in the general population (Slater, Beard & Glithero, 1963). This would seem to indicate that disintegration of cerebral functioning alone may lead to the release of paranoid phenomena, even in the absence of inborn or acquired predispositions.

The form of paranoid symptoms

In the differential diagnosis of paranoid conditions attention paid to descriptive psychopathology may prove useful. Some relevant considerations will therefore be summarized.

Kolle (1957), much of whose life work has been concerned with paranoia and paranoid conditions, accepts the classical differentiation between 'true delusion' (the German *'Wahn'*, for which there is no adequate equivalent in English) and delusional ideas, overvalued ideas, intrusive thoughts, and ideas of reference with full and immediate insight and often an obsessional quality. He quotes Gruhle whose views represent a development of Jasper's seminal ideas: 'Delusion is an interconnecting (an interpreting) without obvious cause or provocation. Delusion

is an immediately present flash of insight without obvious antecedent. Delusional mood is a mood without obvious cause. Delusion does not originate from subliminal wishes or from suppressed emotions. It is a cerebral or organic, not-further-derivable symptom, with which one cannot empathise.' (Gruhle assumed that schizophrenia was a cerebral disease of unknown but specific pathology.) Kolle then approvingly quoted Schneider: 'Where there is true delusion, there is schizophrenic symptomatology and, though not entirely without exceptions, clinical schizophrenia.' Kolle goes on to enumerate four principles: two are classical and two others, which oppose them, are modern. (1) He agrees with Gruhle that true delusions are always incomprehensible and cannot be explained by reference to psychological motives. They are symptoms of a psychosis, usually schizophrenia, but occasionally epilepsy or some other cerebral disorder. Thus, true delusion is a feature of *process paranoia*. (2) The delusional ideas of litigious personalities ('paranoia querulans'), of over-ambitious and overactive ('hyperthymic') personalities, of fanatic 'weaklings', of prisoners, of deaf persons, and of the morbidly jealous, should be distinguished from true delusions. Such 'delusional ideas' are characteristic of *developmental paranoia*. Opposed to these classic principles are two modern ones. (3) There are paranoiacs whose delusions can be understood and explained in terms of constitution, experience or milieu (i.e. there is no disease entity called *paranoia*). (4) Nosology and a medical conceptual framework are inappropriate. Delusions are regarded as products giving meaning to an existence which, without delusions, would be condemned to failure. Delusion is not illness, but a form of existence, a way of life, and a view of the world.

Kolle discusses earlier views concerning the psychological structure, the origin and the outcome of delusion, and its relationship to normal mental life (e.g. to falling in love or to superstitions). He finds rather too obvious to be helpful Bleuler's dictum: 'Illness is only the fixation of the error, out of which arises delusion, and through which the abnormality becomes paranoia.'

In practice it may prove difficult to recognize the finer structure of paranoid symptoms because communication difficulties are very common. Many patients are very reticent about their beliefs, which may only be discovered by accident or at a time of crisis. The experiences are difficult to describe, except for people gifted in language. Many paranoid persons have an incomplete command of the English language, or are deaf or indistinct in diction. Even when the patients' statements are clear and explicit, the fact that the delusion has arisen autochthonously, without motive or explanation, may be very difficult to establish. It is usually only possible to decide that in a given patient the symptom lies somewhere between a true delusion and a delusional idea, but this will be useful in alerting the clinician to the possibility of a basically schizophrenic or organic disorder. True delusions without any other psychotic symptoms, i.e. paranoia, are so rare that a psychiatrist is unlikely to encounter more than two or three cases during a professional lifetime. By contrast, the presence of delusional ideas, using the term to indicate that the mental mechanisms are obvious even during routine history-taking and exploration, will direct the clinician's attention to the exclusion of a depressive, manic-depressive, or early psycho-organic illness. Finally, with few exceptions, paranoid ideas (including ideas of reference), which fluctuate in degree of conviction, and which are clearly related in content to some specific problem or trauma, make the presence of a paranoid reaction in a deviant personality a strong possibility. Contact with the patient is well preserved and the ideas are anchored in real, if idiosyncratically described, conflicts (Pauleikhoff & Mester, 1972).

Prognosis in paranoid disorders

Concerning the course of illnesses with prominent paranoid symptoms, it is generally accepted that they are compatible with life outside psychiatric institutions in the great majority of cases, but precise data on the fate of the paranoid symptoms themselves are hard to come by. For elderly paraphrenics, there have been prognostic studies before the introduction of major tranquillizers (Kay & Roth, 1961; Kay, 1963): patients hardly ever remitted. Pharmacotherapy has improved short- and long-term prognosis markedly (Post, 1966). Only in 8 per cent of cases was there no immediate response to medication; 31 per cent of patients continued to have abnormal experiences and to entertain delusional beliefs, but as their behaviour became more controlled they could return to community living. In 61 per cent, complete remission of symptoms was achieved, and half even achieved some insight into the pathological nature of their recent beliefs and experiences. Over the subsequent three years, and largely dependent on successful maintenance drug therapy, 34 per cent remained without

symptoms or psychiatric disabilities throughout the follow-up period, 38 per cent pursued a fluctuating course, but 28 per cent remained psychotic throughout, though not necessarily continuously in hospital. The most searching prognostic studies of younger subjects are those of Retterstöl (1966, with an excellent summary of the whole subject of paranoid disorders, 1968, 1970).

In later publications, Retterstöl reported on the results of a follow-up of some 300 patients for 5 to 18 years. All the patients were seen by him at the time of follow-up and he had personally assessed many of them during the index admission to a University clinic. They were all regarded as psychotic and suffering from delusions ('incorrect or unreasonable ideas, arising on a pathological basis and given the value of absolute truth by the patient'). Initially there were 52 'process schizophrenics' and 167 'reactive psychotics' according to the Scandinavian terminology (see chapter 4), 76 in whom this differentiation could not be made, and 10 with various cerebral organic conditions, though only one was due to alcohol. At follow-up there were 84 'process schizophrenics', 206 'reactive psychotics', 7 organics, 2 alcoholics, and 2 manic-depressives. Affective psychotics with paranoid delusions had been excluded from the original material, but it should be noted that, although the majority of patients had leading delusions of persecution (178), self-reference (38), and jealousy (21), there were also patients with other types of delusion, especially of a depressive (19) and a hypochondriacal (15) kind.

Seven patients had committed suicide during the observation period and seven had made an attempt. Retterstöl fails to draw attention to the problem of homicide in paranoid psychoses, presumably because it had not arisen in patients seen at a university clinic. Only 10 per cent of the 'process schizophrenics' made complete and lasting remissions, while 90 per cent continued to exhibit schizophrenic symptoms or defects. By contrast, 54 per cent of reactive psychotics remitted completely and lastingly, 36 per cent remitted but had further attacks with good recoveries, and only 10 per cent pursued a chronic course. In the whole sample, systematized delusions remitted somewhat less frequently (60 per cent) than unsystematized delusions (76 per cent). There was some evidence of a better outcome in patients treated since ataractic drugs had come into use. Not unexpectedly, especially when present in combination, favourable prognostic factors were acute onset and the presence of obvious precipitating factors, depressive mood, good emotional contact with the patient when first seen, and an unremarkable or sensitive personality. Unfavourable prognostic factors were an insidious onset, hallucinations, and ideas of influence.

In conclusion, Retterstöl's careful and personal follow-up study confirms that paranoid symptoms occur in a variety of clinical settings and that the prognosis is that of the basic disorder. However, some of the reactive psychotics might have been diagnosed elsewhere as affectives (Berner, 1972). Economically, paranoid illnesses were not usually incapacitating (more than 60 per cent continued at work most of the time), a few required further admissions, and favourable changes in social circumstances could often be shown to have had beneficial effects.

6
Differential diagnosis
ERIK STRÖMGREN

It is highly probable that the concept of schizophrenia comprises a number of disorders with different aetiologies. Since there is much disagreement
concerning the nature of these disorders it is necessary to question whether a diagnosis is worth making.
So far as the central group of syndromes, recognized
by most psychiatrists throughout the world, is concerned, there are several reasons why making a diagnosis can be useful. Such a diagnosis has some relevance for the choice of treatment, for prognosis, and
for research. Moreover, in certain cases a diagnosis
of schizophrenia has relevance for genetic counselling. It is much less clear that some of the more
peripheral conditions discussed in chapter 4 have any
practical significance at the moment.

Before a diagnosis of schizophrenia is made,
some basic requirements should be fulfilled. First, it
is necessary to know whether the patient shows any
sign of disturbed consciousness. If that is the case a
diagnosis of schizophrenia cannot be made with certainty even if there are characteristic schizophrenic
symptoms. Next, it is necessary to make an approximate estimate of the intelligence level of the patient;
in the severely mentally retarded any psychosis may
acquire atypical characteristics. The same is true of
psychoses arising during adolescence, before personality is fully formed. Finally, since peculiarities of
language in a psychotic patient suggest a possible
diagnosis of schizophrenia, it is necessary to discover
whether the patient was ever in command of the local

language and, if so, whether organic defects have affected verbal ability.

Few diagnostic aids are available for differentiating schizophrenia from other conditions. There may well be biochemical abnormalities in some schizophrenic subgroups but none is useful in diagnosis. Nor can other physical findings be regarded of importance for this purpose. The same is true of psychological tests. In spite of the enormous number of publications about the differences in psychological performance between schizophrenic patients and matched controls, no test has been devised which can make a satisfactory allocation to one group or the other. One of the most useful tests is one devised at the beginning of the century, namely Jung's Association Test (1969). The Rorschach test is still widely used, and in some cases it gives useful diagnostic hints, but these are rarely decisive. There is too great a temptation to diagnose 'borderline' and 'latent' schizophrenias which cannot be confirmed in any other way.

Our main tools for the diagnosis of schizophrenia are therefore, as they were a hundred years ago, the history of the disorder, the patient's own account of his experiences, the way he interacts in the clinical interview, and observation of his behaviour over time. With regard to the interview it should be borne in mind that a great number of symptoms and signs are of importance for the diagnosis of schizophrenia, and it is therefore advisable that a comprehensive and systematic technique should be used; one which covers the great majority of relevant symptoms such as the Present State Examination (Wing, Cooper & Sartorius, 1974).

Problems of differential diagnosis will be discussed in the following order: (1) organic disorders; (2) endogenous psychoses; (3) reactive psychoses; (4) neuroses and personality disorders; (5) Kanner's syndrome; (6) mental retardation.

(1) Organic disorders

Many toxic agents can give rise to mental abnormalities which may be more or less like schizophrenia. Few of them, however, completely imitate schizophrenia. The best known of these is amphetamine (Bonhoff & Lewrenz, 1954; Connell, 1958). Some cases of amphetamine psychosis cannot be distinguished symptomatologically from schizophrenia. Delusions and hallucinations are prominent and the emotional change is the same as in schizophrenic autism. In addition, the experiences from the Japanese pervitin epidemics seem to show that some of these schizophrenia-like psychoses continue for years after the cessation of the drug abuse. In such cases only the history and knowledge of the pre-morbid personality can give some diagnostic help.

Marihuana psychoses may mimic schizophrenia (Bernhardson & Gunne 1972) but here the history usually helps to the right diagnosis. Clinically these patients are more emotionally labile than most schizophrenics. When marihuana has been used for years and then discontinued, a chronic deteriorated stage may persist. These patients may be mistaken for hebephrenics but contact is usually better than with true schizophrenics. They may be childish, without ambition, but often also without any definite psychotic symptoms.

In populations where alcohol abuse is widespread many schizophrenics will also be alcoholics. In these cases it may for a long time be impossible to determine which came first. Chronic hallucinosis in alcoholics seems to be of two kinds; some of these patients turn out to be schizophrenics, others preserve good contact with their surroundings and, although they continue to be deluded and hallucinated, do not make an autistic impression during interview. On the contrary, they may seek help, talking vividly and anxiously about their hallucinations, which are often of a schizophrenia-like type; e.g. several voices talking about the patient, one accusing and threatening the patient, another defending him. The patient is dominated by fear, and his whole attitude is clearly different from the often apathetic behaviour of the schizophrenic or the amphetamine addict who experiences hallucinations of a similar kind.

Among *metabolic disorders* myxoedema occasionally gives rise to chronic paranoid states which may be mistaken for schizophrenia. Their physical symptoms may not be very prominent but their general mental inactivity in spite of reasonable contact usually gives a suspicion that it is something else than schizophrenia.

A number of *infectious disorders* can occasionally cause schizophrenia-like states. During the 1920s and 1930s Economo's encephalitis in some cases precipitated schizophrenia-like disorders, especially of the catatonic type. All the classical catatonic symptoms could be seen in pure form. Episodes with hallucinations and illusions could also occur. In these cases there are of course usually some neurological symptoms which can decide the diagnosis, and in addition emotional contact with these patients is usually much better than with schizophrenics; they have more insight and they usually want treatment.

In children with rheumatic encephalitis (chorea minor) the mutism and peculiar movements may sometimes lead to a false diagnosis of schizophrenia. The history and the neurological examination soon disprove this diagnosis.

Among the *degenerative disorders* Huntington's chorea is well known for being able to produce definitely schizophrenia-like symptomatology. Such symptoms may for years be the only expression of the disorder. The family history, however, usually solves the problem. Cases of this kind as well as cases of amphetamine psychosis have given rise to speculations concerning the possibility of a purely organic causation of schizophrenia.

Several cases of *leucodystrophy* (Einarson & Strömgren, 1961) start as a mental disorder, sometimes imitating a mild deterioration with pseudo-psychopathic behaviour. When these symptoms are accompanied by paranoid ideas a diagnosis of schizophrenia is not far-fetched. Here again a close neurological examination will solve the problem. Similar mistakes may arise in early cases of *Pick's disease* (lobar atrophy) where the first symptoms may be emotional blunting, careless or antisocial behaviour without obvious organic syndromes. These patients are, however, more alert and more easy to contact than schizophrenics. As soon as the suspicion of lobar atrophy has arisen CT-scanning will decide the case. Early stages of *Alzheimer's disease* can be mistaken for schizophrenia when the symptoms are mainly paranoid. Very soon, however, the typical disorders of language and of motor behaviour become obvious.

The problem of chronic *epileptic psychosis* versus schizophrenia had been discussed for generations until the investigations of Slater and associates (1963) finally put an end to it through their careful studies of the families of epileptics with chronic schizophrenia-like psychosis. The result was that these psychoses were an expression of the epileptic disorder and not a concomitant schizophrenia. In most cases there is also a symptomatology which in spite of the presence of chronic delusions and hallucinations distinguishes these cases from schizophrenia. The emotional contact with these patients is better than with chronic schizophrenics, and the favourable reaction of these psychoses to drugs like carbamazepine is often striking. In most cases the EEG will also help the differential diagnosis.

(2) Endogenous psychoses

Different kinds of *paranoid psychoses* which probably have nothing to do with schizophrenia can under certain circumstances be mistaken for paranoid schizophrenia. Kretschmer's *'sensitiver Beziehungswahn'* (1966), a sensitive delusion of reference, is a typical example of this group. These patients do not show anything like schizophrenic autism, contact with them is good. The symptoms are fully understandable, speech is quite normal, they do not suffer from hallucinations, although they often are subject to mistakes and illusions in accordance with their delusions of reference. They sometimes respond favourably to psychotherapy. Paranoid psychoses may arise in persons who are isolated with respect to language (Allers' syndrome), for instance immigrants, prisoners of war, and deaf people. Here again the emotional contact is usually easy to obtain, and the symptoms recede as soon as verbal contact is established.

The distinction between schizophrenia and *manic-depressive disorder* has been one of the big issues in psychiatric discussion ever since these two disorders were described as separate entities by Kraepelin. Occasionally manic-depressive phases may be quite atypical, acquiring some of the symptoms which are regarded as characteristic of schizophrenia. This is especially the case when the attacks are of long duration. Manic patients who in the beginning were optimistic and good-humoured may during a long stay in hospital become litigious and paranoid. Some manic-depressive disorders characterized by recurrent attacks with typical affective symptoms may occasionally present with a completely atypical clinical picture, for instance with dominating delusions and hallucinations. If this occurs during the first attack it may be difficult to establish the correct diagnosis. Nevertheless, it is nearly always true that contact with the patients is easy to obtain and that the basic emotional change can be disclosed; the delusions and hallucinations then usually seem to be in accordance with the underlying emotion. Depressives may be predominantly paranoid. On the surface their delusions may seem to be of a persecutory nature, but on closer analysis they turn out to be based on deep dissatisfaction with the patient himself, on ideas of guilt and self-deprecation. In the pre-therapeutic era many manic-depressive patients had to stay for years in psychiatric hospitals and the influence of the hospital environment sometimes produced adventitious symptoms. If the energy of mania was not directed into more useful channels, motor activity could take the form of catatonic-like stereotyped movements. Similarly, mute and stuporous patients with melancholia could be mistaken for catatonic schizophrenics. Although such pictures have now become rare, it is important that they are recognized when they do occur.

When manics are left by themselves, e.g. in a single room in a hospital, they may carry on a dialogue with themselves, giving the impression that they are hearing voices. As soon as they are approached it becomes clear that this is not the case. In acute mania the stream of associations may be so vivid that there is no time to complete sentences, the speech thus becoming more or less disrupted and virtually 'incoherent'. If the patient can be interrupted, however, and persuaded to concentrate, he can often explain what is meant. Grandiose ideas in manics may occasionally seem quite unreasonable, but here again discussion with the patient will usually demonstrate that he can take account of reality. For example, a statement that 'my thoughts come from the sun' might be regarded as a first-rank symptom until the patient explains that he means, 'I am so great that my thoughts could come from the sun'. Similarly, a statement that the doctor is influencing a female patient to have intercourse with him might reflect hypersexuality rather than a delusion of control.

Although in most cases it is possible, on close examination, to find out whether a psychosis is schizophrenic or manic-depressive, there are some cases in which the distinction seems impossible. In some cases which over the years develop into unquestionable schizophrenia the onset may have been of a seemingly typical melancholic nature. After several months or even years the emotional components seem to fade away leaving the delusions and hallucinations as the dominant features. See chapter 19 for further consideration of the differential diagnosis.

(3) Non-organic reactive psychoses

When these psychoses have a strong paranoid component they may be mistaken for schizophrenia. It is, however, characteristic that they arise in immediate connection with a severe mental trauma and that the symptomatology is centered on this trauma. The emotional contact is well preserved, and these patients are usually eager to seek treatment and to discuss their problems. Difficulties may arise in cases where the patient has amnesia for the trauma or for some reason is unwilling to disclose the trauma or does not want to talk about it because this would be too stressful and painful. After some time, however, the patient usually prefers to share his problems with others.

(4) Neuroses and personality disorders

Initially it may be difficult to distinguish pseudoneurotic schizophrenia from true neurosis. The salient point is that pseudoneurotics do not obtain the secondary gain which is characteristic of neurotics. Even if contact with pseudoneurotics usually is much better than with other schizophrenics, and although the pseudoneurotic may be relatively attached to the therapist, a distance remains which is not found in the treatment of neurotics. With regard to pseudopsychopathic schizophrenia, there are especially difficult diagnostic problems, these cases often being blurred by a concomitant addiction to drugs or alcohol and by their conflicts with their surroundings. It usually takes a long-lasting acquaintance with them before the different components in these vary mixed pictures can be separated from each other.

One type of personality disorder has been the subject of unusually lively discussion throughout psychiatric history: the *schizoid personality* which has been supposed to have a special affinity to schizophrenia both as a common pre-psychotic personality and as a common personality variation occurring among the relatives of schizophrenics. It has even been suggested that schizophrenia, schizoidia, and normal personality lie on the same continuum. This was for a long time the opinion of Kretschmer and some of his associates. Others regard this type of personality as a soil favourable to the emergence of schizophrenic psychoses. Others again regard a schizoid type as being mainly of pathoplastic importance in the sense that any psychosis arising in such personalities would have a schizoid colouring. In the ICD 9, 'schizoid personality disorder' (301.2) is defined thus: 'Personality disorder in which there is withdrawal from affectional, social and other contacts with autistic preference for fantasy and introspective reserve. Behaviour may be slightly eccentric or indicate avoidance of competitive situations. Apparent coolness and detachment may mask an incapacity to express feeling.' In spite of detailed descriptions of this kind it is usually very difficult to make the diagnosis of schizoid personality, and the usefulness of the term must be limited in research. Many traits which fit in well with the concept of schizoidia may partly be culturally determined.

In some patients a development may occur which imposes great diagnostic (and theoretical) problems: It happens that patients who during a number of years seem to have been suffering from typically neurotic obsessions and compulsions gradually develop definite schizophrenias. In the beginning they have full insight into the falseness of their ideas and impulsions but very slowly over the years their attitude changes and eventually becomes fully paranoid. It is, however, characteristic that even at this stage contact is reasonably well preserved. For a long time during this development their comments on the symptoms may be very vague, making it quite difficult to discover whether they are neurotic or psychotic. Finally, however, the psychotic development becomes manifest.

(5) *Kanner's syndrome*

The diagnosis of 'infantile autism' is dealt with in chapters 29 and 30. Since this syndrome has only recently been accepted within psychiatry it can happen that the psychiatrist is confronted with adults with this syndrome which was not diagnosed while they were children. At present few lifelong histories of such personalities exist, but some features which are characteristic of these patients in young adulthood are now known. Although nearly all such patients remain odd in behaviour as adults and may for this reason raise the suspicion of schizophrenia, on closer examination they will turn out to be something different. They do not have a broad capacity for contact but some have a great need to explain themselves and to be understood. Most remain severely retarded but a few have an amazing understanding of their own pecularities, their very special form of reaction, and they deeply appreciate understanding shown to them. This is also true of the special form known as Asperger's syndrome (chapter 29). It is unfortunate that the misleading term 'autism' has been attached to these patients.

(6) *Mental retardation*

Psychoses arising in the mentally retarded may, regardless of the origin of the psychosis, acquire a schizophrenia-like picture especially in the direction of catatonic features. Manic-depressive psychoses may easily be mistaken for schizophrenias in patients who have difficulties in describing their experiences. The same is true in oligophrenics with reactive psychoses. Here it may be difficult to discover the mental trauma, which may therefore be overlooked. In addition, many mentally retarded people are especially inclined to repress and forget the mental trauma or at least have only a very vague recollection of it. In these cases it is essential to obtain information about the capacities for intellectual and emotional contact which were present in the patients before the psychosis broke out. The distinction between schizophrenia superimposed on mental retardation ('*Pfropfschizophrenie*') and other psychoses may be extremely difficult. Unusual ideas of a fragmentary or fleeting kind are not uncommon in mental retardation and do not carry any implication of schizophrenic or paranoid psychosis. Some severely retarded people with features of Kanner's syndrome may appear both withdrawn and thought-disordered, as well as severely disturbed behaviourally. The differential diagnosis is discussed in chapter 30.

There are thus a great number of disorders which occasionally or at certain stages may closely resemble schizophrenia. Although some symptoms are of great distinctive value, such symptoms may be difficult to observe and to evaluate. In addition, there are the usual difficulties arising from the prevailing differences with regard to the delimitation of the concept of schizophrenia. Such differences will of course greatly invalidate comparative statistical studies on the frequency of schizophrenia. In addition, the differences can easily be intensified by emotional factors in the observer. A psychiatrist who uses a wide concept of schizophrenia will include in the concept a great number of cases with a favourable prognosis; to this psychiatrist the diagnosis of schizophrenia is therefore not catastrophic. In contrast, the psychiatrist who applies a very narrow concept of schizophrenia and includes only cases with an unfavourable course will often, out of empathy with a patient and his relatives, be reluctant to label the patient schizophrenic; he may, consciously or unconsciously, act as an advocate for a more favourable diagnosis. Being a good therapist he will, however, in spite of his making a diagnosis with less sinister implications, not hesitate to use therapies which he believes to be of help to people with schizophrenia. So in the end it is only the statistics which suffer.

7
Course and prognosis of schizophrenia

J. K. WING

Elements of the course

Three main types of factor are involved in any consideration of the course of a condition, such as schizophrenia, which is defined mainly in terms of its manifestations. The first is clinical, the second social, the third personal.

Clinical factors

Although there is an approximate consensus as to the syndromes that are most characteristic of schizophrenia, there is much disagreement on details, and follow-up studies have rarely specified diagnostic principles precisely enough to allow close comparison of the results. If, as Eugen Bleuler suggested, there are several 'schizophrenias', each perhaps with its own characteristic course, the composition of each sample of patients becomes crucial. In particular, some psychiatrists take course into account when making a diagnosis, excluding those illnesses that they think have a good prognosis.

The elements involved in tracing the clinical course include pre-morbid personality and presence of abnormality in childhood, acuteness of onset of florid schizophrenic symptoms, presence of other symptoms such as depression, duration of initial episode and quality, frequency and type of subsequent acute episodes (not all of which are necessarily characterized by schizophrenic symptoms), and the degree of cognitive and affective impairment ('negative' symptoms) that persists between or following episodes.

All these elements are difficult to define and measure. Each can be influenced by various predisposing, precipitating, modifying, ameliorating, or maintaining factors, many of which can also differ in different samples, making comparison even more difficult.

Social factors

Apart from the importance of social factors in precipitating or modifying the symptomatic course, some social factors (such as a long experience of poverty or prejudice, poor employment opportunities, or lack of family and social support) may be handicapping in themselves. A lower than expected level of social performance is then not necessarily due, either wholly or in part, to any clinical disorder that has previously been present or that is present at the time of follow-up.

Personal factors

Each individual reacts to the experience of illness, impairment, and social disadvantages in his or her own way. Unless florid or negative schizophrenic symptoms are very severe and chronic, in which case they are likely to determine the level of social performance as well as the clinical course, the individual's personal reactions will be an important factor. These, in turn, depend to a considerable extent on the reactions of influential people in the immediate social environment, such as relatives, employers, workmates, and professionals. Some patients are able to support themselves in employment in spite of experiencing almost continuous hallucinations; others find the experience completely disabling. Some prefer to live in a protected environment, such as a hostel or hospital; others refuse to do so even when it might be wise.

Methodological problems

The problems of defining and measuring the clinical, social, and personal factors mentioned above are formidable enough but a further problem is presented by the choice of outcome criteria. A single overall index – e.g. good, moderate, or poor – tends to attract roughly equal proportions into its categories. As Zubin (1978) pointed out, this does not allow comparability between studies or over time. Length of stay in hospital was frequently used as an index in earlier studies, but many people remained in hospital whose clinical symptoms and impairments were quite

mild (Wing & Brown, 1970). Factors such as marital status (Ødegård, 1946), occupation (Cooper, 1961), and whether or not the patient received visitors (Brown, 1959) also determined length of stay. Moreover, discharge from hospital does not necessarily mean that the patient is symptom-free (Brown et al., 1966). More than a century ago, during the era of 'moral treatment', discharge rates were as high as they are now (Bockoven, 1956; Jones, 1972).

The concept of social outcome has also been extensively used but with very varied connotations. (For a criticism of the concept, see: Harris et al., 1956; Shepherd, 1957). Level of social performance can be affected by social disadvantages and adverse personal reactions independently of clinical disability. Length of follow-up period, prospective versus retrospective or combined designs, and the inclusion of patients at different phases of disorder are other factors that are rarely controlled.

A useful summary of methodological difficulties and of the varied solutions adopted by workers who have conducted follow-up studies will be found in the volume devoted to the two-year outcome of patients included in the International Pilot Study of Schizophrenia (WHO, 1979). Another helpful review of studies of course and outcome is given by several authors in section 12 of the report of the second Rochester international conference on schizophrenia (Wynne, Cromwell & Matthysse, 1978).

Follow-up studies
Description of course and outcome

Kraepelin (1913) reviewed a number of early studies which indicated a generally poor outcome in dementia praecox, no matter what the early course had been. His own series of patients admitted to the Heidelberg clinic suggested only about 4 per cent with good recoveries (17 per cent if those with a fairly good 'social adjustment' were included).

Mayer-Gross (1932) followed up 260 patients out of a total of 294 admitted to the same clinic in 1912 and 1913. Sixteen years later, some 35 per cent had made 'social recoveries' and 5 per cent were socially disabled but out of hospital. There was, however, a high death-rate (43 per cent) among those who had remained in hospital.

Most early descriptions of the course of schizophrenia were based on hospital records. Up to the 1930s, about 60 per cent of all patients hospitalized for the first time and given this diagnosis (or that of dementia praecox) were likely to remain there indefinitely, about 20 per cent were said to be severely

Table 7.1. *Five-year outcome of schizophrenic patients*

Five-year outcome	Admitted for insulin therapy to Maudsley Hospital 1945–50 %	First admitted to three mental hospitals 1956 %
Patient independent: no symptoms or only moderately severe	45	56
Patient dependent: no symptoms or only moderately severe	12	16
Severe disturbance, not in hospital	9	17
In-patient	34	11
	(N = 123)	(N = 94)
	Harris *et al.* (1956)	Brown *et al.* (1966)

impaired but could be discharged from hospital, and about 20 per cent made a reasonable recovery.

A series of follow-up studies of patients admitted to hospital before the introduction of reserpine and chlorpromazine, in which the outcome was determined by re-examination as well as case-record data, suggested that 44–66 per cent had a poor outcome (WHO, 1979, chapter 2), although the methodological problems mentioned earlier make a general conclusion difficult to draw. A further study, of 125 schizophrenic patients admitted to the Maudsley Hospital in London for deep insulin treatment between 1945 and 1950, showed that 45 per cent had made a 'social recovery' five years later and 21 per cent were socially disabled but out of hospital (Harris *et al.*, 1956). The series reported by M. Bleuler (1972, 1978) is given more extended consideration below.

Achtè (1967) studied two series of patients, one first admitted in 1950, the other ten years later. He found that five years later (when most patients were re-examined by the author) 62 per cent of the earlier series and 41 per cent of the later were either unable to work or were in hospital, and concluded that the course had definitely improved.

Brown and his colleagues (1966) studied 111 schizophrenic patients first admitted to three British mental hospitals in 1956. Five years later, 56 per cent were regarded as 'social recoveries', 34 per cent were socially disabled, and only 11 per cent were still in hospital. A comparison with the results of the study conducted by Harris and colleagues (1956) gives some indication of a possible change in the course of schizophrenia (table 7.1).

Brown and colleagues described the five-year pattern of course of their cohort of first admitted patients as follows: no problem during the final four years – 35 per cent; no, or only minor, problems during final two and a half years – 11 per cent; episodic course throughout the five years – 27 per cent; chronic course – 28 per cent.

The International Pilot Study of Schizophrenia (IPSS), carried out under the auspices of the World Health Organization, included consecutive series of patients contacting psychiatric services, most of whom were admitted to hospital in nine centres. There were 1200 patients in all (WHO, 1973). All were aged under 45 years and had had an onset within the previous five years. The results of a five-year follow-up study are not yet available but the two-year course has been reported in detail (WHO, 1979). One-third were asymptomatic at follow-up. More than half were either completely well or had only minor problems. On the other hand, nearly 20 per cent suffered severe social disablement, with the remainder intermediate. In spite of the wide diversity of cultural and clinical settings, the overall results were not very different from those of Achtè (1967) and Brown and colleagues (1966). The differences between centres will be considered in chapter 9.

The personal series reported by M. Bleuler

Manfred Bleuler has reported a unique series of 208 patients, personally followed for 20 years or more, who were admitted to the Burghölzli hospital, Zurich, after 1942. He also described other series, less intensively studied and followed up (Bleuler, 1972,

1978). The author states that borderline conditions – personality disorders, pseudoneurosis, etc. – have been excluded and that the diagnosis has been made on symptomatic criteria independently of any knowledge of course. He concludes that 25 per cent of schizophrenic patients recover entirely and remain recovered for good. The criteria for full recovery include lack of psychotic symptoms, normal social integration, and ability to work. These people do not require drug treatment or social care. Bleuler does not regard the attainment of full 'insight', in the sense of a completely objective attitude to all the past symptoms and experiences, as a useful criterion for recovery. The essays presented in *Schizophrenia from Within* provide an illustration of the reasonableness of this decision (Wing, 1975). Approximately two-thirds alternate for decades between acute psychotic phases and phases of improvement or recovery. About 10 per cent remain severely psychotic permanently.

Bleuler considers that the psychotic condition rarely progresses after a period of about five years. If anything it tends to improve after that. Statistically speaking, rather over 50 per cent will appear to have recovered at any given cross-section of the course followed by a cohort of patients, but many of these will, of course, be subject to future relapses. Some patients recover from active psychotic symptoms but 'remain underactive, lack personal initiative and have somewhat apathetic colourless personalities'.

Over all, Bleuler agrees with a general clinical impression that the course of schizophrenia has improved during this century, particularly because an acute severely psychotic episode in adolescence is now very rarely followed by a severe chronic psychosis that lasts a lifetime, and because the course has become much more episodic, with good periods of remission more common. On the other hand, the proportion of long-standing recoveries does not seem to him to have increased, nor the number of eventual severe chronic psychoses to have diminished.

Differentiation of the course of schizophrenia from that of other disorders

The course of the affective psychoses is described in chapter 20, and the specific problem of schizo-affective disorders is discussed there and in chapters 4 and 17. If a standard interview procedure is used, in which all acutely psychotic patients admitted to hospital are asked about a comprehensive list of symptoms, as was the case in the US–UK Diagnostic Project (Cooper *et al.*, 1972) and the IPSS

(WHO, 1973), it is found that acutely schizophrenic patients manifest a wide range of symptoms other than those regarded as specific for the diagnosis (Wing, Cooper & Sartorius, 1974). Depressed mood and other characteristics of the depressive syndrome – including hallucinations and delusions based on the affect, pathological guilt, psychomotor retardation, early morning waking, and subjective anergia – are quite common. As the patient improves, the schizophrenic symptoms disappear first, leaving the other symptoms behind. These observations suggest a hierarchical element in diagnosis and course (Wing, 1978c) and make it likely that patients who experience multiple episodes will occasionally have attacks which are purely depressive or manic. Such a course has indeed been observed (Sheldrick *et al.*, 1977; WHO, 1979). Patients also commonly experience 'non-specific' symptoms such as anxiety, irritability, muscular tension, and worrying between episodes or as the sole clinical outcome (Brown *et al.*, 1966).

Kraepelin (1913) observed that the course of schizophrenia could be differentiated from that of manic-depressive psychosis because of the usual development of cognitive and affective impairment ('dementia' as he called it) in the former but not the latter. He actually, for a time, incorporated this impairment into his criteria for diagnosing schizophrenia, although he subsequently regretted doing so.

In fact, acute schizophrenia can be distinguished reasonably well from manic or depressive psychotic episodes on symptomatic criteria (see chapters 6 and 19) and symptomatic acute schizophrenia may or may not lead to chronic deficit. Manfred Bleuler (1972) has pointed out the disadvantages of making course a criterion of diagnosis.

Astrup and Noreik (1966) carried out one of the few follow-up studies of patients first admitted with 'functional psychoses' whose outcome was determined in most cases by personal re-examination. They found that much larger proportions of patients with manic-depressive psychosis, reactive depressive psychoses, and hysterical psychoses were recovered or improved five to twelve years later than was the case with the schizophrenic psychoses. Paranoid psychoses were intermediate. Norris (1959) and Shepherd (1957) found that schizophrenic patients tended to stay longer in hospital than patients with affective psychoses.

The two-year outcome of patients in the IPSS (WHO, 1979) shows the 'movement down the hierarchy' already referred to, symptomatic differences between the various diagnostic categories tending to become less marked at follow-up. Where there was a further psychotic episode during the two year period, it tended to take the same symptomatic form as the episode of inclusion. Out of 59 cases in which the original episode of inclusion had been manic or psychotic depressive, the subsequent episode was also one of affective psychosis in 49. Out of 174 cases in which a schizophrenic patient had a further psychotic episode, this was also schizophrenic in 131. There was, however, a considerable overlap between diagnostic groups in terms of non-symptomatic measures of course and outcome. This was particularly true of schizophrenia and depression. However, the study was not well designed for an investigation of differential course and outcome because of its lack of an epidemiological base and the cut-off age of 45.

Mortality

Long-term hospital care has, in the past, been associated with excess mortality from diseases such as tuberculosis (Baldwin, 1979; Ekblom & Frisk, 1961; Mayer-Gross, 1932) but it has not been demonstrated that people with schizophrenia were specifically at risk. Ekblom and Frisk (1961) found that mortality rates in more recent cohorts were not significantly in excess. Modrzewska and Böök (1979) pointed to a possibly lower death risk from cancer among mental patients but Fox (1978) suggested that the results of many of the earlier studies varied according to the statistical index used. Interpretation is, in any case, difficult when the subjects are hospitalized patients. Baldwin (1979) reviewed the literature and concluded that the evidence for an excess or deficit in morbidity or mortality from any specific disease was inconclusive. The World Health Organization is currently sponsoring studies which should provide more adequate data.

Tsuang and colleagues (1978, 1980) found a significant excess of unnatural deaths (suicides, accidents, and homicides) among the schizophrenic members of a cohort followed up for 30 to 40 years. More recent studies of chronic schizophrenic patients have also found high rates (Lindelius & Kay, 1973; Saugstad and Ødegård, 1979; Wing, L., *et al.*, 1972; Wykes & Wing, 1981). The two-year IPSS follow-up gives minimal rates for suicide or possible suicide of 7 out of 552 men and 4 out of 650 women (WHO, 1979). Compared with the rates for Europe (May, 1972) these are very markedly higher than expected.

Prognosis
Pre-morbid factors and type of onset

In an extensive review of factors predicting outcome in schizophrenia, Zubin and his colleagues (1961) found that one of the most robust results was that sudden onset suggested a good prognosis while an insidious onset suggested a bad one. This correlation has held up in subsequent studies (Brown *et al.*, 1966; Simon & Wirt, 1961; Stephens, Astrup & Mangrum, 1966; Vaillant, 1962, 1964; WHO, 1979). Acute onset is associated with a number of other factors which also predict a favourable outcome, notably a good previous personality and record of social achievement, the presence of depression, and florid rather than negative symptoms (e.g. paranoid rather than simple or hebephrenic subgroup). Precipitating factors are also mentioned in several studies but methodological problems have rarely been overcome sufficiently to make the results convincing.

Brown and his colleagues (1966) pointed out that different factors might well predict different types of outcome. For example, their best predictor of employment during the last two years of the five-year follow-up period was employment during the two years before first admission. Clinical disturbance at follow-up was much less easy to predict (being separated or divorced before first admission made the only sizeable contribution) and it proved impossible to predict whether a patient would receive hospital care during the last two years of the follow-up period.

The five factors best predicting a poor two-year outcome on a composite index in the IPSS study (WHO, 1979) were: social isolation, long duration of episode before examination, history of past psychiatric treatment, being widowed, divorced or separated, and abnormal behaviour before admission. Only 19 per cent of the variance was explained by these factors.

Clinical factors

The attempt to differentiate symptom-complexes which lead to different outcomes has taken two main forms; the delineation of classes of schizophrenia and the demarcation of a 'schizophreniform' (reactive, atypical, acute, exogenous, etc.) group separate from the 'true' schizophrenias. (See also note on *bouffées délirantes*, chapter 1, page 7.)

Insofar as the simple and hebephrenic subtypes of schizophrenia are characterized by an insidious onset with increasing social withdrawal and affective flattening, in someone with a poor past history of social performance, the diagnosis is likely to be associated with an unfavourable course and outcome. The IPSS follow-up did show a small relationship of this kind though not sufficient to be of clinical value. Similarly, paranoid psychoses are more likely to occur later in life in people with some record of social achievement, and are less likely to be associated with severe cognitive impairment.

Langfeldt has made the strongest case for isolating a schizophreniform psychosis as a separate entity. In his first monograph (1937) he analysed, retrospectively, the initial characteristics of 100 patients whom he had followed for ten years or more. In his second monograph (1956), he summarized his views on the differences between the two groups. Factors associated with a favourable outcome were: good previous personality, precipitating events, acute onset, and a clinical picture characterized by clouding of consciousness and/or affective symptoms and an absence of affective flattening. These characteristics were absent in 'typical schizophrenia', in which the clinical picture was dominated by delusional experiences of influence and control which were incomprehensible to the observer. Catatonic symptoms were also associated with a poor prognosis.

Other workers associated with Langfeldt reached similar conclusions from subsequent studies. Welner and Strömgren (1958), however, in a study of patients originally diagnosed as suffering from schizophreniform psychoses, found nine years later that the clinical course required them to re-classify the condition as chronic schizophrenia in 30 per cent of cases.

The more heterogeneous the range of disorders considered to be 'schizophrenic' in the first place the easier it is to include a group with a favourable outcome. This may be one reason for some of the discrepancies in the literature. Brown and his colleagues (1966) found that psychiatrists at one of their three hospitals were far more likely to diagnose some form of schizophrenia than those at the other two. Much of the difference was due to symptoms such as depersonalization, apathy, odd somatic sensations, and ideas of reference. 'Depersonalization' was the term used by Langfeldt to describe delusional experiences of influence and control, although it is better restricted to non-delusional experiences common in affective disorders and anxiety states (Stengel, 1960). The US–UK Diagnostic Project (Cooper *et al.*, 1972) showed that American hospital diagnoses of schizophrenia were much more widely based than British

and included some conditions (for example, mania and psychotic depression) that might be expected to have better prognoses, and others, such as severe personality disorders, that would not be expected to have a favourable course.

Schneider (1971), who described the syndrome of 'first-rank symptoms', did not claim that these had any particular significance for the prognosis. The IPSS follow-up study (WHO, 1979) demonstrated no particularly adverse implications for the overall course when such symptoms were present.

Precipitating and modifying factors
Disease, trauma, and toxicity

Slater and his colleagues (1963) reviewed the occurrence of schizophrenia-like psychoses associated with epilepsy. Davison and Bagley (1969) made a systematic review of associations with conditions such as epilepsy, porphyria, cerebral tumour or trauma, and Huntington's chorea. Childbirth is another frequently reported precipitant as are amphetamine, bromide, and alcohol (see volume 2, chapters 5 and 14). Florid schizophrenic symptoms may be completely typical, although accompanied by other symptoms indicating the underlying diagnosis. Cutting (1980), however, found that first-rank symptoms were rare in his series of patients with physical illness accompanied by cerebral dysfunction.

There is some evidence that the chronic 'negative' symptoms are less evident when acute schizophrenic syndromes are precipitated in such ways. In Slater's series of 69 cases of epilepsy, for example, delusions in clear consciousness occurred in 67 but loss of affective responsiveness in only 28. Acute amphetamine psychosis is also less likely to be followed by chronic impairments (Connell, 1958).

Pasamanick and Lilienfeld (1955) suggested that there were predisposing as well as precipitating factors; in particular, prenatal or perinatal brain damage. (For a recent review, see McNeil & Kaij, 1978.) The evidence is statistical only but some confirmation may be derived from the fact that in identical twin pairs discordant for schizophrenia, the schizophrenic co-twin has often had a low birth weight and poor school performance (Kringlen, 1967; Pollin *et al.*, 1966; Tienari, 1963). Genetic predisposition is reviewed in chapter 11.

Social and cultural factors

The substantial role played by social and cultural factors in precipitating acute attacks of schizophrenia and in modifying the subsequent course is considered in chapter 9.

The influence of such factors in modifying the clinical picture also needs to be considered. Examples taken from the IPSS (WHO, 1973, pp. 275–6) include a Taoist priestess living in Taiwan who developed a psychosis characterized by 'delusions of influence and possession' which were, in fact subcultural in origin (diagnosis: hysterical psychosis), and an Indian villager who developed a psychosis with elation, grandiose ideas, and over-activity, but also complained that 'the ghost Braham Dev' possessed him and 'abused others through my voice' (diagnosis: mania).

Other types of social modifying factors are illustrated by cases of 'socially-shared psychopathology' (Guenberg, 1957; Lasèque & Falret, 1877; Sims *et al.*, 1977). Pathoplastic features are common in psychiatric disorders everywhere in the world. Small subcultural groups with a religious or other ideological motivation, small family groups like those described by Gruenberg and Sims, and individual patients who derive their attitudes from more remote contacts with such ideas, often contribute puzzling features to the clinical picture and psychiatrists need to be aware of the total social context before reaching a diagnosis. Otherwise, a diagnosis of schizophrenia will be made more frequently than is justifiable and will cloud the issues of course, outcome, and prognosis.

Age of onset, sex and intelligence

The age of onset is usually taken as the time that schizophrenia is first diagnosed. It is relatively easy to estimate when psychosis suddenly develops in someone of ordinary personality and social performance. When the development is insidious and the individual has 'always' been odd or withdrawn it becomes somewhat arbitrary to assign a date of onset. Several studies have suggested that children who later developed schizophrenia as adults have scored lower on intelligence tests than other children or their own siblings, though the differences are not large and could be due to motivational factors, as maladjustment is also common. Watt and Lubensky (1976), for example, state that boys who later became schizophrenic were negativistic, egocentric, unpleasant, and antisocial, while equivalent girls were quiet, introverted, and egocentric. Hanson and colleagues (1976) described three characteristics which, if present together in childhood, might indicate a very high risk of schizophrenia developing

subsequently: poor motor skills, high variability in psychological test results, and 'schizoid' behaviour (emotionally flat, withdrawn, distractable, passive, irritable, and negativistic) when observed at age four *and* at age seven. Only the presence of all three factors together is likely to be predictive according to these authors. Lee Robins (1970) considered that a combination of neurotic and antisocial behaviour during childhood could presage adult schizophrenia but not that a shy, withdrawn personality was predictive. Lewine and colleagues (1978) found a pattern of 'emotional instability, insecurity, introversion, submissiveness and inconsiderateness/egocentricity'.

These conclusions confirm clinical experience that many schizophrenic patients present with a history of unusual behaviour reaching back into childhood. It may be that such a history explains part of the association, described above, of an insidious onset with a poor prognosis. Schizophrenia can also begin acutely during childhood, usually in the immediately pre-pubertal years. The symptoms are then typical except for the obvious pathoplastic effects of age and the prognosis can be quite good (Eggers, 1978). The psychoses of early childhood, which have a generally poor prognosis, are not to be confused with schizophrenia, although psychiatric disorders, including also mania and severe depression, do occasionally supervene later. The differential diagnosis is considered in chapter 30 and the genetics in chapter 36.

Age of onset is also associated to some extent with type of symptom. Post (1966) points out that paranoid personality traits and symptoms are commoner in later life and exaggerated by loneliness, deafness, mild dementia, and belonging to a socially isolated group. Schizophrenic psychoses beginning after the age of 45 tend to be predominantly paranoid in colouring. In adolescence and young adulthood these paranoid features are less noticeable and the negative syndromes tend to be predominant ('hebephrenia'). Delusional and hallucinatory states are still, however, quite common.

Age of onset also differs to some extent between the sexes. The inception rates for younger men (up to the age of 34) are higher than those for younger women, whereas after 35 the rates are higher in women (Wing & Fryers, 1976). The explanation may be that women are better able to cope with the condition and therefore come into contact with services later or, more probably, that the age of onset is delayed in women compared with men. If so, the reason is unknown. A further difference between the sexes is that at the time of onset, women are more likely to be married than men. This is partly due to the later age of onset in women and partly to the fact that women are better able to carry on their social roles after the onset than are men, because of different social expectations. The clinical picture of schizophrenia beginning in women at the time of the menopause has long been thought to have characteristic features: pressure of talk, affective symptoms, and a sexual content to the delusions (the pre-senile delusional psychosis of Kraepelin). Such features can be found at all ages and in men as well as women but there does seem to be some relationship to age and sex.

Conclusions

Although methodological problems make it necessary to be cautious when interpreting the many studies of course and outcome in schizophrenia, a few generalizations can be made. The first is that the outcome is not uniformly unfavourable, with an inevitable progression to permanent disablement. On the contrary, several recent studies which meet minimum methodological criteria suggest that about one-quarter of all patients given a diagnosis of schizophrenia (fairly strictly defined and not excluding those thought to have a good prognosis) will recover completely. Another two-thirds will continue to have occasional acute relapses and may develop mild to moderate affective and cognitive impairment, while only ten per cent will become totally disabled. According to Manfred Bleuler, the best and the worst outcomes have not changed much since the introduction of the physical therapies. To this extent, the concept of a 'natural' history applies. The major change lies in the fact that, for most patients, the course is now fluctuating rather than continuous, and the experience of lifelong hospitalization which formerly was common is now rare.

This conclusion suggests that further improvement can be expected, both from new developments in physical treatment and from the better application of principles of social prevention. It also suggests that the new pattern of course presents risks, both to the individual patient (seen most clearly in the suicide rate) and to the families who have to share the responsibility when a patient remains partially disabled or is liable to unpredictable relapses. These questions are considered in more detail in chapter 14.

So far as clinical prognosis is concerned, two strands need to be separated. One is the acute episode characterized by florid delusions and hallucinations and accompanying behaviour disorder. This may be intermittently or frequently repeated, with periods of more or less complete remission between. There is no consistent evidence that the frequency or timing of such attacks can confidently be predicted, early in the course, from the characteristics of the mental state or by factors in the social or personal history. However, the five years following the first attack are likely (at least statistically) to provide an indication of what the subsequent course will be. Symptomatically, episodes tend to be similar to each other, but there can be episodes of symptoms (e.g. mania, depression, or anxiety) lower in the hierarchy. The question of social precipitation of acute episodes is considered in chapter 9.

The other strand in clinical course and outcome is provided by the cognitive and affective impairment which, though it may be exacerbated at times when florid symptoms relapse, tends to be more chronic and predictable. A cluster of factors, identifiable at the time of first diagnosis, is associated with a chronic course. By and large, these can all be linked with the earlier 'onset' of precursors of symptoms later identifiable as flatness of affect and thought disorder. These include poor educational performance, consistent emotional flatness, poor social relationships and lower than expected social achievement (all of which are likely to be taken into account when assessing previous personality), and a slow insidious development of more overt and diagnosable symptoms. The reverse side of the same coin is the absence of a sudden (often precipitated) appearance of florid symptoms with an admixture of affective elements responding relatively rapidly to physical and social treatments and leaving little residual impairment.

If these two strands are designated 'acute florid' and 'chronic negative', recognizing that this is a considerable oversimplification, we can say that like predicts like. In each case, the earlier course suggests what the later development will be. Matters are made more complicated, however, by the fact that the strands can come together or remain separate. In the 'typical' Kraepelinian schizophrenia, acute episodes are superimposed upon, or followed by, chronic impairment. Acute episodes without chronic impairment make up the pattern sometimes called 'schizophreniform'. However, there are intermediate patterns as well, since each of the main strands may be more or less prominent in the clinical picture. When precipitating and modifying factors, and the influence of social disadvantage and personal responses, are taken into account as well it is understandable that so many subgroupings have been suggested.

A better understanding of the course of schizo-phrenia, and a better ability to predict, during its early stages, what the course and outcome is likely to be, now awaits more precise knowledge of the multiple aetiology and pathology and a more rational basis for treatments.

Section 2

CHAPTERS 8–12

Aetiology and pathology

8
Epidemiology of schizophrenia

EDWARD HARE

Introduction

The present review is based mainly on English-language publications of the decade 1969–78. Previous reviews on the subject include those of Rosenthal and Kety (1968), Yolles and Kramer (1969), Cooper and Morgan (1973), Babigian (1975), Schwab and Schwab (1978), and Cooper (1978). For the general principles of epidemiology, consult (for example) MacMahon and Pugh (1970) or Barker and Rose (1976).

Epidemiological studies of schizophrenia are hampered by the lack of any objective diagnostic test and by the fact – or at least the probability – that schizophrenia is not a single condition but a group of disorders of varied cause.

Genetic and environmental factors

Studies made during the 1970s (Gottesman & Shields, 1972) have firmly established the importance of genetic factors in the aetiology of schizophrenia. In contrast, nothing certain is yet known about the nature of the environmental causes. The fact that monozygotic twin pairs are not always concordant for schizophrenia has commonly been taken to mean that there must be environmental causes, though the possibility remains that such causes may be simply the unavoidable stresses of ordinary life (Bleuler, 1978, p. 430). The epidemiological search for preventable causes is based on the hope, rather than the assurance, that there are such causes to be discovered. Nevertheless, the mode of inheritance in schizophrenia is very similar to that in tuberculosis (Kallmann & Reisner, 1943) in which environmental factors are undoubtedly of importance. The fact that there are genetic factors in schizophrenia in no way excludes environmental factors of decisive effect.

The frequency of schizophrenia
Rates of incidence and prevalence

Measures such as incidence, prevalence, expectancy and risk are the technical tools of epidemiology, but Kramer (1978) has properly drawn attention to the fact that they have been used imprecisely and in various senses, and that there is a need for standard definitions.

The *prevalence* of a disorder is the number of cases in a particular population at some point or over some period of time. It is an index primarily of concern for the planning of health care. Estimates of the prevalence rate of schizophrenia have ranged from about 2 to about 9 per 1000; tables are given by Yolles and Kramer (1969) and by Babigian (1975). But schizophrenia is a disorder of very varied outcome; the date at which a patient is considered to be cured is often arbitrary and may depend on the adequacy of follow-up care; there are problems of differential mortality; and different outcomes may reflect schizophrenias of different aetiology. For these reasons prevalence is a much less useful measure than incidence in the search for preventable causes.

The *incidence* of a disorder is the number of new cases which develop in a population during a particular period of time. In general, the number of new cases found in any study will depend on the method of case-finding. For large-scale studies of schizophrenia, the oldest and simplest method is based on first-ever hospital admissions. This has the advantage that diagnosis can be based on a period of close observation, but has the disadvantage that not all new cases may be admitted and that the proportion admitted is likely to reflect the local standards of health care.

For England and Wales, first admission rates for schizophrenia (including schizo-affective disorder and paranoia) per 100 000 population (all ages) per year for the five years 1970–74 were 16, 14, 13, 12 and 11 (Department of Health, 1977). Before concluding that the real incidence was falling, we should need to consider such questions as: was the population changing (e.g. in its age structure); was the age-incidence of schizophrenia changing; was the diagnosis of schizophrenia being made less often (without any change in the nature of the cases); was the system of reporting becoming less complete; or were new cases being less often admitted to hospital? Such questions, to which there may be no satisfactory answers, reflect the limitations of the hospital method, particularly on a national scale. It has been argued that most cases of schizophrenia will eventually be hospitalized; but while this may have been true for some countries during certain periods, it is not true everywhere, and a tendency towards treatment outside hospital probably accounts for much of the recent decline in first admission rates for schizophrenia in England and Wales.

Another method of case-finding is to include cases coming to the attention of any psychiatric service (i.e. to include those from out-patient clinics, private practice, general hospitals, etc.). L. Helgason (1977) made such a study in Iceland, and found a schizophrenia incidence rate of 27 per 100 000 per year for the years 1966–7; he also found that 56 per cent of the males and 28 per cent of the females had not been hospitalized. Psychiatric Registers for smaller areas have yielded equivalent rates of about 30 in Salford during 1959–63 (Adelstein, Downham, Stein & Susser, 1968) and about 70 in Monroe County, New York, in 1970 (Babigian, 1975). The high rate in Monroe County may partly be explained by the broad criteria likely to have been used for the diagnosis of schizophrenia there in 1970. The first-ever contact rates calculated from the Camberwell and Salford Registers during 1969–73 were much lower: 14 and 11 per 100 000 per year (Wing & Fryers, 1976).

In comparing these rates with those from in-patient admissions, we need to consider that they have been based on relatively few cases, that the non-admitted cases are likely to have been studied less carefully, and that the local Register populations may differ from the general population in such factors as age-distribution, social class, ethnicity, and the proportion of immigrants.

The incidence of schizophrenia may also be expressed in terms of *risk* or *expectancy*, usually as the cumulative risk to an individual who lives to a given age. Thus, using the data from the Camberwell Register, Shields (1978) found a cumulative risk of 0.86 per cent up to 55 years and 0.90 per cent up to 60 years. For hospital admissions, a number of European studies yield a mean risk of about 0.85 per cent (Slater & Cowie, 1971). In Iceland, a study by T. Helgason (1964), based on a cohort of births, gave a risk of about 0.75, and the later study by L. Helgason (1977) of about 0.45.

The incidence rates found for schizophrenia must be considered against the limitations of method. But they may be taken as providing a broadly reliable rate for the major industrial countries of the Western World during the past 40 years or so.

Variations in incidence with age and sex

Since Kraepelin's time it has been generally accepted that the over-all incidence of schizophrenia is about equal in the sexes, though in Monroe County in 1970 Babigian (1975) found a male/female ratio of 1.40 in the white population.

To study variations of incidence with age, the age of onset rather than the age at first attendance should be known; but as the onset of schizophrenia is often insidious, this may be problematic. Using data from Norwegian hospitals, where age of onset had been routinely recorded, Noreik and Ødegård (1967) found a *median* age of onset which rose from 25.5 to 28.3 years in males between 1926 and 1960, and from 28.9 to 33.3 in females. The *mean* age will be higher than the median: thus Lindelius (1970) – who noted that the onset was acute in 21 per cent, insidious in 38 per cent – found a mean age of onset for hospital admissions in South-west Sweden during 1900–10 to be 27.1 in males and 32.3 in females; the corresponding medians were 25.3 and 31.3 years.

The reason for the sex difference in age of onset is not known, though it is of much theoretical interest. An explanation in terms of brain maturation has been suggested by Flor-Henry (1974).

Variations with time and place

The study of variations in the incidence of a disorder is one of the primary functions of epidemiology, as it commonly leads to the formulation of causal hypotheses. If environmental factors are important in schizophrenia, then variations in incidence would be expected because such factors are unlikely to be uniform either in space or time. However, the evidence for such variation, other than that which can be attributed to age or to selection for genetic risk, is sparse, and the opinion has often been held that there is in fact little variation in incidence either in place or time (Dunham, 1971).

Böök, Wetterbergh, Modrzewska and Unge (1978) confirmed a previous finding of high incidence in an isolated North Swedish population: studies in 1949 and again in 1977 showed a risk of 3 per cent compared with 1 per cent in Sweden as a whole. But they considered the explanation was selection for high genetic risk. Crocetti, Lemkau, Kulcar and Kesic (1971) cautiously confirmed their earlier report of a high incidence of schizophrenia – and other psychoses – in the Istrian peninsula of Yugoslavia. A series of studies from South Ireland (e.g. Kelleher, Copeland & Smith, 1974) have shown the first-admission rate for schizophrenia there to be three or four times as high as in England and Wales, which apparently is not due to diagnostic differences.

The question whether schizophrenia is of universal occurrence has been discussed by Torrey (1973a). He suggests there is evidence that schizophrenia with a poor prognosis is rare in countries which have had little contact with the industrialized world, and his study in New Guinea (Torrey, Torrey & Burton-Bradley, 1974) supported this. There have been many other reports of raised incidence in particular communities (e.g. Murphy, 1968), but the findings tend to be plagued by problems of diagnosis and of differences in the local psychiatric services and the use made of them. Further discussion will be found in chapter 9.

If a satisfactory comparison of incidence rates in different places has proved difficult, it has proved still more difficult to make comparisons in time. This is because any real change in incidence rates may be masked by changes in procedures for data collecting, in attitudes to health care, and in diagnostic practice. One of the puzzles in the history of psychiatry is that descriptions of a disorder corresponding to Kraepelin's schizophrenia are almost unknown in the literature before about 1812 (when Rush referred to auditory hallucinations in the insane). Either the disorder was unrecognized as a separate condition before then (Altschule, 1976) or it had been rare and only became common in the nineteenth century, a view taken by Cooper and Sartorius (1977) who suggested a social explanation, and by Torrey and Peterson (1976) who suggested a viral cause.

The general study of incidence rates during the past 50 years suggests no substantial change in industrialized countries.

Fertility and mortality

There is convincing evidence that the fertility of patients with schizophrenia is low, though under modern conditions of community care this is mainly due to the high proportion who never marry (Stevens, 1969; Larson & Nyman, 1973). A major problem for genetic theories is to account for the persistence of schizophrenia in spite of this overall low fertility. One possibility is that the presumed carriers of schizophrenia genes have a biological advantage, but several studies (e.g. Rimmer & Jacobsen, 1976) have shown no increased fertility in the close relatives of schizophrenics. On the other hand, increased energy and creativeness in relatives has been reported (e.g. Heston & Denney, 1968; Schulsinger, 1976).

Schizophrenia is not a disorder which leads to death from any directly associated pathological changes, but its mortality rate is high from indirect effects. Infectious disease, particularly pulmonary tuberculosis, was a common cause of death during the custodial era but is much less important now. Under the system of community care, however, suicide has become commoner (Lindelius & Kay, 1973). Studies indicating an excess mortality in schizophrenia are those of Weiner and Marvit (1977), Giel, Dijk and Weerden-Dijkstra (1978), Tsuang and Woolson (1978), and Saugstad and Ødegård (1979). In these studies suicide and accident were found to be the principal causes, but when these were allowed for the death rate was still significantly higher than expectation.

There is some evidence that the incidence of malignant disease is below expectation in schizophrenia (Giel *et al.*, 1978; Modrzewska & Böök, 1979).

Environmental factors

Hypotheses of causal relation between schizophrenia and environmental factors are commonly divided into social, psychological, and biological, although the division is somewhat arbitrary.

Migration

Ødegård's finding (1932) of a high schizophrenia rate among migrants from Norway to Minnesota has been repeatedly confirmed in other migrant groups – in the UK by Hemsi (1967), Rwegellera (1977) and Cochrane (1977), for example – and his explanation in terms of *selection* (i.e. that persons with schizophrenia or at risk for it will be over-represented in migrant populations) has been widely accepted. The alternative hypothesis of acculturation stress as a causal factor has received only occasional support.

More recent studies indicate that the proportion and type of unstable persons in a migration will depend on the conditions of the migration. Thus Rosenthal and his colleagues (1974) found the emigration rate in their Danish schizophrenics to be less

than in their controls and attribute this to the strictness of modern migration laws and so to greater selection for health in migrants. When immigration was less restricted, the real or fancied opportunities attracted unstable persons – and, one could add, the emigration of such persons might be actively encouraged by their relatives. Murphy (1977) reached similar conclusions.

Urban conditions

Faris and Dunham (1939) found higher rates of schizophrenia, in terms of admission to hospital, in the central 'hobo' area of Chicago than in the suburbs, and this began a search, especially in the United States, for social causes of schizophrenia. The excess of schizophrenia in the centre of large cities was repeatedly confirmed, and the question then was: did social conditions there cause schizophrenia or was there a 'drift' of individuals with schizophrenia, or at risk for it, to the city centre where living was cheaper and oddities of behaviour more tolerated? Dunham's later study in Detroit (1965), comparing areas with a high and a low rate of schizophrenia, led him to attribute the different rates to the greater mobility of the population in the high-rate area rather than to any direct causal effect of social conditions. Rowitz and Levy (1968) replicated the earlier study in Chicago and found no clear ecological pattern for the distribution of schizophrenia when first admissions only were considered.

Reviewing the subject, Dunham (1976) concluded there was no satisfactory evidence that schizophrenia could be caused by social pressures in the community and that the findings could be better explained in terms of mobility and selection. The studies of Wing and his colleagues (Wing, 1978b) strongly suggest that the *relapse* of a schizophrenic illness may be precipitated by social pressures, particularly those found in some families, but there is no evidence so far that these factors are more associated with urban than with rural conditions (see chapter 9).

Socio-economic conditions

It has long been observed that schizophrenia is commonest among those in the least skilled occupations, and the observation has been repeatedly confirmed. Unskilled work is usually associated with low income and poor social conditions, and the question then was: were poor social conditions (e.g. low social class) causal for schizophrenia, or was it rather that people handicapped by schizophrenia or by a schiz-oid constitution could manage only unskilled jobs (i.e. were *selected* for low social class)? Because such occu-pational handicap will not have been operant during childhood, the social class of the patient's father dur-ing his childhood should be a decisive test in respect of these alternatives. All recent studies have shown the social class distribution of the fathers of schizo-phrenics to be similar to that of the general popula-tion; and studies of particular cases have generally shown that schizophrenics either fall in occupational level because of their illness or never achieve their expected occupational level because of the early onset of the illness or because of the constitutional handicap (Goldberg & Morrison, 1963; Dunham, Philips & Sri-nivasan, 1966; Turner & Wagenfeld, 1967; Grünfeld & Salveson, 1968; Heston & Denney, 1968; Lindelius, 1970; Hare, Price & Slater, 1972; Wender *et al.*, 1973). Brown, Birley and Wing (1972) found no relation between social class and risk of schizophrenic relapse. A more general effect of illness-induced handicap in lowering occupational status has been shown by Harkey, Miles & Rushing (1976).

Reviewing the evidence, Dunham (1976) con-cluded that 'social class is not an aetiological factor in the development of schizophrenia'. Although some workers have continued to maintain that low social class has a causal effect (Kohn, 1973), the weight of evidence today must very decidedly favour the selec-tion explanation rather than the causal one. On the other hand, it is still not unreasonable to postulate that social factors – not necessarily those associated with low social class – may play a part in precipitating onset or relapse, or in maintaining chronic impair-ments. The effects of social and psychological stress are discussed in chapter 9.

Family influences

Although only about 10 per cent of schizo-phrenics have had a schizophrenic parent, it is likely that some peculiarity of behaviour will be common in the non-schizophrenic parents. The studies of Bateson, of Lidz, and of Wynne, suggesting abnor-malities in family communication, have been criti-cized on technical grounds and have not been con-firmed by other workers (Hirsch & Leff, 1975; Leff, 1978). Fischer (1973) found no difference in the risk of schizophrenia between the children of monozygotic twins themselves discordant for schizophrenia, and Bleuler (1978, p. 138), in a longitudinal study, con-cluded that home-contact with a schizophrenic parent played no important part in a subsequent schizo-phrenic illness in the offspring. The consistent con-clusion from studies of fostered and adopted children is that the development of schizophrenia has not been shown as attributable to any particular psychological conditions in the rearing family (see chapter 9).

Family size and birth rank are factors which might influence the risk of schizophrenia either by psychological or biological pathways. Hare and Price (1970) found no difference in the sibship size of schizophrenic patients and of patients with other psychiatric conditions. Birtchnell (1972), and Hare and Price (1974), showed that the birth-rank distribution of schizophrenic and other psychiatric patients reflected those found in random samples of the gen-eral population. There seems at present no good evi-dence that family size or birth rank are of significance in schizophrenia.

Another family factor which might influence the risk of schizophrenia by psychological or biological means is the age of parents at the time of the patient's birth. A raised maternal age in schizophrenia has been found in several studies, and Dalén (1977) sug-gested this might be a cause of the high rate of first admissions for schizophrenia in South Ireland (where late marriage is common). The subject has been stud-ied and reviewed by Hare and Moran (1979), who found both paternal and maternal ages to be raised (compared with expectation from the general popu-lation or a control group) in all main categories of psychiatric disorder, though most markedly in schiz-ophrenia. The higher age of the father was the pri-mary factor, and Hare and Moran concluded that this was best explained as due to constitutional traits in the parents, leading to late marriage.

Obstetric complications

Functional psychoses, including schizophrenia occur with more than chance frequency in women during the puerperium, even in the absence of any complications. A study by Kendell, Wainwright, Hailey and Shannon (1976) suggested this was due to physiological rather than psychological causes; but the nature of the causes is unknown (see volume 2, chapter 5).

The association between schizophrenia and the occurrence of obstetric complications at the patient's birth has been much studied during the past 10–15 years; the term 'obstetric complication' being con-veniently used to cover complications of pregnancy, birth and the neonatal period. In a review and further study of the subject, McNeil and Kaij (1978) concluded that obstetric complications probably interact with genetic disposition to increase the risk of schizophrenia. On the other hand, Gottesman and Shields (1976) and Shields and Gottesman (1977) pointed out that the incidence of schizophrenia in the offspring of schizophrenic mothers is no higher than in the offspring of schizophrenic fathers, which implies that obstetric complications are unlikely to be a specific causal factor. Hanson, Gottesman and Heston (1976) found a combination of poor motor skills and schizoid traits to occur in 17 per cent of children with a schizophrenic parent, and concluded this was not due to obstetric complications but was part of the schizophrenic inheritance and probably associated with a high risk for schizophrenia. 'High-risk' studies in the relatives of schizophrenics are particularly considered in chapter 9.

The general question of the relation between schizophrenia and the health of parents before the patient's birth is probably worthy of more attention than it has received. MacSweeney, Timms and Johnson (1978) reported an excess of thyroid disorder in the mothers.

Season of birth and season of admission

With the development of national systems of health care and the centralization of data, birth dates of patients can be compared with those of a general population. Such comparisons confirm earlier findings that schizophrenics show an excess of births in the winter months, and this has been replicated in a number of countries in the northern hemisphere and also (though perhaps less clearly) in the southern (Dalén, 1975; Torrey, Torrey & Peterson, 1977; Jones & Frei, 1979). Two main explanations have been put forward: first, an abnormality in the seasonal conception habits of the parents; second, a foetal or neonatal factor, maximum for the winter-born, causing constitutional damage of a kind which increases the risk of later schizophrenia. On the first hypothesis, the same seasonal birth distribution should occur in the sibs of the schizophrenics; but the findings have been conflicting (Buck & Simpson, 1978). The present weight of evidence is perhaps towards the damage hypothesis (Kinney & Jacobsen, 1978).

A high rate of admissions to mental hospitals during the summer months has long been observed; and this is true for schizophrenia as well as for affective psychosis. The phenomenon is generally attributed to biological rather than social factors. Abe reviewed the topic in 1963; and Hare and Walter (1978) suggested a common factor in season of birth and season of admission.

Nutritional factors

Schizophrenia-like psychoses occur in pellagra, and although this disease is now rare (Roe, 1973), the discovery of the nutritional cause of pellagra (and so of its prevention) remains one of the triumphs of epidemiology (Terris, 1964).

Dohan noted that admissions for schizophrenia during the Second World War declined in many countries but increased in the United States. He suggested that the decline was due to dietary causes, especially to a fall in the consumption of wheat protein. In line with this suggestion was the reportedly high incidence of schizophrenia in coeliac disease, a disease of intolerance to wheat gluten. Work on this hypothesis has been summarized by Dohan (1978).

Schizophrenia associated with organic disorders

Davison and Bagley (1969), in a comprehensive review, established that schizophrenia-like states were not uncommon in many types of brain disorder and that, in view of the evidence that there was no increased incidence of schizophrenia in the relatives, such cases were probably phenocopies of genetic schizophrenia. Deafness, particularly that due to middle ear disease, has been established as a probable causal factor in late paraphrenia (Cooper, Garside & Kay, 1976).

There have been occasional reports, dating at least from the influenza pandemic of 1918, of schizophrenia-like illnesses due to viral infection. The hypothesis of a viral cause in some types of common schizophrenia has received support on epidemiological grounds (Torrey, 1973b; Torrey & Peterson, 1976; Kety, 1978). Direct evidence of a virus-like agent in the cerebrospinal fluid of schizophrenic patients has been reported by Tyrrell and colleagues (1979). If this is confirmed, much light may be thrown on many puzzling features of the history and epidemiology of this disease.

Conclusion

This brief review of a major field of study is necessarily coloured by the reviewer's predilections. Although the epidemiological study of schizophrenia is greatly hampered by lack of an objective diagnostic test, the history of epidemiology suggests that precision in diagnosis is not essential for progress. There was no great precision in the diagnosis of dementia paralytica or of pellagra when epidemiological studies pointed strongly to particular environmental factors in their aetiology, thus encouraging the search for confirmation by laboratory and clinical work. Another, less obvious, consideration may complicate present research in schizophrenia. The prognosis of schizophrenia has improved over the past 40 to 50 years (Cottman & Mezey, 1976; Wing, 1978a) and its clinical manifestations have been changing (Grinker, 1973; Morrison, 1974; Kuriansky *et al.*, 1977). Whether such changes are the result of better care and treatment, or of an increasing host resistance to the (unknown) environmental causes, remains undecided. But there is no reason to suppose that the manifestations of schizophrenia are not continuing to change, and this is a circumstance which must increase the difficulty of diagnostic precision by any formal set of subjective criteria (Hogarty, 1977).

9
Psychosocial factors influencing the onset and course of schizophrenia

J. K. WING

Introduction

The work reviewed in section 1 indicates that although the schizophrenic and paranoid psychoses have certain syndromatic similarities there is a broad range of clinical manifestations of varying severity, course, and outcome. It is inevitable that an equally wide range of theories of aetiology and pathology has been suggested. There are reviewed in section 2. The evidence that psychosocial factors can modify the clinical picture in the early stages, and thus confuse the prognosis, has been considered in chapter 7. The epidemiological evidence that factors such as social isolation or poverty are contributing causes is dealt with in chapter 8. The present chapter is concerned with theories that microsocial and societal factors predispose to the later development of schizophrenia, precipitate acute psychotic episodes, or influence the severity of chronic impairment. The evidence will be considered under four headings – family factors, societal factors, precipitants of acute breakdown, and factors influencing chronic impairment.

Family factors in causation

Most of the theories that posit an abnormality in the social environment provided for the infant by its parents, determining the later development of schizophrenia, are derived from psycho-analysis. Hajdu-Gaines (1940), after analysing four women patients, concluded that their mothers were cold and aggressive and their fathers indifferent and passive.

Fromm-Reichman (1948) used the term 'schizo-phrenogenic mother' to describe features that she regarded as specifically harmful to the child. Much research has been undertaken in order to clarify the concept and demonstrate its relationship to the subsequent onset and course of schizophrenia. Section 10 of the *Rochester Symposium* (Wynne, Cromwell & Matthysse, 1978) is devoted to abnormalities of family relationships and communication. Leff (1978) has provided a detailed review of the evidence for the main theories, which are associated with the names of Gregory Bateson, Theodore Lidz, and Lyman Wynne.

The double-bind

Bateson and his colleagues suggested that the specific factor is an ambiguity of communication between parents and child which they called the 'double-bind'. This consists of an overt negative command which is at the same time countermanded (e.g. by tone of voice or gesture, or at a more abstract level), both commands being accompanied by threats of punishment if they are not obeyed. The child is not able to escape from the situation nor to point out the contradiction, which is denied by the parents. The only technique for dealing with the situation is to respond with ambiguous or incomprehensible statements which avoid making a choice. In this way, the child learns an abnormal pattern of communication which is regarded by the authors as the fundamental basis of schizophrenia (Bateson *et al.*, 1956; Haley, 1959; Watzlawick *et al.*, 1968).

Two empirical studies have been undertaken to test the theory (Haley, 1968; Ringuette & Kennedy, 1966) but it proved impossible to recognize a double-bind situation reliably or to show any difference between the parents of schizophrenic and non-schizophrenic patients. The possibility that parents respond to an abnormality in the schizophrenic patients' communication could not, however, be ruled out.

Schismatic and skewed families

Lidz and his colleagues have based their theories on an intensive study over many years of a small number of families, mostly middle-class and affluent, containing an overtly schizophrenic member (Lidz, 1975). They suggest that two types of family are unable to provide an adequate social environment for the developing child. The first is the schismatic fam-

ily, 'in which the two parents are in abiding conflict, undercutting the worth of the other to the child, and the child is not only used to complete a parent's life and salvage the marriage but his psychic structure is torn apart by the internalization of two irreconcilable parents' (Lidz, 1978). The second is the skewed family, 'in which one parent, usually the mother, does not establish boundaries between herself and the child, uses the child to complete her life, and continues to be extremely intrusive into the child's life though impervious to the child's needs and feelings as a separate individual'. The other parent is too passive to counteract this influence.

Schizophrenia is formulated as 'a failure to differentiate properly between the self and others and between what arises within the self and what is outside the self'. This is regarded a form of egocentricity, which is learned from egocentric parents. The crisis point comes during adolescence when the child has to meet the demands of the world beyond the family.

The evidence produced for his theories by Lidz himself is entirely descriptive and does not constitute a proper test. However, a number of comparative studies have been carried out (Ferreira & Winter, 1965; Sharan, 1966; Winter & Ferreira, 1967) without providing support for predictions derived from the theories. Where abnormalities of the kind predicted have been found, they have also occurred in families with a non-schizophrenic member or containing no one with a psychiatric disorder.

Laing's theories are similar, in many respects, to those of Bateson and Lidz, though he emphasizes societal attitudes more (Laing, 1960, 1967). No studies have been reported that undertake a critical test of hypotheses derived from his work.

Parental communication deviances

Wynne and his colleagues have put forward the theory that families containing a young adult schizophrenic patient are distinguished by abnormal styles of communication. These abnormalities are particularly influential at the time when 'the basic phase of focusing attention and sharing foci of attention begins'. In families containing a member with some other psychiatric disorder, or with no disordered member at all, there are fewer communication problems, which develop later and in less damaging ways. The communication abnormalities include ambiguous, distracting, fluctuating, vague, and odd remarks. A useful and reliable technique of measurement is based on an objective system of rating samples of speech obtained by presenting Rorschach cards and recording the responses.

The authors have recently reviewed the empirical research designed to test their hypotheses (Singer, Wynne & Toohey, 1978; Wynne *et al.*, 1977), which is empirical compared with that of the authors cited earlier in this chapter. They claim to have demonstrated, and that others have confirmed, that a very high proportion of the parents of people with schizophrenia show communication deviances compared with matched control groups. Hirsch and Leff (1975), who closely replicated their techniques, were unable to substantiate the finding, although they did find that the fathers of schizophrenic patients used more words to describe the Rorschach blots than the fathers of the controls. There was no difference between the mothers in the two groups. The explanation for this failure may lie in the tighter experimental design of the London workers, who investigated a consecutive series of patients rather than a personally collected one, but it is likely to be due, in large part, to the fact that the American workers used a much looser definition of schizophrenia. In other words, there may well be conditions, such as certain personality disorders, where a strong association of the kind posited by Wynne and his colleagues exists, but they do not include schizophrenia strictly defined. Rutter (1978) has given a useful review of the subject.

Conclusions

The theories reviewed above have similar disadvantages. They are complex, difficult to translate into testable hypotheses and fail to explain all the known facts about schizophrenia, for example, why *all* the siblings who have been exposed to 'schizophrenogenic' parents do not become schizophrenic. Where aspects of the theories have been tested independently, using adequate controlled designs, they have usually not passed the test. Even if the results had been more positive, it would be impermissible to extrapolate from studies of young adults to influences in infancy and early childhood. Even if it were permissible, the results could as readily be explained in terms of a genetic hypothesis or, just as plausibly (since there are empirical pointers in this direction), of an influence of the offspring upon the parent.

Hirsch and Leff (1975), who conducted an extensive survey of the family literature, concluded that very few results emerged consistently from studies meeting reasonable standards of design and method. Parents of schizophrenic patients are more likely to have psychiatric disorders than parents of normal children and more likely to be at odds with each other. Mothers of schizophrenic patients show more concern and protectiveness than mothers of normals. 'Pre-schizophrenic' children are more likely to show physical ill-health or mild disability early in life than normal children. These few facts could be explained in several different ways.

Societal factors

Two American sociologists, Erving Goffmann (1961) and Thomas Scheff (1966), put forward theories concerning the origin of schizophrenia which were more radical than those discussed above. They used a very broad and vague concept of schizophrenia, virtually equating it with severe mental illness. Scheff, in particular, derived his theory from that of Lemert (1951) on social deviance. In Scheff's view, relatively minor disturbances in childhood, such as head-banging, which could not be explained in terms of generally accepted concepts such as delinquency would, if referred to specialists, become labelled as psychiatric. Subsequent 'treatment' and, in particular, institutionalization, led to a societal definition of the individual as 'mad' and to the individual's acceptance of this label; 'mental illness' thus being created by the process of diagnosing and treating it. There is virtually no evidence that this process does actually occur. Follow-up studies of children who attended child guidance clinics (O'Neal & Robins, 1958; Waring & Ricks, 1965) suggest that most of them do not become severely mentally ill in adulthood. More specifically, labelling theory fails to account for most of the known facts concerning schizophrenia (Wing, 1978c, chapter 5).

Both Goffman and Scheff made observations on the effects of long-term hospitalization on people admitted for mental illness during the 1950s. These will be considered in a later section.

Social precipitants of acute schizophrenic breakdown

Life events

It has long been observed clinically that an acute episode of schizophrenia has begun shortly after a period of intense stress in the patient's life but until recently no systematic studies have been made to check the hypothesis. A number of studies, using different methods of measuring 'stress', and investigating various medical conditions were summarized in a recent publication (Dohrenwend & Dohrenwend,

1974). G. W. Brown developed an interview technique whereby 'life events', usually involving threat or actual danger, could be dated in a fairly reliable manner and classified as to whether they were independent of changes occurring in the subject's mental state. Brown and Birley (1968; Birley & Brown, 1970) estimated the frequency and type of events occurring during the three months preceeding the onset of an episode of schizophrenia (whether the first onset or a relapse) and during the three months before interview with a group of normal people. Some 60 per cent of the patients had experienced an independent or possibly independent event during the three months before onset, compared to about 15 per cent of control subjects. Some of the apparently precipitating events were life changes (such as becoming engaged to be married) which would ordinarily be supposed to be positive. This contrasts with the position in depression, where precipitating events tend to be mainly threatening and connected with loss (Brown, Bhrolcháin & Harris, 1975).

In an earlier study of rehabilitation of long-stay schizophrenic patients with no evident florid symptoms, it was observed that several broke down within a week of beginning to attend a centre, used mainly by physically disabled people, where the expectations were considerably higher than those they had experienced in hospital (Wing, Bennett & Denham, 1964).

Expressed emotion

Workers from the Medical Research Council Social Psychiatry Unit have conducted three studies of the relationship between key relative (usually parent or spouse) and schizophrenic patients at the time of hospitalization during an acute episode and the extent to which this predicts short-term outcome (Brown *et al.*, 1962; Brown, Birley & Wing, 1972; Vaughn & Leff, 1976). The third of these was a replication of the second, using a specially developed measure of the emotional expression to the patient by the key relative (Brown & Rutter, 1966; Rutter & Brown, 1966) which could be reliably derived from tape-recordings of standardized interviews. Ratings were made of hostility, warmth, and emotional involvement and the number of critical comments made by the relative (judged on content and tone of voice) were counted. Relapse during the nine months after discharge was found, in both studies, to be significantly associated with three of the measures of emotional expression – critical comments, hostility, and over-involvement. The relapse rate of patients in

'high-emotion' families was significantly higher than that of patients living in 'low-emotion' families. When previous work history and past history of behavioural disturbance were controlled, the strength of the association between emotional expression and relapse was not much diminished. Controlling for emotional expression, however, reduced the association between the earlier factors and relapse almost to zero.

When data from the two studies were combined, it was shown that two other variables were important in predicting relapse – the amount of face-to-face contact between key relative and patient, and whether the latter was taking phenothiazine medication. There was an interaction between the three predictive factors such that, when all three were unfavourable (high emotion, high contact, no medication), the relapse rate was over 90 per cent. When two were unfavourable, it was 40–50 per cent. For patients living in high-emotion homes but taking medication and in relatively low face-to-face contact with the key relative, the relapse rate was only 15 per cent, much the same as for those living in low-emotion homes. The last group had a low relapse rate whether or not they were taking medication.

Vaughn and Leff (1976) also made a content analysis of the critical comments made by key relatives. They found that these were not chiefly directed at florid symptoms such as delusions or hallucinations which, in general, were seen as abnormal and beyond the patient's control. Criticism was more frequently directed at longer-term aspects of the patient's personality – laziness, slowness, lack of conversation, and unfriendliness – which were not regarded as symptoms of an illness although probably correlated with negative symptoms. Sensitivity to the emotional expression of the relative is not specific to schizophrenia. Vaughn and Leff (1976) found that depressed patients also were more likely to relapse when critical comments were relatively frequent. The threshold, however, was much lower in depression than in schizophrenia.

The practical implications of this work will be considered in chapter 14 and its theoretical implications at the end of the present chapter.

Factors influencing chronic impairment

Many pioneers of modern psychiatry, from Pinel and Tuke to Kraepelin and Eugen Bleuler, emphasized that factors in the social environment of the patient could increase or decrease the severity of long-term incapacity. Much emphasis was placed on the preventive and therapeutic value of work but education, family life, constructive leisure activities, and self-control were also regarded as important elements in 'moral treatment' (Bennett, 1975; Lewis, 1957; 1962). The harmful features of certain institutional regimes were documented in several studies during the 1950s and 1960s, which will be considered in chapter 14, but the descriptive nature of the studies rarely allowed the isolation of factors that were specifically associated with an increase in chronic schizophrenic impairments.

A study carried out in two psychiatric hospitals near London, made use of a behaviour-rating scale completed by nurses, and a standard interview with a representative sample of long-stay patients (Wing, 1961) to measure the negative symptoms such as social withdrawal, slowness, underactivity, flatness of affect, and poverty of speech. This 'clinical poverty' syndrome was found to be more marked in the hospital with the poorer social environment and to be more severe, in both hsopitals, the longer the patient had been resident (Wing, 1962).

A further study was undertaken in three psychiatric hospitals, chosen because their social regimes were reputedly very different. Additional indices were constructed to measure the quality of the environment. Again it was found that the hospital with the most socially stimulating regime contained patients with the least severe impairments. Moreover, within each hospital, patients in the most restrictive and understimulating wards had the greatest disability. The single most important environmental factor associated with symptoms such as flatness of affect and social withdrawal was length of time doing nothing.

Because of the difficulties associated with a cross-sectional design the three cohorts of patients were followed up on several occasions between 1960 and 1968. It was found that, as the social regimes in the hospitals improved, so the clinical condition of the patients improved concomitantly. More important, when, in one of the hospitals, the social environment actually became more impoverished for a time, the patients exposed to this deterioration became more underactive, slow, and withdrawn (Wing & Brown, 1970).

An experimental study of the effect of introducing and withdrawing social stimulation in two hospital workshops showed that negative schizophrenic symptoms became more or less severe in close association with the environmental change (Wing &

Freudenberg, 1961). The effect was quite different from the negatively accelerated learning curve that would be expected, for example, in people with Down's syndrome with a rather lower general intellectual level. Moreover, there was no 'transfer of training' from workshop to ward.

A marked lack of social stimulation is not, of course, characteristic only of impoverished hospital environments. It can occur in other residential or day settings and in the patient's own home (Brown *et al.*, 1966). It is particularly evident among patients who live alone or who become destitute (Leach & Wing, 1980).

The results of these studies, and of the rehabilitation trials considered in chapter 14, suggest that chronic schizophrenic patients suffer from a specific form of impairment which makes them particularly vulnerable to social understimulation when impairment is severe. They are unable, without external help, to generate sufficient internal motivation to remain active. Mild to moderate degrees of impairment are, of course, much commoner than severe forms.

Cultural factors

Very few of the follow-up studies of schizophrenia carried out in different parts of the world have met minimal criteria of methodological adequacy. Techniques of sampling, diagnosis, measurement, and follow-up have been deficient. Three studies do deserve mention. Murphy and Raman (1971) followed up for twelve years schizophrenic patients in the island of Mauritius and concluded that they had fewer relapses and a more favourable outcome than an English group (Brown *et al.*, 1966). Kulhara and Wig (1978) followed up, for five years, a group of schizophrenic patients admitted for the first time to the psychiatric hospital in Chandigarh, India. They found that the course and outcome were similar to the English series and less favourable than the Mauritian group. The two-year follow-up of the IPSS series (WHO, 1979) indicates a substantially better course and outcome in patients in the Ibadan, Agra and Cali series (in that order) compared with those in London, Moscow, Prague, Taipei, or Washington, while those in Aarhus had the most unfavourable course of all. The very different sampling procedures used in the various centres and the different conditions of follow-up make it difficult to interpret these results with confidence, but there are clear grounds for further studies.

If further investigations showed that course and outcome are indeed more favourable in some areas than others, it would be worth while looking at the factors discussed earlier in this chapter to discover whether the social environments in which people with schizophrenia live in developing countries makes their impact less obtrusive. The family structure may make a concerned but neutral attitude easier for relatives to adopt. A lower expectation for occupational performance may result in less anxiety. Afflicted people may be less often labelled as socially incompetent and thus be better able to maintain an acceptable self-image.

Relationship between factors precipitating relapse and those influencing chronic impairment

It appears, from the work reviewed above, that too much, or too intrusive, social stimulation can precipitate an episode of florid schizophrenic symptoms, whether for the first time or as a relapse. On the other hand, too little stimulation can result in an increase in the negative schizophrenic impairment. Venables and Wing (1962) found that the severity of social withdrawal, slowness, and underactivity was highly correlated with central and peripheral measures of 'arousal' (two-flash and two-click threshold, and skin conductance), the most withdrawn being the most 'aroused'.

More recently, patients from the study conducted by Vaughn and Leff (1976) have been tested in their own homes, using skin conductance and pulse rate as measures of 'arousal'. After a period of 15 minutes to establish a baseline, the key relative was asked to enter the room and stayed for a further 15 minutes. A control group of normal people showed a short-lived increase in arousal on entry of the relative. Schizophrenic patients showed a higher level of baseline arousal than the controls but the entry of a relative who previously, and independently, had been found to express high emotion resulted in a significantly higher increase than the entry of a 'low-emotion' relative. Moreover, the group of patients with a 'high-emotion' relative present remained highly aroused while the group with a 'low-emotion' relative present showed a decrease towards normal levels (Tarrier *et al.*, 1978).

The relation between arousal levels, medication, and social environment deserves further investigation, since it has both theoretical and practical implications. It can be hypothesized that, although there is little evidence that social factors during childhood contribute to the aetiology of schizophrenia, there is a psychophysiological reactivity shortly before onset, and often continuing throughout the course, which makes the patient vulnerable, in different ways, to overstimulating and understimulating social environments (Wing, Leff & Hirsch, 1973). Since, as suggested by the follow-up studies reviewed in chapter 7, most patients with schizophrenia are now likely to experience a fluctuating course, with occasional acute psychotic episodes and mild to moderate chronic impairment, an understanding of their sensitivity to factors likely to exacerbate or ameliorate each type of symptom is of the first importance. The implications will be reviewed in chapter 14.

10

Psychological deficits in schizophrenia: information processing and communication problems

THOMAS F. OLTMANNS
JOHN M. NEALE

The recent literature on psychological deficit in schizophrenia, although showing much diversity, is focused primarily on cognitive processes and language. Two principal questions are asked: (1) Which cognitive processes are dysfunctional in schizophrenics? (2) What specific aspects of the language of schizophrenics impair their ability to communicate? We shall first examine current research on these topics and then consider the literature on psychological deficit more generally.

Cognitive processes and language

Prior to 1960, cognitive processes were not an important concern to most mainstream psychologists. Behaviourism was in its heyday and little was known about cognition even in normal people. Psychological theories of schizophrenic behaviour were based either on the perceptual theory of the Gestalt school (e.g. Goldstein, 1939) or on non-cognitive principles derived from various learning models (e.g. Lang & Buss, 1965; Mednick, 1958; Broen & Storms, 1966). These theories have met with very limited success and have not provided an adequate account of schizophrenic cognition.

Information processing and linguistic performance

In more recent years, experimental psychologists have abandoned the 'antimentalistic' constraints of radical behaviourism and begun to explore the complex phenomena of human information processing and psycholinguistic abilities. Many of the methods and concepts developed within this area of research have been applied to the study of schizophrenia. This development, too, has had its problems. Consider, for example, the investigation of selective attention in schizophrenia. In 1958, Broadbent published the first general model of human information processing, suggesting that mental activity could be seen as a limited capacity channel which processes a continuous flow of information. Limitations were conceptualized in terms of the amount of information and the speed with which it could be handled. To protect this system from overloading, Broadbent proposed the existence of a hypothetical 'filter' immediately preceding the limited capacity portion of the nervous system.

Shortly after the publication of this seminal volume, it was suggested that schizophrenics' cognitive problems might stem from a failure of this perceptual filter (McGhie & Chapman, 1961; Payne, Matussek & George, 1959; Weckowicz & Blewett, 1959). Encouraged by the subjective reports of the patients themselves, who often mentioned attention-related problems (Freeman, 1974), investigators sought to confirm this hypothesis using more objective measurements. Reaction time, size estimation, and various competing information tasks were all popular indices of attention during the 1960s (Neale & Cromwell, 1970). Schizophrenics indeed performed poorly on these and other tasks, but the results of the studies were difficult to interpret because the measures were only loosely tied to the theoretical constructs they were meant to test. (See Oltmanns & Neale, 1978, for a review of conceptual and methodological difficulties associated with psychological deficit research.)

A large proportion of recent studies have been plagued by the same problems but a number of interesting reports have revealed specific areas of cognitive deficit. These studies have been concerned both with information processing and with linguistic performance. Over all, the data indicate that schizophrenics encounter difficulty at the level of controlled, or conscious, cognitive processes. Operations which are automatic in nature (or do not require conscious processing) seem to be relatively intact.

In a series of studies, McGhie and his colleagues demonstrated that schizophrenics' performance on various perceptual and cognitive tasks was seriously impaired by the introduction of irrelevant stimuli (see McGhie, 1970). These investigators suggested that the locus of this dysfunction occurred after the initial registration of the stimulus in a more advanced stage of memory. Their hypothesis was based on Broadbent's original theory which included the notions of a filter and relatively discrete stages of memory. Although more recent theories of information processing have questioned the value of the filter hypothesis and moved toward a more flexible model of memory, the basic distinction between levels of processing and the amount of effort involved in a particular operation still seems to be useful (Schneider & Shiffrin, 1977). Yates (1966), on the other hand, argued that the problem in schizophrenics' performance occurred immediately after the peripheral reception of sensory information. Subsequent studies have tended to favour the view expressed by McGhie. For the most part, schizophrenics' search operations in sensory memory appear to be similar to, although perhaps somewhat slower than, those of normal subjects (Davidson & Neale, 1974; Koh, Szoc & Peterson, 1977; Russell & Knight, 1977). Thus the principal difficulty that schizophrenics experience must lie somewhere beyond this initial level of processing.

Further clues to the nature of this deficit have come from the study of organizational factors in short-term memory. Several studies have found that while schizophrenics could *recognize* previously presented words as well as could control subjects, their performance was significantly impaired if they were asked to *recall* the items without the aid of cues or prompts (Bauman & Murray, 1968; Nachmani & Cohen, 1969). One explanation for this differential deficit involves the ability to organize the to-be-remembered units (e.g. into conceptually similar categories) – a strategy which facilitates recall.

This kind of active processing may be crucial for recall but unnecessary for recognition. In an effort to explore this possibility, a number of investigators have employed tasks that evaluate, both directly and indirectly, the ability of schizophrenics to utilize strategies for organizing or imposing structure on to-be-remembered material. The results indicate that schizophrenics are inefficient in the use of mnemonic aids (Bauman, 1971; Koh, Kayton & Berry, 1973; Larsen & Fromholt, 1976; Traupmann, 1975). This deficit is apparently not the result of a failure to recognize or encode the relevant stimulus attributes at the point of recognition (Koh, Kayton & Schwartz, 1974; Koh & Peterson, 1978; Russell & Beekhuis, 1976; Traupmann, Berzofsky & Kesselman, 1976) but seems to lie in the active organization of information once it has reached the level of conscious experience and short-term memory. It seems to be at this level that schizophrenics become inefficient and perhaps confused. They are less able to recall words on the basis of semantic attributes and less consistent in the construction and utilization of systems for organizing or categorizing words.

The data regarding short-term memory fit recent evidence pertaining to selective attention. Many studies carried out in the 1960s demonstrated that distracting stimuli were particularly disrupting for schizophrenics performing cognitive tasks. A possible explanation is that distraction interferes with the sensory registration of relevant stimuli. On the other hand, although schizophrenics may register and identify items appropriately, distraction may impair their ability to perform control operations which are also necessary for efficient performance of some tasks. Tentative indications favour the second possibility. Signal detection analyses have shown that the stimulus sensitivity of schizophrenics is not impaired in the presence of distracting noise (Korboot & Damiani, 1976) but schizophrenics' performance on competing information tasks is impaired if recall is required (Hawks & Robinson, 1971; Oltmanns & Neale, 1975). Thus, distraction seems to present special problems for schizophrenics only on tasks which require higher level processing. (See also the review by Venables, 1978.)

This hypothesis has been supported by two further studies. Oltmanns (1978) found that distraction had a specific effect on schizophrenics' performance of a serial recall task; it interfered with their ability to remember words presented early in a list but did not affect their recall of later items. Since the advantage ordinarily enjoyed by the early items (they are remembered more easily than later items) generally depends on the utilization of rehearsal and related controlled processes, these data indicate that schizophrenics become inefficient users of active organizational strategies in the presence of irrelevant stimuli. Pogue-Geile and Oltmanns (1980) have extended this hypothesis on the basis of data collected using a dichotic listening paradigm. They found that distraction interfered with schizophrenics' ability to remember the content of a story that they had shadowed (repeated aloud as it was presented) but that it did not disrupt their shadowing performance. This result necessitates a revision of the hypothesis that distraction disrupts all controlled processing. Since

distraction did not significantly disrupt schizophrenics' ability to shadow relevant passages, it seems that distraction does not impair all aspects of active information processing. As in the memory studies reported by other investigators, schizophrenics were able to anticipate and recognize the words in each story but unable to encode the meaning in memory so that it could be retrieved efficiently. Thus, the impairment associated with distraction may be an exacerbation of already existing deficiencies in specific controlled processes.

The use of linguistic rules

How do these findings relate to speech disturbance and thought disorder? The organization of meaningful communication is affected by grammatical rules. Sentences are encoded and decoded according to the syntactic structure, or constraints, of the language. Early investigations (e.g. Lawson, McGhie & Chapman, 1964) concluded that contextual constraints did not aid schizophrenics in their recall of verbal passages. Taken together with the data on organizational factors in memory, these studies might indicate that schizophrenics are deficient in their knowledge of syntactic rules. Given this deficiency, they might be unable to take advantage of organizational properties inherent in verbal discourse. As a result, their ability to process information and to communicate would be impaired. Several studies have tested this hypothesis and the results are largely negative (Carpenter, 1976; Gerver, 1967; Rochester, 1973; Rochester, Harris & Seeman, 1973). If the problem is not one of *competence* (or knowledge of linguistic rules) it must involve *performance;* the ability to use these rules in combination with information processing skills. The periodic nature of thought disorder makes it seem likely that schizophrenics sometimes have trouble using their grammatical knowledge rather than that they alternate between periods of competence and incompetence. Several recent empirical studies have helped to elucidate the nature of the relationship between information processing and communication skill.

Referential speech

Cohen and his colleagues have focused on the performance of referential communication tasks in which one subject, the 'speaker', is asked to communicate information to another person, the 'listener'. In a single-word task, reminiscent of the game 'Password', Cohen and Camhi (1967) found that schizophrenics were as accurate as normals in the role of listener, regardless of whether clues were provided by schizophrenic or normal speakers. As speakers, however, the schizophrenics were significantly less effective than normals. Since schizophrenics were efficient listeners, their problems did not seem to be due to deviant associative hierarchies. Cohen and Camhi argued that the schizophrenics' impaired performance as 'speakers' indicated that they had trouble disregarding, or editing, inappropriate clue words which were generated as associates to the referent word. This hypothesis was subsequently explored using a task which elicited longer verbal responses, thus being more closely related to actual discourse (Cohen, Nachmani & Rosenberg, 1974; Kantorowitz & Cohen, 1977). Subjects were shown sets of coloured discs which varied in similarity of hue and intensity and were asked to produce a verbal description which would allow another person to determine the stimulus which was the referent. Cohen and his colleagues reasoned that as the discs became more similar in colour, subjects would have to reject their initial responses (e.g. 'red') and generate more detailed descriptions (e.g. 'late-autumn-leaf red turning brown'). If schizophrenics are poor editors, they should have special difficulty with stimuli that are very closely related. This is what was found. For easily distinguished colours, schizophrenics were as accurate in their descriptions as normals. But with increasing levels of display similarity, schizophrenics encountered more and more difficulty. Many of their responses repetitively emphasized dominant stimulus characteristics while they failed to touch upon the subtle distinctions which were necessary for accurate listener comprehension. This problem could not be traced to a complete disregard for the hypothetical editing process because schizophrenics actually took longer than normal subjects to initiate their responses to difficult stimuli. The investigators argued that the data could be viewed in terms of a perseverative-chaining model. According to this model, schizophrenics continue inappropriately to sample already rejected responses during the editing process. As this perseverative sampling proceeds, the probability that the inappropriate response will be emitted increases. After the inappropriate response is said aloud, the schizophrenic continues to produce associates to this word rather than to the original referent.

Cohen's studies clearly indicate that referential speaking presents special difficulty for schizophrenics, particularly when it is necessary to use care in editing their verbal responses with due regard to the listener's needs. But do schizophrenics also have trouble encoding sentences during less structured conversation? And can we identify more specifically the problems which their communications present for the listener? Cohen's studies indicate general inaccuracies but they do not provide a specific description of the distinctions between the speech of schizophrenics and normals.

Analysis of speech samples

These questions can be answered by a series of studies reported by Rochester and her colleagues. They have carried out detailed analyses of speech samples obtained from normal subjects and two groups of acute schizophrenic patients (Martin & Rochester, 1975; Rochester, Martin & Thurston, 1977). Each patient in one group of schizophrenics was rated as being 'thought-disordered' by two psychiatrists. These ratings were based on perseveration, echolalia, blocking, incoherence and other traditional criteria for thought disorder. None of the patients in the second group showed overt evidence of 'thought disorder'. The analyses were concerned with non-structural variables which are particularly relevant to the listener's task in verbal discourse: cohesion and reference. Schizophrenics' speech was characterized by a failure to provide the listener with necessary information (noun phrase referents), the use of ambiguous noun phrases, and the infrequent use of logical links (conjunctive ties) between sentences. Rochester's data provide a useful confirmation and extension of Cohen's studies. Taken together, these two lines of investigation clearly demonstrate that the communication difficulties of some schizophrenics stem from a failure to encode or consider information which will be required by the listener.

Hesitation patterns in speech

The difficulties which schizophrenics have in considering the needs of their listeners may be related to impairments in controlled processing which have been indicated in studies of memory and selective attention. The translation of covert thoughts into verbal communications requires a complex interaction of linguistic knowledge and information-processing abilities. Unfortunately, psycholinguists have made much more substantial progress in studying speech comprehension than they have in identifying the manner in which speakers encode messages. The cognitive processes which intervene between a thought and its expression are poorly understood (Cairns & Cairns, 1976). One of the few clues which is available involves the hesitations which speakers make prior to and during spontaneous utterances. These pauses tend to occur either before major clausal units or within clauses before particular words. Clark (1971) has labelled these pauses 'conventional' and 'idiosyncratic', respectively. Conventional pauses seem to reflect major decision points at which the speaker is considering structural variables and the direction of discourse. Idiosyncratic pauses accompany lexical decisions. Changes in the pattern of such hesitations may provide some indication of the cognitive operations which may mediate disordered speech.

Rochester, Thurston and Rupp (1977) have studied hesitation patterns in speech samples collected from 'thought-disordered' and 'non-thought-disordered' speakers (defined as in the previously cited Rochester studies). All subjects participated both in an unstructured interview and a cartoon interpretation task. Speech was recorded and the form and duration of all hesitations were later analysed. Rochester and her colleagues found that 'thought-disordered' schizophrenics differed significantly from other schizophrenic patients and normal subjects in the duration of initial silent pauses; their conventional hesitations were longer than those of the other two groups. There were no differences between groups in the nature or duration of idiosyncratic pauses. Subjects who produced less coherent messages paused longer before speaking. Apparently the cognitive operations which occupy those initial pauses are somehow inefficient or disrupted in many schizophrenics.

Several explanations might account for these results. Conventional pauses may reflect major planning stages. In the terminology of Cohen and his colleagues, this may be the point at which self-editing takes place. These workers also found that schizophrenics paused longer than normal subjects before offering deviant descriptions of their coloured discs. Another possibility is that schizophrenics are distracted during interclausal hesitations. Maher (1972) has offered an attractive hypothesis which elegantly integrates the data on selective attention and language. He suggests that inappropriate associative intrusions occur at terminal points in an utterance. While normal speakers are able successfully to inhibit the intrusion of such distractions into their speech, schizophrenics cannot. This suggestion is, in many ways, similar to Cohen's hypothesis.

Rochester (1978) has outlined another alternative which is more closely related to the data regarding organizational processes in short-term memory. She suggests that the poor referential clues provided by thought-disordered speakers may reflect a deficiency in the controlled processes of short-term memory. This is the point at which the speaker must keep in mind what has already been said and what will be said shortly. The frequent production of noun phrases which are not supported by informative referents may reflect the fact that schizophrenics forget that these have not been provided or that they need to be provided. Inordinately long conventional pauses may be the result of disturbances in such organizational processes.

All these alternatives are reasonable and others will certainly emerge. None has been tested empirically, yet each is consistent with the major sets of data we have considered. They represent the possibility of an integration of contemporary knowledge concerning psycholinguistics and information processing. Such a development will be required if we are to unravel the puzzle of thought disorder which has occupied such a prominent position in the study of schizophrenia and which has eluded myriad attempts to define it.

Other aspects of psychological deficit

The recent work reviewed above has been concerned mainly with identifying a specific abnormality in the language of schizophrenic patients. The passage of time has seen some prominent areas of deficit research continue and others fall by the wayside. The reaction time crossover effect, first noted by Rodnick and Shakow (1940), continues to be pursued by Steffy and his colleagues (Steffy & Galbraith, 1974; Bellissimo & Steffy, 1975). Similarly, studies of intelligence have persisted and revealed that the low IQ found in schizophrenics (e.g. Foulds & Dixon, 1962) is also characteristic of pre-schizophrenics (e.g. Lane & Albee, 1968). In contrast, Rodnick and Garmezy's (1957) social censure formulation, which spawned so many investigations in the 1950s and 1960s, is no longer being actively studied. Likewise, earlier theories which proposed that some schizophrenics are overaroused and others underaroused (e.g. Venables, 1964) are no longer generating empirical research. But psychophysiological research, which formed the basis for these arousal theories, has continued to flourish, albeit with a different focus.

Many psychophysiological studies had focused on assessing tonic levels of skin conductance or heart rate in an effort to assess general arousal levels. But a contradictory pattern of findings and growing dissatisfaction with the concept of general arousal (see Neale & Oltmanns, 1980) have led contemporary researchers to a more intensive study of the orienting response (OR). Early studies of the OR had revealed contradictory findings. Zahn (1964) and Zahn *et al.* (1968) reported that schizophrenics' OR failed to habituate while Bernstein (1964, 1970) found that schizophrenics failed to show an OR. More recently, Gruzelier and Venables (1972, 1974) have found what appear to be two distinct groups of schizophrenics – OR responders emit ORs and fail to habituate; non-responders do not emit ORs. Furthermore, the responsive schizophrenics have higher amplitude responses from their right than their left hands. This latter finding has generated a neurophysiological theory of schizophrenia (Venables, 1977). Assuming that the OR is ipsilaterally controlled by the limbic system and that low amplitude ORs are abnormal, the OR pattern of responsive schizophrenics would then reflect a left hemisphere, limbic dysfunction. Other research also supports the notion that some schizophrenics may have a left hemisphere dysfunction. Electroencephalograms and neurological tests reveal a pattern consistent with this theory (e.g. Flor-Henry, 1976), as does performance on some psychological tests (e.g. Gur, 1978). This lateralization theory of schizophrenia, although highly speculative, is currently being actively pursued. (See Lishman, 1978, for further discussion.)

Some general issues in deficit research

The findings we have discussed thus far have typically been interpreted as being specifically relevant to schizophrenia. But in studies which have compared the performance of schizophrenics with that of other psychiatric patients, it has proved difficult to find deficits that are unique to schizophrenics. Breakey and Goodell (1972), using Bannister's Grid Test for thought disorder, failed to distinguish between schizophrenics and manics. Manics are also as distractible as schizophrenics on laboratory measures of selective attention (Oltmanns, 1978) and appear to be even more over-inclusive than schizophrenics (Andreasen & Powers, 1974).

Depressed patients may also show impairments on measures of cognitive abilities. Ianzito, Cadoret and Pugh (1974) interviewed groups of schizophrenic and depressive patients within three days of hospital admission and rated various categories of thought disturbance which are included in the Present State Examination (Wing, Cooper & Sartorius, 1974).

Schizophrenics clearly displayed more communication problems but, in accordance with the assumptions of the system, depressives also showed signs of cognitive disturbance. In fact, they were rated as having more difficulty in concentrating than schizophrenics. Some laboratory measures have also indicated that schizophrenics and depressives share similar problems. Depressives have difficulty in utilizing contextual constraints in the same way as schizophrenics (Levy & Maxwell, 1968), and they are less accurate than normals on tests of short-term memory (Sternberg & Jarvik, 1976) and selective attention (Hemsley & Zawada, 1976). Depressive patients' problems affect many other areas of perceptual and cognitive functioning (Miller, 1975). Harrow & Quinlan (1977) have argued on the basis of results from Rorschach, sorting, and proverbs tests that disordered thought is not a unique feature of schizophrenia. They suggest that it is a continuous rather than a discrete phenomenon and that it is a general concomitant of acute psychopathology.

Are there unique features of schizophrenics' information processing or linguistic performance? A definitive answer is not currently available and difficult issues surround the search for conclusive data. The failure to distinguish between patient-groups with particular instruments may indicate that hopes of identifying special anomalies in schizophrenics' performance have been in vain. But they could also mean that the indices employed were crude and insensitive. Accepting the null hypothesis has never been a defensible logical position. At best, we may say that there is some reason to believe that schizophrenics are not the only group of psychiatric patients who have trouble in speaking or in processing information. Future investigations must clearly allow for this state of affairs in their research designs and take clinical knowledge into account. Schizophrenic and normal subjects are not sufficient; heterogeneous 'non-schizophrenic' groups are of little additional help. The most satisfactory projects will include multiple, specific diagnostic categories and simultaneously allow for the consideration of task performance as it relates to specific symptoms (Bannister, 1968; Neale & Oltmanns, 1980).

Aside from the issue of specificity, what can the study of psychological deficit tell us about schizophrenia? One possibility is that the specification of performance anomalies may provide clues to the mechanisms involved at physiological and biochemical levels. For example, Snyder (1974) has outlined an intriguing model which unifies many of the data pertaining to selective attention and dopaminergic dysfunction. His speculations are consistent with the results of an investigation we conducted which concerned the effects of phenothiazine medication on distractibility (Oltmanns, Ohayon & Neale, 1978). We found that these therapeutically effective drugs have a specific cognitive effect of reducing susceptibility to irrelevant, competing stimulation. Thus, the biochemical dysfunction outlined in the dopamine hypothesis, and the difficulties of information processing considered in this chapter, may eventually be integrated in a more comprehensive network of relationships which will expand our understanding of the schizophrenia construct.

Psychological variables may also play an important role in defining early phases of the disorder, particularly vulnerability (Zubin & Spring, 1977). Meehl (1962) proposed that several subtle cognitive anomalies play an important role in preschizophrenic behaviour. 'Cognitive slippage', for example, was described as an important schizotypic sign (Meehl, 1964). Several currently ongoing high-risk projects, studying children of schizophrenic parents, have hinted that these offspring may differ from other normal children in subtle but important ways. In the realm of attention, Asarnow and colleagues (1977) have reported that children of schizophrenics show a deficit on the span of apprehension task which Neale (1971) has used in studies of adult schizo-

phrenics. Similarly, Rutschmann and colleagues (1977) found that high-risk children perform poorly on a continuous performance task. In the field of cognition, Oltmanns and colleagues (1978) reported that children of schizophrenics show a deficit in object-sorting performance which parallels the pattern of data found among adult schizophrenics. If these indications turn out to be reliable, they may serve several practical and theoretical functions. They may become useful signs for early detection of schizophrenia and may also provide a better picture of the relationship between cognitive processes and subsequent clinical symptoms.

The utility of linguistic and cognitive data in constructing a picture of schizophrenia have been hampered by the almost exclusive use of cross-sectional designs. But the significance of the role that psychological processes play in schizophrenia will not be meaningfully understood until we have determined their relationship to other symptomatic and biological variables over the course of the disorder. Very few data of this sort have been collected. Longitudinal studies are difficult and expensive to complete. But the necessity for causal inferences in the context of correlational designs demands their adoption. As the results of such investigations begin to be reported, cognitive processes will probably constitute an important aspect of our knowledge and may occupy key positions in the emerging nomological network.

11
Genetics of schizophrenia

JOHN D. RAINER

Introduction

The results of genetic studies in psychiatry have been interpreted in two quite different ways. At one level, the age-old nature–nurture controversy has persisted, each side claiming that the balance of evidence is strongly in its favour and that the burden of proof lies with the other side. However, there has also been a more scientific level of presentation. Psychiatric genetics has become the enterprise of research workers who are knowledgeable and experienced in all aspects of psychiatry, including the social and developmental as well as the neurochemical and chromosomal. This enterprise involves the concepts of liability, of interaction, and ultimately of the biological substratum of mental disorder – what is inherited, and how it operates throughout normal and disordered development.

Over the past six decades or so there have been applied, successively or concurrently, a number of paradigms in psychiatric genetic research. Studies of pedigrees, of family risk data, and of twins have established to many people's satisfaction the fact of heritable aetiological factors in the major psychoses. More currently, investigations of neurochemical abnormalities, chromosomal linkage, and association with genetic markers have tentatively suggested what some of the mechanisms might be and the loci of their operation, while longitudinal observations from early age of persons at high risk focus on pre-morbid phenomena and add the dimension of time.

Genetic strategies need to complement one another, since no one method can answer every question. Diagnosis, interaction with environment, modes of transmission, course, and biological substrate are all interlocked. With tentative agreement on diagnostic criteria, older family studies suggested modes of inheritance, but only with arbitrary 'penetrance' parameters thrown in. More recently, liability models that incorporate environmental and genetic factors with thresholds make it possible to match parameters of various genetic hypotheses with actual risk data to determine best fit and most likely mode of transmission. Meanwhile biochemical studies of enzyme variants and other 'markers' work toward determining objective measures of liability as well as likely biological pathways (Rieder & Gershon, 1978). Adoption studies hope to tease out the details of environmental interaction or at least to rule out certain environmental factors, while high-risk studies aim to trace the ontogenesis of illness from early days.

The application of these methods to the study of the genetics of schizophrenia requires a critical review of some of the currently popular strategies. There is, however, some common ground. It may be said that, in spite of uncertainties about diagnosis (and hence validity of research) and about the nature of interaction with environment, the mode of inheritance, the development of the syndrome in individuals at risk, and ultimately the biological nature of the genotype, the evidence for a necessary genetic vulnerability in schizophrenia is generally accepted. The data are consistent with an essential genetic component and have not been adequately explained in any other way. The reader is referred to the texts by Roberts and Pembrey (1978) and Emery (1976) for a general introduction to the ideas and techniques of genetics and to recent reviews of their application to psychiatric conditions (Slater & Cowie, 1971) and more specifically to schizophrenia (Rosenthal & Kety, 1968; Shields, 1978).

Research strategies

Strategies used effectively in research on the genetics of schizophrenia include, in historical order, (1) analysis of pedigrees; (2) determination of the risk of schizophrenia in specified groups of relatives of schizophrenic patients, compared with the risk in the general population; (3) determination of the rate of schizophrenia in monozygotic twins of patients, compared with that in dizygotic twins and in other brothers and sisters; (4) determination of the rate of schizophrenia in schizophrenic patients' offspring who were adopted early in life by non-relatives, compared with that in adoptees born to healthy parents; (5) determination of the rate of schizophrenia in biological and adoptive families of schizophrenic and healthy adoptees; and (6) longitudinal investigations searching for early differences in children at high risk, usually those who have one or two parents with schizophrenia.

Pedigree studies

Simple pedigree observation, useful in rare syndromes, has been of limited use in psychiatric genetics in general, and in the study of schizophrenia in particular. Early reports were based on biased studies of a few families and were naive both genetically and psychiatrically. The quantitative science of genetics had not yet developed, psychiatric diagnoses were global, and non-genetic familial causes were not ruled out. There is information in pedigrees, however, that is not available in pooled population risk data, and the method has lately come into prominence again because of new techniques of segregation analysis aimed at defining mode of inheritance (Spence, Elston, Namboodiri & Rainer, 1976; Elston, Namboodiri, Spence & Rainer, 1978). If schizophrenia is heterogeneous genetically, individual pedigrees, large ones if possible, will also provide for further investigation groups with presumably uniform aetiologies and pathophysiology. Although neither of these approaches has yet yielded a definitive mode of inheritance or specific genetic markers, there could be much gain from supplementing population studies by methods which focus on individual families.

Family risk studies

Family risk studies were originally designed to determine the expectancy of schizophrenia in people with various degrees of relationship to patients as compared with the expectancy in the general population. One of the largest of the earlier studies was reported by Kallmann (1938). The charts of 1087 patients (all those admitted to two Berlin hospitals around the turn of the century) were reviewed and carefully rediagnosed. Their siblings and descendants were then traced. For siblings, the risk of schizophrenia was 11.5 per cent; and for children 16.4 per cent. In both cases there was a higher risk for the relatives of catatonic and hebephrenic patients than for those with paranoid symptoms or simple schizophrenia, an early indication of the relation of genetic risk to type or severity of illness.

Second degree relatives (grandchildren, nephews and nieces, first cousins) showed a risk of about 4 per cent in Kallmann's material. Pooled results of other family studies (Slater & Cowie, 1971) yield figures somewhat lower than Kallmann's (9 per cent in sibs, 12 per cent in children, 2 to 3 per cent in second degree relatives). For children of two schizophrenic parents, the risk pooled over a number of studies is in the neighbourhood of 40 per cent.

All these figures involve an estimate of lifetime expectancy based on weighting each individual in the sample according to his age from what is known about the general age-of-onset distribution of the disease – Weinberg, Strömgren or similar method (Larsson & Sjögren, 1954, pp. 40–51) – or on life-table techniques (Deming, 1968; Kramer, 1961). They can be compared with the risk in the general population, measured by various epidemiological techniques, which is remarkably constant at from slightly under 1 per cent to as high as 2 per cent (see chapter 8).

These data on family risk are not specific to any form of inheritance. Recessive inheritance is unlikely, although Kallmann at first interpreted his data in terms of a single autosomal recessive gene, subject to modification by other genes conferring a greater or lesser degree of resistance (Kallmann, 1938). Other proposals have included a dominant mode of inheritance with incomplete penetrance in heterozygotes (Slater & Cowie, 1971; Elston & Campbell, 1970) a polygenic form of inheritance with a threshold (Gottesman & Shields, 1972), and a heterogeneity model specifying a variety of separate genes, dominant or recessive, any one of which might be involved in the aetiology of schizophrenia (Erlenmeyer-Kimling & Paradowski, 1966).

Moreover they by no means preclude – in fact they almost require – the operation of non-genic and environmental factors. 'It is too often forgotten that only predispositions are inherited and never attributes as such, and that the phenotypical manifestation of the trait in the individual depends on the sum of all the given environmental conditions' (Kallmann, 1938).

Nevertheless a unique effort to separate genetic and a particular set of environmental factors appeared to rule out the effect of early total deafness, a severe sensory deprivation, upon the vulnerability to schizophrenia. Altshuler & Sarlin (1962) collected 138 families of patients with both schizophrenia and deafness. Although the schizophrenia rate among the general deaf population had been estimated at no more than 2.5 per cent (Rainer & Kallmann, 1959), that among the siblings of deaf schizophrenics was 11.6 per cent. This figure was significantly higher than that for the general population and was similar to that observed for siblings of hearing schizophrenics. Of major importance was the fact that the schizophrenia rates of deaf siblings (15.8 per cent) and hearing siblings (11.2 per cent) did not differ significantly. For parents of deaf schizophrenic index cases, the rate was 7.3 per cent. These findings confirmed the genetic transmission of schizophrenia without significant interaction with severe communicative defect.

Two important corrolaries emerged from conventional family data: first, that the children of schizophrenic mothers had the same risk as the children of schizophrenic fathers; second, that the children of two schizophrenic parents showed a risk as *low* as 40 per cent. Neither of these might have been predicted from a hypothesis of strictly intrafamily environmental causation. Otherwise, the data have been of use chiefly as empirical risk figures, of value in genetic counselling.

Liability-threshold models

It currently remains for more complex models of transmission to differentiate among various modes of inheritance. One of the more promising approaches (Gottesman & Shields, 1967; Kidd & Cavalli-Sforza, 1973) is to consider the liability for schizophrenia (genetic and environmental) as distributed among the population in a regular fashion (e.g. a normal distribution under a polygenic hypothesis or three overlapping normal distributions for two classes of homozygotes and heterozygotes respectively under a single gene hypothesis). A threshold may then be specified cutting off the group of phenotypically well from that of affected persons in the general population; a threshold is also determined for the similarly distributed group of relatives. The positions of the thresholds along the distributions are related to the areas under the distribution curve which they cut off; these areas are a measure of the population risk and the risk for relatives respectively. An elaboration of this method is based on two (or more) thresholds for narrow (severe) and wide (less severe) forms of the disease (Reich, James & Morris, 1972). With large enough samples, it may be possible to distinguish between the various forms of transmission by fitting the observed data successively to various models and determining a unique fit. Of course if an empirical measure of liability – biochemical, behavioural, psychophysiological, etc. – were to be found which would reasonably specify such a model, it would go a long way toward determining not only modes of inheritance but basic mechanisms as well; hence the importance of these new approaches.

Meanwhile, since the study of standard families confounds genetic and rearing influences, the complementary strategies of studying twins (genetic differences, same families) and adoptees (genetic sameness, different families) became prominent tools for research.

Twin studies

The major twin studies in schizophrenia may be divided into two groups: the older ones (1928–61), in which the twins had severe and usually chronic schizophrenia and were found in hospitals, and the more recent ones (1968–72), which included patients with milder illness and non-hospitalized patients. In the older studies the concordance rate for monozygotic twins ran from 60 to 70 per cent with a mean of 63 per cent; for dizygotic twins of the same sex, from 13 to 18 per cent with a mean of 12 per cent. Since the mean risk for siblings in studies at that time was about 9 per cent, the somewhat increased effect of dizygotic twinship could have been environmental or based on ascertainment biases, but the greatly increased effect of monozygotic twinship appeared to be genetic.

The largest investigation of that group was conducted by Kallmann in New York who reported overall concordance rates of 69 per cent for monozygotic twins and 10.3 per cent for dizygotic twins (1946). Examination of his data by Gottesman and Shields (1966) indicated that there was a spread of from 26 to 100 per cent in the monozygotic rates with a similar spread from 2 to 17 per cent in the dizygotic, depending on the severity of illness in the hospitalized twin.

These trends were maintained in the more recent studies of twins which included non-hospitalized index cases and a wider range of pathology. While the absolute concordance rates were lower, the monozygotic rates were appreciably higher than the dizygotic, and were higher for more severely ill twins than for those with milder course.

Among these studies, Gottesman and Shields (1972) studying all schizophrenic twins treated at the Maudsley Hospital in London as out-patients or short-stay in-patients, found an over-all concordance of 50 per cent for monozygotic pairs and 10 per cent for dizygotic pairs. The rates of the monozygotic pairs rose to 77 per cent, however, if the index twin had spent two or more years in the hospital. Kringlen (1967) studied a group of Norwegian twins, culled from a total twin registry, and found schizophrenia concordance rates of 25 to 38 per cent for monozygotic pairs and 4 to 10 per cent for same-sex dizygotic pairs, variations again based on the severity of illness as well as on the strictness of diagnostic criteria.

A noteworthy finding in a Danish study by Fischer (1971) was a review of the children of monozygotic twins, from pairs with schizophrenia in one or both members. The risk of schizophrenia in such children was similar to the known risk for children of one schizophrenic parent and did not vary significantly whether the child's parent was schizophrenic or not, or came from a concordant or discordant pair.

In the minds of many, twin studies have done more than any others to date to establish the necessary role of heredity in schizophrenia but they have not succeeded in achieving Kallmann's main purpose, which was 'not to show concordance but to study those pairs that differ in onset or production in order to prevent or heal the condition'. They have failed to shed much light on what is inherited, how it is inherited, and what the significant environmental factors are. And there were still some diehards who tried to explain the increased concordance rates of monozygotic twins entirely on the basis of psychological closeness or greater similarity in parental treatment.

Adoption studies

The second 'experimental' strategy for separating genetic and environmental variables exploits data derived from adoption in early infancy. Studies of families and twins were being criticized for not fully disentangling genetic and experiential influences. The ideal experimental situation – pairs of monozygotic twins randomly selected for separation at birth and for rearing by families bearing only a random resemblance to the biological ones – existed only anecdotally, and the converse paradigm – monozygotic twins, dizygotic twins, sibs, half-sibs, and step-sibs variously reared in the same families – did not satisfy those who felt there were experiental or even prenatal influences which differed among these groups. Adoption studies were calculated to contribute to both the problem of diagnosis and that of gene–environment interaction. In the diagnostic area, they have been concerned with the concepts of diathesis, of spectrum diagnosis, of continuous versus discrete classification of psychopathology, of psychotic equivalents, and of borderline states; in the area of interaction, with the importance, or unimportance, of the roles of stress, rearing, and parent-child relationships, and the specificity or lack of specificity of such factors. Heston (1966) reported a study of 47 children born to schizophrenic mothers and separated at birth. Fathers were not known to be hospitalized and the children never lived with maternal relatives. A group of 50 controls matched for sex, placement, and time in institutions, with no record of mother in a hospital, was chosen. There were two serious difficulties with this study: first, the illness of the mother preceded and continued during her pregnancy with the given child, making for the possibility that some intra-uterine noxious factor played a role; second, connected with the above time table, the adoptive parents knew of the psychiatric illness of the biological mothers. This represented a particular interaction and suggested a self-fulfilling prophecy, though Heston said that no adoptive parent refused to adopt on these grounds. A number of other interaction experiments were built into this study. First, it turned out that half of both experimental and control groups were reared up to the age of 5 years in foundling homes, the other half starting life in foster homes usually with paternal relatives. Second, the social class of the subjects' childhood homes showed a broad variation. The results of Heston's studies bore out the necessary role of genetic transmission. The experimental group of 47 offspring had an age-corrected rate for schizophrenia of 16.6 per cent (uncannily close to Kallmann's 16.4 per cent) with none in the control group. Other significant differences between the two groups were in sociopathic personality, spending more than one year in a penal or psychiatric institution, and discharge from armed forces on psychiatric or behavioural grounds. Those experimental subjects who showed no psychosocial impairment were said not only to be successful adults, but to be more spontaneous and to have more creative, colourful jobs and more imaginative hobbies. The study showed no evidence that adult adjustment of the adoptees was affected by the social class of the childhood home, by whether the child was reared in a foster or a foundling home, or by the length of time the latter remained in a foundling home before being adopted. Thus no interactions between genes and

these particular aspects of environment were demonstrated. Anticipating criticisms candidly acknowledged by subsequent investigators, Heston said that there remained tremendous scope for other environmental variables of a less obvious kind, but regarded it as extremely unlikely that such elements could have been distributed so conveniently between the two groups.

Heston's study was followed by a series of studies, some still ongoing, under the direction of Rosenthal, Kety, Wender, and others, conducted mostly in Denmark but also in the United States. These were of three basic designs. The first was like Heston's in which the children of schizophrenic biological parents reared by adoptive parents were compared with a matched control group of adoptees whose biological parents had no psychiatric history. In the second design, the biological extended families of schizophrenic adoptees were compared for rates of psychopathology with the biological families of matched non-schizophrenic control adoptees. In the third, biological and adoptive parents of schizophrenic patients were studied for disturbed behaviour.

The first design was an improvement on Heston's in that (1) the adoptees were chosen from a total sample of adoptees in Copenhagen (and currently in all of Denmark), (2) the illness of the biological parent usually began a considerable number of years after the birth and subsequent adoption of the given child, and (3) the adoptive parents were not aware of the illness of the child's biological parent.

In the first design (Rosenthal *et al.*, 1968; Rosenthal, 1972) the rate of spectrum diagnosis was significantly increased in the offspring of affected parents over that in the offspring of control parents. In the second design, it was found that chronic and borderline schizophrenia and inadequate personality occurred significantly more frequently in the biological relatives of the chronic and borderline adoptees than in the other three groups of relatives (biological relatives of controls and both groups of adoptive relatives) (Kety, Rosenthal, Wender & Schulsinger, 1968; Kety *et al.*, 1975). Moreover, a highly significant increase in schizophrenia pathology was found in the biological paternal half-siblings of these schizophrenic adoptees, as compared with the biological paternal half-siblings of the controls. This finding was important in ruling out intra-uterine and other prenatal influences. No instances of schizophrenia spectrum disorder were found in the biological relatives of the acute schizophrenic reaction probands, supporting the tendency to consider that syndrome genetically unrelated to the others. In the third design (Wender *et al.*, 1977), the biological parents of schizophrenics showed a higher rate of spectrum disorders and a lower rating on the Menninger Mental Health Rating Scale than the adopting parents of schizophrenics or a group of parents burdened by rearing a mentally retarded child.

A refinement of Rosenthal's adoptee study was provided by Wender and colleagues (1974) in a cross-fostering study aimed at further clarifying the role of experiential factors. Three groups were compared: adopted-index, with biological parent in the schizophrenia spectrum, the adoptive free to vary; adopted-control, with no recorded psychiatric diagnosis in the biological parent and the adoptive free to vary; and the cross-fostered, with the biological parent free of illness but the adoptive parent's diagnosis in the schizophrenia spectrum. Here the adopted-index group showed significantly greater psychopathology than either of the other groups. Actually, the chief 'environmental' factor ruled out by this study is schizophrenia or severe psychiatric disorder in a parent.

Some nosological considerations

Genetic studies of families, twins, and adoptees have made tentative inroads on problems of nosology, distinguishing for example between nuclear, endogenous, typical, or process schizophrenia on the one hand and peripheral, exogenous, atypical, or reactive on the other (e.g. Mitsuda, 1967). Paranoia (delusional disorder) was found to breed true in an Iowa study (Winokur, 1977) while genetic studies of borderline conditions have thus far been limited and inconclusive (Siever & Gunderson, 1979).

High-risk studies

Hypotheses and data on the transmission of schizophrenia may be supplemented by studying the development of pathology through life-history observation of children into adulthood, thus eventually charting the interplay of gene products and environmental demands in the course of that development. Longitudinal studies make it possible to avoid confusing early or precursor changes with symptoms caused by the effects of illness. Such studies may be retrospective or prospective. Retrospective studies in schizophrenia have considered the home and school backgrounds of patients and have compared these patients with their twins, their siblings, or their classmates. Poor school records and a history of withdrawal or of bizarre, delinquent behavior have been described, but it is hard to avoid bias based on distorted memory influenced by subsequent events. In prospective studies, the most economical approach is to use high-risk populations. With a 10 to 15 per cent risk for the offspring of one schizophrenic parent and a 40 per cent risk for the offspring of two schizophrenic parents, the study of these children may yield valuable clues about pathogenesis as well as help to spot early difficulties and suggest preventive measures in this vulnerable but potentially salvageable group.

A number of major longitudinal studies are presently ongoing and only preliminary results are available. Erlenmeyer-Kimling and her colleagues, for example, are investigating the offspring of one or two schizophrenic parents in intact families where the children are between the ages of seven and twelve at the beginning of the study (Erlenmeyer-Kimling, Cornblatt & Fleiss, 1979). Among the forms of investigation in their study are psychiatric and neurological examinations and psychophysiological and psychological tests; children of hospitalized non-schizophrenic patients and of normal parents are used as controls. The selection of measures is based on the idea that schizophrenic individuals are unable to filter out excessive or irrelevant stimuli. Hence the investigation concentrates on measures of attention, distractibility, response latency, and neurophysiological functioning. In early results, high-risk subjects as a group did poorly in a continuous performance test demanding sustained attention, they were unable to ignore irrelevant stimuli, and were more disturbed by external distraction. Group differences occurred also in the Bender Gestalt and Draw-A-Person test.

Moreover a large subgroup of the high-risk subjects showed extreme deviance on a composite of five test indices. Although it is too early to say that these measures predict future outcome, most of the subjects who have already been in psychiatric treatment are in the high-risk group.

Genetic markers

Probably the most important contribution to genetic studies would be the detection of biochemical genetic markers, making it possible to separate aetiologically distinct syndromes, and to detect vulnerable pre-clinical and subclinical cases within families. The search today is mainly for enzymes which may be controlled quantitatively or qualitatively by genetic mechanisms and which may show differences in schizophrenics. Monoamine oxidase (MAO) activity as measured in blood platelets has been shown to be heritable. While the results are still inconclusive, a decrease in enzyme activity has been found in some chronic schizophrenics as compared with controls, and a significant correlation has been reported between members of discordant twin pairs (Wyatt, Potkin & Murphy, 1979).

Heredity counselling

The application of genetic knowledge to heredity counselling in psychiatry represents the clinical application of the data accumulated in research. Such counselling requires accurate evaluation of the clinical picture, communication with hospitals and other physicians, physical and mental examinations, psychological investigations, and laboratory procedures. In addition, skill is required to obtain accurate family pedigree material, including information about all family members, even that often repressed or conveniently forgotten, as well as about environmental effects on parents, especially on mothers during pregnancy.

In schizophrenia, the most significant empirical risk, about 40 per cent, is to the offspring of two schizophrenic parents. If one potential parent is schizophrenic, the risk is in the 10 to 15 per cent range, while with only collateral relatives affected, the couple can usually be reassured that the risk is not appreciably greater than for the general population. There is evidence from the twin and adoption studies that acute or paranoid schizophrenia carries a lower risk than the chronic or undifferentiated form.

In all cases the genetic counsellor needs to help the patient and his family evaluate the future personal burden, a quantity which is the result of many factors including the genetic risk, the nature of the clinical condition, the couple's potential as parents, and the effect of a healthy or unhealthy child upon the parents' own difficulties. For these reasons, many feel that providing genetic advice on schizophrenia and other mental disorders must be left to psychiatrists. At least it needs to be in the hands of professionals who can combine a knowledge of the frontiers of genetic research, an appreciation of the clinical course and heterogeneity of the illness, an experience with family management and the ability to communicate empathically with each family that comes for help.

12
Biochemistry and pathology of schizophrenia

RICHARD RODNIGHT

This chapter surveys recent investigations into organic factors that may be involved in the aetiology of schizophrenia. The main emphasis is on recent developments in the biochemical field, where there has been an increasing interest in central neurotransmitters and the enzymes responsible for their metabolism. Recognition of the importance of 'transmitter balance' (see Domino & Davis, 1975) in regulating normal behaviour has naturally led to the concept of 'transmitter imbalance' as the ultimate basis for abnormal behaviour. Imbalance in neurotransmission may arise from diverse primary causes – inherited metabolic abnormalities, degenerative processes, viral infections, auto-immune mechanisms, nutritional factors, drugs – to name a few. Thus for the schizophrenias the concept encompasses the possibility of multiple aetiologies all leading to a final common disordered pathway.

On the basis of knowledge of the chemical anatomy of the rat brain, it seems likely that the human brain uses a minimum of 12 transmitter substances for neuronal communication. Only a few of these have been investigated in schizophrenia, and of these only the catecholamines and indoleamines have received more than cursory consideration. There are of course many problems inherent in the investigation of central transmitter function by the conventional approach of body fluid analysis and these have led some investigators to turn to the study of brain tissue taken post-mortem from patients. Here the problems of interpreting results are different: for example, post-mortem stability of the brain chemistry and provision of suitable control material. Surprisingly, for some transmitter systems at least, these are proving less intractable than once suspected (McGeer & McGeer, 1976; Wyatt *et al.*, 1978; Spokes, 1979; Rodnight, 1980).

Catecholamine systems
Dopamine

The suggestion that some disturbance of dopaminergic function exists in schizophrenia stems largely from two observations from pharmacology: that high doses of dopamine-releasing agents (amphetamine and methylphenidate) can precipitate in normal subjects a psychosis closely resembling paranoid schizophrenia (Connell, 1958; Griffith *et al.*, 1972; Crow *et al.*, 1976) and that with few exceptions the neuroleptic drugs possess the property of blocking dopamine receptors with a potency that parallels their therapeutic efficacy (Crow *et al.*, 1976; van Praag, Korf & Dols, 1976). The fact that areas within the limbic forebrain are relatively rich in dopaminergic nerve terminals has added weight to the hypothesis (Stevens, 1973; Torrey & Peterson, 1974). The subsynaptic site of the suspected abnormality in dopaminergic function is unknown. Originally hyperactivity of dopamine pathways, resulting in an abnormally high rate of release of the amine from pre-synaptic terminals, was proposed. However, the available evidence indicates that dopamine turnover is either normal or depressed in schizophrenia. The urinary excretion of dopamine and its metabolites is normal in the condition (Crowley *et al.*, 1978). More to the point, accumulation in the lumbar CSF of homovanillic acid (the main metabolite of dopamine in the brain) after administration of probenecid was either significantly lower (Bowers, 1974) or normal (Post *et al.*, 1975) in cases of acute schizophrenia compared to non-psychotic controls; in fact the accumulation tended to be even lower in the more severely ill patients (Post *et al.*, 1975). Further, the dopamine synthesis inhibitor α-methyl-*p*-tyrosine is devoid of neuroleptic action and in one study failed to potentiate the clinical actions of neuroleptic drugs in chronic schizophrenics (Nasrallah *et al.*, 1977). Dopaminergic hyperactivity (unless highly localized in the brain) would be expected to decrease the concentration of prolactin in the blood since release of this hormone is tonically inhibited by dopamine; however, blood prolactin levels were found to be normal in schizophrenia and

were increased by dopamine receptor blockade equally in normals and patients (Gruen *et al.*, 1978). Two studies (Bird, Spokes & Iversen, 1979; Crow, Baker *et al.*, 1979) have demonstrated a modest increase in the concentration of dopamine in post-mortem brain tissue from patients dying during a chronic schizophrenic illness (compared to matched control tissue), but the absence of any parallel increase in homovanillic acid concentration excludes abnormal turnover as an explanation of this finding.

An alternative to dopamine hyperactivity at pre-synaptic receptor sites could be an abnormality in post-synaptic receptor function resulting in super-sensitivity to the transmitter. One consequence of experimentally-induced supersensitivity of the dopamine receptor in animals is an increase in the activity of the dopamine-stimulated adenylate cyclase linked to the receptor; however, the activity of this enzyme in post-mortem tissue from schizophrenics could not be distinguished from controls (Carenzi *et al.*, 1975). Another approach is represented by receptor binding studies in post-mortem tissue, and here several groups (Lee *et al.*, 1978; Mackay *et al.*, 1978; Owen *et al.*, 1978) have shown an increase in schizophrenic subjects in the density of dopamine receptors in the striatum and nucleus accumbens (a limbic area), which is interpreted as indicating supersensitivity. Although animal experiments have shown that treatment with dopamine blocking agents increases dopamine receptor density and sensitivity, preliminary evidence (Owen *et al.*, 1978) suggests that prolonged therapy with neuroleptics only accounts for part of the observed 'supersensitivity' in patients. However, more data are required to establish the meaning of the phenomenon for the schizophrenic process.

For the present therefore we must conclude that there is no firm evidence for either hyperactivity or receptor supersensitivity of dopaminergic systems in schizophrenia. Yet the evidence that the antipsychotic actions of the neuroleptics are related to their capacity to block dopamine receptors is very strong (Johnstone *et al.*, 1978), and the discrepancy has led to the suggestion that transmitter imbalance in schizophrenia stems from a disturbance in another neuronal pathway normally regulated by the dopamine system. Neuroleptics are then viewed as creating a new balance by decreasing the dopaminergic input to the disordered system. Neurones known to interact with dopamine pathways include those utilizing acetylcholine or γ-aminobutyric acid as transmitters, but current research (McGeer & McGeer, 1977; Perry *et al.*, 1979; Bird *et al.*, 1979; Cross, Crow & Owen, 1979; Bennett *et al.*, 1979) has so far failed to provide convincing evidence for an abnormality in these pathways.

Noradrenalin

There is no firm evidence at present that noradrenergic function is abnormal in schizophrenia. Recent work (Wyatt *et al.*, 1978; Crow, Baker *et al.*, 1979) failed to confirm an earlier report (Wise *et al.*, 1974) of a deficit of dopamine-β-hydroxylase in post-mortem brain from schizophrenics. A raised noradrenalin concentration in post-mortem tissue confined to the putamen (Crow, Baker *et al.*, 1979) or specific parts of the limbic forebrain (Farley *et al.*, 1978) has been reported, but as with dopamine it seems likely this is iatrogenic in origin. The urinary excretion of 3-methoxy-4-hydroxyphenylene glycol (the major metabolite of noradrenalin metabolism in the brain) was normal in chronic patients, although within the schizophrenic group the rate of excretion of the conjugated form correlated inversely with severity of illness (Joseph *et al.*, 1976).

Transmethylation and indoleamine systems

The possibility has often been considered that transmitter imbalance in schizophrenia results from a disturbance in the widespread process of transmethylation (Osmond & Smythies, 1952; see Gillin, Stoff & Wyatt, 1978 for a recent review). Both ring hydroxyl groups and amine groups in certain transmitters are subject to methylation in reactions using *S*-adenosylmethionine as methyl donor; generally *O*-methylation results in inactivation and *N*-methylation in a change in function.

Current research has focused on the *N*-methylation of certain indoleamine precursors to yield products possessing psychotomimetic properties when administered in relatively high doses to normal subjects (Domino, 1975; Rodnight, 1975; Gillin *et al.*, 1976). Of particular interest is the *N*-methylation of tryptamine in the brain and other tissues by the enzyme indoleamine-*N*-methyltransferase to give the potentially psychotoxic substance dimethyltryptamine (DMT). The normal function of DMT is unknown, but its potency as a psychotomimetic is about four times that of mescaline; the symptoms it produces are characterized more by 'inward withdrawal' than by frank hallucinations (Kaplan *et al.*, 1974). Normal human subjects excrete traces of DMT in their urine (Carpenter *et al.*, 1975; Oon *et al.*, 1977) and the possibility that its metabolism may be disturbed in schizophrenia has aroused considerable interest. The evidence is equivocal. Discounting work published before 1975 because of inadequate methodology, urinary excretion of the substance appeared normal in one qualitative study (Carpenter *et al.*, 1975), whereas other workers (Rodnight *et al.*, 1976; Murray *et al.*, 1979) have consistently reported a two- to three-fold increase in the 24-hour excretion rate in about 50 per cent of acutely ill psychotic subjects including drug-free patients with a hospital diagnosis of schizophrenia. In the latter work all patients received a Present State Examination and from the ratings it appeared that the raised DMT excretion was associated with psychotic rather than neurotic psychopathology in which syndromes suggesting elation, perceptual abnormalities and difficulty in communicating were prominent. However, it is far from clear whether the phenomenon of raised DMT excretion has aetiological significance in the genesis of psychotic symptoms or whether it represents a response to some aspect of the stress of the illness. Thus abnormal excretion (when present) was only observed in acutely ill subjects; as the symptoms receded during drug treatment the excretion tended towards normal, with rapid changes in mood and mental state failing to correlate with daily fluctuations in DMT excretion (Checkley *et al.*, 1980). Moreover, a raised DMT excretion of the same magnitude as seen in psychosis has been observed in some psychiatrically normal patients with severe liver disease (Checkley *et al.*, 1979). Attempts have been made to measure the concentration of DMT in blood (Angrist *et al.*, 1976; Walker *et al.*, 1979) and CSF (Corbett *et al.*, 1978) from schizophrenia patients, but present results are inconclusive. Likewise, because a non-specific assay method was used, an attempt (Erdelyi *et al.*, 1978) to measure the activity of the DMT-synthesizing enzyme in autopsy brain tissue from patients must be discounted.

There have been many attempts to demonstrate a more general disturbance in indoleaminergic pathways in schizophrenia. However, numerous studies of the metabolism of serotonin, its precursor tryptophan and its main metabolite 5-hydroxyindoleacetic acid in the CSF and body fluids, have failed to reveal any consistent abnormalities in schizophrenia. In one study of post-mortem brain tissue from nine schizophrenic subjects the serotonin content of the putamen was significantly raised, but without evidence of increased turnover (Crow, Baker *et al.*, 1979); the authors considered that this result was probably iatrogenic in origin. More interesting perhaps is a recent report (Bennett *et al.*, 1979) of a 40–50 per cent decrease in the binding of [³H]LSD to serotonin receptors in post-mortem frontal cortex tissue from schizophrenic subjects, although the authors point out that their results do not necessarily imply a decline in receptor density.

The monoamine oxidase (MAO) story

In a search for possible genetic markers for vulnerability to schizophrenia MAO has attracted particular attention for several reasons: the enzyme is present in blood platelets, is relatively easy to assay, and is involved in the inactivation of the amine transmitters, as well as potentially toxic amines such as DMT and phenylethylamine. There are now more than 26 independent studies of platelet MAO activity in schizophrenia (reviewed recently by Wyatt, Potkin & Murphy, 1979) the majority of which report significantly decreased activity, particularly in chronic patients. There have also been persistent reports of low activity being mainly confined to patients with paranoid symptoms (Orsulak *et al.*, 1978; Potkin *et al.*, 1978). However, reduced platelet MAO activity has often been observed in non-psychotic psychiatric populations (Buchsbaum *et al.*, 1978) as well as in physical conditions and occasionally in normal subjects (Murphy *et al.*, 1976). While the activity appears to be partly determined by genetic influences (Wyatt *et al.*, 1973; Winter *et al.*, 1978; Wyatt *et al.*, 1979; however see Becker & Shaskan, 1977), it is also conditioned by a variety of endogenous and environmental factors including drug status (Murphy *et al.*, 1977). It is noteworthy that in a study of chronic schizophrenics who were free of drugs (Owen *et al.*, 1976) platelet monoamine oxidase activity was normal. It remains possible, however, that in some schizophrenic subjects an abnormally low activity of platelet MAO may have minor aetiological significance as a predisposing factor. The association in normal populations of a low activity of this enzyme with a higher than normal risk of developing psychiatric problems (Buchsbaum *et al.*, 1978) supports this conclusion.

In contrast to studies on platelet MAO an attempt to demonstrate an abnormality of MAO activity in post-mortem brain samples gave negative results (Crow, Baker *et al.*, 1979).

Plasma creatine phosphokinase (CPK) activity

Acutely psychotic patients often exhibit remarkably high concentrations in the plasma of the muscle enzyme CPK (Meltzer, 1973, 1976; Soni, 1976). Neuromuscular abnormalities in schizophrenic patients have also been described (Meltzer, 1976) but when present these were not necessarily associated with raised plasma CPK levels. The latter response is relatively non-specific and appears to be a stress-related phenomenon, like the increase in urinary DMT, since it is confined to acutely ill patients exhibiting florid symptoms; however, excessive muscular activity *per se* does not seem to account for the abnormality although it may contribute (Goode *et al.*, 1979).

Histopathology and gross pathology

There have been many reports (reviewed by Roisin, 1972; Corsellis, 1976, see also Fisman, 1975) of abnormal histopathology in the brain of subjects dying with schizophrenia, but there is very little evidence at present to justify ascribing any of the reported abnormalities specifically to schizophrenia, mainly because it has proved difficult to exclude non-specific changes due to ageing, long-term drug treatment, or even many years of living in an institution. It remains possible, of course, as in other areas of schizophrenia research, that the putative pathology is of a type not revealed by current procedures.

Rather better evidence is available for a mild form of cerebral atrophy in schizophrenia. By means of CAT (computerized axial tomography) scans two groups (Johnstone *et al.*, 1976; Weinberger *et al.*, 1979a) have reported enlargement of the lateral ventricles in a proportion of chronic schizophrenic subjects, an observation which, in the absence of any obstruction of the CSF flow, is generally interpreted as implying some degree of cerebral atrophy. CAT scans have also detected other structural abnormalities (fissure widths and sulci dimensions) in the brain of some schizophrenics (Weinberger *et al.*, 1979b), but the occurrence of these did not correlate with ventricular enlargement. In the later study of ventricular size (Weinberger *et al.*, 1979a) the increase was present in patients in the 3rd, 4th and 5th decades of life, although in all cases the mean volumes (expressed as ventricle/brain ratios) were still within the normal range for subjects in their 8th decade, and considerably less than values commonly found in Alzheimer's dementia. However there was no correlation with length of stay in hospital, and type of treatment. Clearly the possibility that an atrophic process is characteristic of some forms of schizophrenia (possibly the 'unremitting type') needs to be taken seriously, even though it is difficult to reconcile with the absence of a specific histopathology.

The viral hypothesis

One possible cause of cerebral atrophy is a long-existing viral infection. Several authors have debated this possibility (Torrey & Peterson, 1976; Crow, 1978; Matthysse & Matthysse, 1978), but only recently has it been seriously investigated. In a study of 47 patients with acute schizophrenic illnesses the lumbar CSF of 18 contained a virus-like agent which exerted a cytopathic effect on cultured cells (Tyrrell *et al.*, 1979; Crow, Ferrier *et al.*, 1979). An agent with similar properties was detected in CSF from 8 out of 11 patients with serious neurological disease, but only in one out of 25 patients with general medical conditions. The virus-like agent has yet to be propagated serially but in all other respects it resembles a virus.

Envoi

Numerous reviews have been written on the biochemistry and pathology of schizophrenia over the past 25 years. Many interesting and apparently significant deviations from 'normality' have been described, but for the great majority of sufferers from the disease no definite pathology has yet emerged. The occasional reports of schizophrenic illnesses occurring in subjects with certain well-defined inborn metabolic errors (e.g. homocystinuria, metachromatic leucodystrophy, porphyria) only serve to highlight our general ignorance. Nevertheless much has been learnt and an optimistic view of future developments is justified. The probability that schizophrenia has a multiple aetiology is now recognized and this should encourage investigators to pay more attention to biological variations within broad diagnostic groups (Buschsbaum & Haier, 1978). Only by this approach can variation that is specific to the psychiatrists' diagnosis of "schizophrenia" be distinguished from variation associated with other psychiatric conditions that sometimes exhibit symptoms. The importance of longitudinal variation in individual patients at different stages of their illness also needs to be borne in mind.

In the biochemical field there is increasing awareness of the wide range of genetically determined biochemical variation in normal populations, which may eventually help to identify predisposing biological factors. However, the most significant development for the future is the enormous growth over the past decade in fundamental knowledge of neurochemistry and of the molecular bases of behaviour. This basic knowledge is essential if investigations are to move away from the old empirical approach towards the study of specific hypotheses.

Section 3
CHAPTERS 13 AND 14
Treatment and management

13
Medication and physical treatment of schizophrenia
STEVEN R. HIRSCH

Effectiveness of neuroleptics
Clinical trials

The first effective medications for schizophrenia were the neuroleptics, chlorpromazine (Delay & Deniker, 1952) and reserpine (Kline, 1954). Neuroleptics are drugs with pharmacological features similar to chlorpromazine, having relatively strong antipsychotic tranquillizing effects relative to their hypnotic effect, but also causing extra-pyramidal side-effects, which were originally thought to be relevant to their antipsychotic action.

Davis and Garver (1978) have summarized the results of 207 double-blind comparisons between neuroleptics and placebo; the former were found to be superior in 86 per cent of trials. Reserpine, promazine and mepazine had weak antipsychotic activity and barbiturates had none.

In a large-scale trial of acutely ill patients (Cole, Klerman & Goldberg, 1964), 75 per cent of patients receiving active medication showed considerable improvement compared with 25 per cent of those receiving placebo. Nearly 90 per cent of those treated with phenothiazines improved, while less than half of those on placebo did so; most of the latter actually became worse. Similar responses to treatment have been observed in one-year catchment-area-based sample (Knight, Hirsch & Platt, 1980).

Neuroleptics compared with other medication for acute psychotic disorders

Compared with other types of medication, neuroleptics have three characteristic types of ameliorative effect on patients with psychoses:

(1) On delusions, hallucinations, thought disorder, psychomotor retardation, mannerisms, and catatonic symptoms.

(2) On agitation, restlessness, and excitement. This effect is obtained with markedly less sleepiness than is the case with opiates, barbiturates, or benzodiazepines.
The combined effects of (1) and (2) lead to improvement in other features of schizophrenia, including withdrawal, self-neglect, negativism, uncooperativeness, hostility, belligerence, bizarre behaviour, and insomnia.

(3) On the prevention of new symptoms arising in recently treated acute patients whose florid symptoms have not yet remitted (Goldberg, Klerman & Cole, 1965) and in successfully treated patients who no longer have psychotic symptoms or whose symptoms are stabilized and relatively quiescent (Hirsch *et al.*, 1973; Leff & Wing, 1971). No other group of drugs is known to have this action.

In addition, neuroleptics have an unspecific sedative effect in non-psychotic individuals who tend to be much more dose-sensitive to the sedative and hypnotic effect of these drugs – for this reason they can be used to quell any form of excitement. It must be appreciated that none of these effects is entirely specific for schizophrenic psychoses, as florid psychotic symptoms in mania and depression, as well as organic psychosyndromes, also respond to neuroleptic medication, though the preventive effect in other disorders has not been investigated to any great extent.

Various forms of neuroleptic compared

Davis and Garver (1978) evaluated the results from 134 double-blind comparisons between 21 different neuroleptics and chlorpromazine. No drug was superior to chlorpromazine in any trial. Mepazine, promazine, and phenobarbitone were consistently inferior except when chlorpromazine was used in insufficient dosage, usually below 400 mg per day. These comparisons taken with their earlier comprehensive review of double-blind studies of antipsychotic medication (Klein & Davis, 1969) and a review of 16 reports each involving more than 250 patients

(Hollister, 1974) lead to the conclusion that it is impossible to establish any consistent difference between the effectiveness of different antipsychotic drugs on specific schizophrenic symptoms or subgroups. There are differences in the number and severity of side-effects, however, as we shall see later.

When differences between drugs on individual symptoms are reported, they probably arise from the large number of statistical comparisons used in the analysis – in no case have such findings been consistently revalidated in subsequent studies. Nor has it been possible to identify a pattern of symptoms, signs, or demographic variables which can be used to predict the response of an individual patient to any given drug. Beliefs about differences between drugs, for example that chlorpromazine is better for excited, disoriented, or hostile patients and fluphenazine better for paranoid or thought-disordered ones, can be explained in terms of differences in their side-effects when drugs are compared at doses necessary to achieve equal antipsychotic effects.

In short, if given in the right dosage, neuroleptics are similar in their effect on psychotic symptoms. All the evidence points to the fact that they can control or affect the florid features of the disease, but not the chronic negative ones, and that they do not effect a cure.

Time course

There are important differences in the time course of the specific antipsychotic effects. The sedative action is immediate as soon as adequate blood levels are reached. Agitation and excitement which have been controlled by treatment can re-emerge quickly when medication is omitted. Though less potent and more hypnotic, barbiturates, paraldehyde, and high-dose benzodiazepines can often substitute for neuroleptics in this respect.

Comparisons of neuroleptics with placebo in recently admitted patients suggest that improvement in the first two to three weeks is a non-specific effect of treatment, because up to this time patients on placebo improve at nearly the same rate as those on neuroleptics. After two to three weeks, active medication shows a significantly better action on psychotic features (Davis & Garver, 1978; Johnstone *et al.*, 1978), generally reaching a plateau of maximum benefit over six to twelve weeks. Some patients run an erratic course, slowly improving over six months or more, but for such patients it is difficult to be sure that medication is a definite factor leading to further recovery, although it probably prevents deterioration.

Numerous well-controlled trials have confirmed the observation (Leff & Wing, 1971) that relapse can occur any time after discontinuing prophylaxis but about half can be expected to relapse within three to ten months, depending on the chronicity of the patients studied and whether they are in hospital or the community (Davis, 1965).

Potency

Some of the reported differences between treatments may be due to a failure to ensure that drugs are used in equivalent dosage. If the *effectiveness* of drugs is defined as their ability to achieve the desired antipsychotic effect, *potency* can be defined in terms of minimum amount of drug in milligrams required to achieve this. In terms of milligram dosage chlorpromazine and thioridazine are low in potency, that is, they require high dosage as compared with fluphenazine, haloperidol or pimozide.

The relative potency of some commercially used neuroleptics is shown in table 13.1 (after Davis, 1976a). Davis estimated each drug's mean clinical daily dose by averaging the doses compiled from all the double-blind comparisons of drugs with chlorpromazine which allowed for flexible adjustment of dosage to obtain an optimal clinical response. In some cases the relative potency was calculated indirectly from studies which compared a drug of unknown potency with one whose potency relative to chlorpromazine had been established. The mean dose of chlorpromazine determined by this method may be biased on the high side because prescribing was blind and studies of chronic patients were not separated from those of acute. However, the method is so far the best approximation available using clinical data to establish the *relative* potencies of different neuroleptics even if absolute dose levels are high. Other methods yield different results, particularly in regard to the relative potencies of the low-dose neuroleptics which may rank in a slightly different order and be one-half or one-third as potent in comparison with chlorpromazine as this table suggests.

It does not follow that because there are no consistent differences in group responses to drugs individual patients will not respond better to one than to another. Neuroleptics differ considerably in clinical structure, and one-hundred-fold differences in plasma concentrations have been observed between individuals taking equivalent doses of oral chlorpromazine, though plasma concentrations account for less than 10 per cent of the variation in clinical response (Lader, 1979). Variation in plasma concentration could

Table 13.1. *Relative potencies of neuroleptics compared to chlorpromazine set at 100*

Drug	Mean daily dose	dose (mg)	Range of clinical daily dose (mg)
Chlorpromazine	100	734	75–2000
Thioridazine	97 ± 7	712	75–800[a]
Thiothixane	4.4 ± 1	32	6–120
Trifluoperazine	2.8 ± 0.4	21	5–60
Haloperidol	1.6 ± 0.5	12	1.5–100
Fluphenazine	1.2 ± 0.1	9	1.5–120[b]

[a] Upper limit set to avoid retinal pigmentation.
[b] One study used 1200 mg/day (Quitkin *et al.*, 1975). (Based on Davis, 1976a.)

be due to differences in absorption, carrier state, metabolism, or excretion (Davis, 1976b). Recently Kulhanek and colleagues (1979) have reported that neuroleptics rapidly form insoluble complexes with coffee and tea. This may account for the wide variation in blood levels with oral medication and the fact that there is much less variation in blood-level when medication is given by the parenteral route. When excitement and agitation cannot be controlled after a few days, or psychotic thought content does not respond after three or more weeks, a change to a drug of a different chemical class or parenteral administration should be considered.

Relative effects of different drugs and their pharmacology

Pharmacology

The main effects of neuroleptics are due to competitive inhibition of adrenoceptors on postsynaptic neurons, thereby blocking the action of the neurotransmitter substance. Each neuroleptic has its own profile of effects on different neurotransmitter systems, thus explaining its sedative, antipsychotic, and extrapyramidal effects. Inhibition of α-noradrenergic transmission centrally is thought to account for sedation, and peripherally to account for hypotension. Inhibition of dopaminergic transmission in the mesolimbic system is thought to account for the antipsychotic action and in the nigro-striatal system to account for extrapyramidal side-effects. However, the effect on nigro-striatal dopaminergic systems, and therefore Parkinsonian side-effects, tend to be modified by any blocking of acetycholine transmission centrally (i.e. the anticholinergic effect) because dopaminergic and cholinergic systems balance each other.

Sedation and neuroleptic quotients

The differences between the clinical effect of drugs can usefully be considered in terms of their effects on different transmitter systems when given in doses necessary to control the florid symptoms of schizophrenia. Their effect on α-noradrenergic transmission may be weak or strong relative to their effect on dopamine transmission. A *sedation quotient* can be defined as the sedative effect of a drug when prescribed at doses necessary to control psychoses. As table 13.2 shows, chlorpromazine has a high sedation quotient when given at average doses. Haloperidol has a low sedation quotient. At clinically effective doses, say 500 mg, chlorpromazine has a strong anti-α-noradrenergic effect, while haloperidol at comparable doses (8–15 mg) is only weakly sedative in an excited patient. It has a low sedative quotient. Similarly a *neuroleptic quotient* can be defined as likelihood of extrapyramidal side-effects when the drug is given at clinically effective doses. This is a function of the anticholinergic potency of the drug. Haloperidol is weakly anticholinergic in the 8–15 mg (antipsychotic) dose range, but has as strong an antidopamine activity as chlorpromazine. As could be expected it has an equally strong antidopamine action in the nigro-striatal system and because it is weakly anticholinergic at this dose it has a strong tendency to cause Parkinsonism. Thus it has a high *neuroleptic quotient*.

The antipsychotic potency, sedation quotient, and neuroleptic quotient of different drugs given in table 13.2 are based on research reports and clinical impression. The differences between the effects of drugs are only relative to their antipsychotic effective dose. When given in very high doses, say ten times the usual clinical range, their effect on dopamine systems will have maximized because of saturation of the receptor sites. Extrapyramidal side-effects due to dopamine blockade will therefore not increase. They may even decrease, because drugs such as fluphenazine or haloperidol build up a stronger anticholinergic effect at higher doses. This explains the so-called 'paradoxical' decrease in severity of some side-effects when neuroleptics are given in very high dosage. It also explains the fact that, at very high dosage, fluphenazine and haloperidol have a sedative

Table 13.2. *Antipsychotic potency, sedation and neuroleptic quotients at average effective antipsychotic dosage*

Drug	Anti-psychotic potency	Sedation quotient	Neuro-leptic quotient
Chlorpromazine	low	++++	++
Thioridazine	low	+++	+
Trifluoperazine	high	++	+++
Fluphenazine	high	++	++++
Haloperidol	high	++	++++
Pimozide	high	+	+

action on psychotic agitation. The curvilinear dose-response relationship does not apply to toxic effects of drugs on the liver and heart which depend on other mechanisms.

Clinical use

Applications in psychiatric emergencies

The high-potency neuroleptics offer advantages in psychiatric emergencies when rapid and massive sedation is wanted. At very high doses their sedative action can be equal to large doses of chlorpromazine, but there are fewer problems with hypotension, excessive anticholinergic action, or excessive hypnotic effect, and there are no more extrapyramidal side-effects than would be observed on lower dosage (Ayd, 1978). Sedation begins about 30 minutes after oral haloperidol or fluphenazine administration and in 10 to 20 minutes after an intravenous injection. After the initial 10 or 20 mg intravenous or intramuscular dose 10 mg can be given every half hour until the desired calming effect is achieved. Large doses, up to 100 mg per day, of haloperidol have been used safely in post-heart-surgery patients with no effect on arterial pressure, pulse pressure, pulmonary atrial pressure, cardiac rhythm or respiratory rate or ECG. Haloperidol and other butyrophenones have no untoward effects on cardiac, hepatic, or ectodermal tissue, so it is a useful drug when treating the elderly or patients with other forms of physical illness.

Dose-response relationships

Our knowledge about dosage depends largely on clinical observation and further detailed studies are required. Toxicity limits the dose range for most drugs in medicine, but neuroleptics are remarkably

Table 13.3. *Antipsychotic effect of chlorpromazine*
(CPZ) at different doses in comparison with placebo

Mean dose mg/day	Number of studies showing CPZ	
	more effective	the same or slightly more effective
<300	11	15
301–400	4	4
401–500	4	1
501–800	14	0
>800	12	0
	45	20

(Based on Davis & Garver, 1978.)

safe over a wide therapeutic range – up to 1000 times
the minimal therapeutic dose. The comprehensive
reviews of controlled therapeutic trials by Davis and
his colleagues have contributed to our understanding
of dose-response relationships (Klein & Davis, 1969,
Davis & Garver, 1978). Table 13.3, which is based on
65 double-blind studies summarizes their findings.
While chlorpromazine was significantly more effective
than placebo in doses less than 300 mg in some studies, in the majority it was not. On the other hand,
every study using a mean dose of chlorpromazine
above 500 mg per day showed the drug to be superior
to placebo. Thus there is an increasing likelihood of
a good response as dosage increases from 300 to 600
mg per day.

Gardos, Cole and Orzack (1973) reviewed
twelve carefully controlled studies, seven dealing with
unspecified groups of chronic schizophrenics and five
limited to treatment of refractory cases. Prien and Cole
(1968) randomized 838 chronic schizophrenics to 2000
mg of chlorpromazine, 300 mg of chlorpromazine,
'current treatment' and placebo. The very high-dose
group did not improve more than the other active
treatment groups except for a subgroup consisting of
25 per cent of the sample who were under 40 and had
less than 10 years' treatment. The younger group
responded significantly better to high-dose treatment,
a finding that was replicated in one other study. The
remaining five studies did not show any advantage
of doses above 600 mg for unspecified groups of
chronic patients. However, of the studies limited to
treatment of refractory patients, in four out of five the

high-dose regime was significantly more effective
although the treatment was associated with more
side-effects. A small but notable minority did better
without any medication. These findings give support
for Davis's suggestion that the dose-response curve
is roughly sigmoidal in shape with an increasing
response between doses of 300 and 600 mg of chlorpromazine per day, or the equivalent, reaching a
gradual plateau between 600 and 2000 mg, doses
above 600 mg mainly being used for refractory cases.
Hollister (1978) points out that because of variable
absorption from the GI tract and metabolism during
passage through the liver (first pass effect) parenteral
administration can increase potency almost four-fold.
A consequence of this would be a much deeper dose
response gradient by the parental route, achieving a
maximal antipsychotic response at a lower dossage.

Mega-dose studies
Quitkin, Rifkin and Klein (1975) compared 1200
mg of oral fluphenazine-hydrochloride daily (equivalent to 100 000 mg of chlorpromazine; cf. table 13.1)
with 30 mg of fluphenazine (equivalent to 2,500 mg
chlorpromazine) in the treatment of refractory
patients. McClelland and colleagues (1976) compared
250 mg of depot fluphenazine with 12.5 mg intramuscularly per week over six months, and others have
compared 600 mg trifluoperazine (equivalent to 21 400
mg chlorpromazine) with 60 mg (Wijsenbeek *et al.*,
1974). None of these studies showed an advantage
for the mega-dose regime. Doses above 600 mg of
chlorpromazine give better response rates than lower
doses, but there is a diminishing return for doses
much higher than this. More data are needed on this
problem, especially in respect to speed of response
in acute studies. However, since medication is relatively safe in high doses for brief periods and trials
have only considered average effects between groups
it is advisable to try a treatment-resistant patient on
very high dosage.

Whom to treat
There are many reasons why patients should
be offered a period off treatment at all stages of
schizophrenia. Contrary to traditional views schizophrenics rarely show progressive deterioration after
five years (Bleuler, 1972) unless it is due to harmful
treatment or environmental influences (see chapter
9). There is no evidence that early treatment prevents
or minimizes deterioration. Up to 25 per cent of
unselected schizophrenic admissions to hospital show

a remission even without medication (Cole, Klerman & Goldberg, 1964).

While spontaneous remission is more likely to occur among the group traditionally recognized as having a good prognosis – first illness, acute florid onset, good previous personality etc. – it is not possible to identify patients who will spontaneously recover unless they are first tried without medication. Moreover, patients improve at similar rates during the first two to three weeks after admission, whether on active medication or placebo; after that period those on drugs do better. Once treatment has begun the patient is likely to remain on it for months even after discharge. Therefore, there is much to support the practice of having a period of unhurried observation before starting medication, in order to make an accurate diagnosis to identify patients who will remit spontaneously and spare a sizeable number of patients the disadvantage of side-effects and unnecessary medication. However, the advantages of such an approach are often counterbalanced by practical considerations in the treatment setting and the pressures for rapid management and discharge.

This rule applies equally to chronic patients stabilized in an unstressful environment. While some chronic patients require neuroleptics for sedation, and others need them to control or prevent the emergence of florid symptoms, a sizeable proportion of chronic patients – 30 per cent to 70 per cent – are unchanged in the short run when medication is withdrawn (Prien & Klett, 1972). Given the risk of developing tardive dyskinesia and the fact that treatment can be rapidly restarted in patients under observation, consideration should be given to a period off treatment in most chronic cases. A proportion even of the very disordered will actually improve – probably due to withdrawal of side effects such as akinesia. The quality of the social and psychological environment should be carefully considered before deciding on drug withdrawal (see chapter 9).

Maintenance treatment

The prophylactic action of neuroleptics in preventing the recurrence or recrudescence of schizophrenic symptoms has now been well established in 24 double-blind trials dealing with chronic in-patients and out-patients (Davis, 1975). Only one study reported a relapse rate as high as 34 per cent with active medication, but the relapse rate on placebo was generally more than 55 per cent. Summing across studies, 65 per cent of 1068 patients on placebo relapsed compared with 30 per cent of 2127 patients on medication. A powerful prophylactic effect has been demonstrated for out-patients maintained on long-acting *depot injections* (Hirsch et al., 1973). Though the value of oral medication had been confirmed earlier (Leff & Wing, 1971) a strongly-held view has developed among clinicians, especially in Britain, that depot injections are more successful in preventing relapse. The development of special clinics and district psychiatric nurses for administering injections has improved patient care and follow-up, but the route of administration does not prove to be a critical factor when treatments are compared under similar conditions. Large controlled studies comparing oral neuroleptics such as penfluridol (Quitkin et al., 1978) or oral fluphenazine (Rifkin et al., 1977) with depot fluphenazine decanoate injections found relapse rates below 10 per cent over one year for both oral and depot medication. About 65 per cent of patients relapsed on placebo. In another study the difference between those treated with pimozide tablets and fluphenazine injections was not significant (Falloon, Watt & Shepherd, 1978). In practice one is likely to achieve better results with long-acting depot injections because many patients are unreliable when left to administer their own medication and the close nursing supervision associated with depot injection clinics assures regular contact with services. The problems associated with poor compliance with follow-up may not be reflected in clinical trials, in which patients are highly selected and more closely observed.

Side-effects on maintenance treatment

As with oral medication, the claim that depot neuroleptics differ in their specific actions has not stood up to scrutiny. Knights and colleagues (1979) were unable to find any differences in the response or outcome of 57 schizophrenic patients randomly assigned to fluphenazine and flupenthixol and followed for six months after leaving hospital. Of those completing the trial 7 per cent relapsed, 53 per cent experienced depressive symptoms and 89 per cent experienced extrapyramidal side-effects (EPSEs) at some time, but only a smaller number were affected at any one time. This study emphasizes the high frequency of EPSEs during the first six months of treatment with depot neuroleptics. Frequent expert assessment by specially trained community psychiatric nurses is required. One patient working with hot molten iron fortunately realized that he needed to take a few days off work after each injection because of shaking in his hands, which lasted only a few days.

When they occur, extrapyramidal symptoms can be abated by reducing the dose or increasing the frequency of injections using smaller doses. Anticholinergic medication is rapidly effective but the necessity for long-term administration after control of the acute symptoms has been called into question (Johnson, 1978; Mindham, 1976). At any point in time about 20 per cent of patients on depot maintenance neuroleptic treatment will have Parkinsonian symptoms, but there is a constant interchange between those affected and those not. In one study only 4 per cent of patients showed an increase of Parkinsonian symptoms after discontinuing anticholinergic medication (McClelland, 1976). Thus, patients may not require anti-Parkinsonian medication on a prolonged basis. At the same time, prolonged use may increase the dose requirement of antipsychotic treatment as a result of enzyme induction and more rapid metabolism of neuroleptics (Lader, 1979). They may cause discomforting and, rarely, life-threatening anticholinergic side-effects, such as paralytic ileus and, in high doses, cerebral toxicity and delirium. They may also increase the risk of tardive dyskinesia. The general conclusion can be drawn that anti-Parkinsonian medication has a definite value when quick relief of side-effects is necessary but prolonged use after 6–12 weeks is generally not warranted.

Discontinuing maintenance treatment

Maintenance treatment can be withdrawn from many in-patients or out-patients for some months without adverse effects (Hirsch *et al.*, 1973; Hogarty & Ulrich, 1977; Letemendia & Harris, 1967). After withdrawal, relapses accumulate with time at a rate which decreases exponentially.

The longer the patient has survived withdrawal from treatment without relapse the more the risk declines. In the first month, the risk of relapsing on placebo or drug was 13 per cent and 4 per cent respectively; by month 24 the probability had declined to 3 per cent and 1.5 per cent. This is probably due to the fact that those most at risk relapse first.

Hogarty and Ulrich have used life-table methods to calculate long-term survival without relapse rates for 374 patients treated with oral chlorpromazine or placebo. Extrapolating their results beyond three years they estimated that eventually 65 per cent of patients on medication and 87 per cent on placebo would relapse. Thus 13 per cent of patients did not need treatment and in 22 per cent medication could indefinitely prevent relapse, while in the remaining 65 per cent relapse was only postponed. They might have achieved a stronger treatment effect with depot injection instead of oral maintenance treatment. In any case the eventual relapse rate does not reflect the large reduction in frequency and severity of relapse observed in patients on maintenance treatment (Denham & Adamson, 1971).

These figures demonstrate the continuing benefit to patients of maintenance medication compared with placebo, but they do not answer a more practical question: What is the likelihood of relapse if medication is withdrawn after several years treatment? Two groups report relapse rates of about 65 per cent for patients withdrawn from treatment after surviving two or three years on medication (Hogarty *et al.*, 1976; Johnson, 1976). The survival rate was only marginally improved (about 7 per cent) by social therapy (Hogarty *et al.*, 1976). If medication is withdrawn during the first year after discharge the relapse rate is particularly high (Hirsch *et al.*, 1973). More research is necessary, but the indications from such studies suggest that patients who have been well controlled on maintenance medication continue to have a high risk of relapse if withdrawn from treatment, even after several years. The possibility that long-term maintenance medication creates dependence on drug treatment in the sense that it increases the risk of relapse if treatment is withdrawn provides an alternative interpretation of these studies and has not been investigated.

Disadvantages of long-term treatment include Parkinsonian side-effects, tardive dyskinesia, and a subtle extrapyramidal symptom, akinesia, which alters the patient's social performance and causes symptoms suggesting distress and depression. (Rifkin *et al.*, 1975). In an effort to reduce the use of medication two alternatives to complete withdrawal were examined in large in-patient trials, reducing the amount and frequency of dosage. Caffey and colleagues (1964) randomized patients to three groups: daily treatment; treatment Monday, Wednesday, and Friday, (i.e. 43 per cent of original dose); and placebo. Within four months the relapse rates were 5 per cent, 16 per cent and 45 per cent respectively. Prien and colleagues (1973) compared daily treatment to treatment 3, 4 and 5 times a week. After four months the relapse rate was 1 per cent and 6–8 per cent respectively, the dose reductions being 19–43 per cent. It is clear that dose reduction in this manner carries less risk of relapse than completely discontinuing treatment, but more risk than full treatment. The risks and benefits of treatment must be assessed for each individual patient but particular attention should be paid to patients in older age groups who are more at risk to develop tardive dyskinesia.

Relative contribution of experimental factors, drug treatment, and psychosocial therapy

The effect of antipsychotic medication on acute and chronic symptoms and on relapse rates is lower than psychiatrists generally appreciate. Davis (1976a) calculated from two large acute treatment placebo studies that the use of active medication versus placebo correlated reasonably well with improvement or deterioration ($r_p = 0.60$). However, this means that drugs explain only 36 per cent of the variance between patients who improve or not. Vaughn and Leff (1976) report correlations or $r_p = 0.39$ between continuation on maintenance medication or not, and relapse or not, explaining only 15 per cent of the variance. The interaction between medication and the important influence of environmental factors is considered in chapter 9.

Other forms of medication

Antidepressants in schizophrenia

Depressive symptoms are very common at all stages of schizophrenia. In the International Pilot Study of Schizophrenia sponsored by the World Health Organization, depressive syndromes were almost as common in the acute schizophrenic attack as they were in acute depressive psychoses or neuroses (WHO, 1973, p. 294). However, depression is less evident than the florid psychotic features and usually remains unnoticed until the latter have settled. It has been explained as a psychological reaction of the patient to his condition, as a pharmacological sequel of neuroleptic treatment, and more recently, as an extrapyramidal side-effect – akinesia (Rifkin, Quitkin & Klein, 1975). Knights and her colleagues (1979) found that 53 per cent of 37 patients closely followed for six months after discharge from hospital had depression at some time during that period, but symptoms improved whether or not patients received antidepressants. In an unpublished study of a year's admissions from a defined catchment area we observed that depressive symptoms were more common during the florid stages of the illness than after discharge; their prevalence and severity decreased

following neuroleptic treatment for florid schizophrenia. Bowers and Astrachan (1967) also noticed a high frequency of depressive symptoms in the acute phase of schizophrenia – furthermore, depressive symptoms present on admission did not improve in patients given imipramine or ECT.

Antidepressants have been combined with neuroleptics to treat chronically inactive, apathetic and withdrawn patients, but most studies do not identify what proportion of the sample were affected by depression. Collins and Dundas (1967) found a significant improvement in all syndromes in 58 per cent of 58 chronic schizophrenics given perphenazine after a two-week interval without medication, as compared with 29 per cent of patients given placebo. Half the perphenazine-treated group also had amitriptyline; they showed significant improvement in flatness of affect and other subscores on the Wing scale but did not improve significantly more than patients given perphenazine by itself. Casey and colleagues (1961) did not find that combining imipramine, isocarboxozid, or trifluoperazine with chlorpromazine gave additional benefit to chronic schizophrenics, and amphetamines made some patients worse. Thus the value of tricyclics for withdrawn chronic patients as such is slight or non-existent.

There are remarkably few studies limited to depressed schizophrenics. In chronic patients it is difficult to differentiate between flatness of affect, apathy, and withdrawal on the one hand and symptoms of depression on the other. Because of improved social milieu and stimulation, patients must appear to respond to the drug when in fact they are only responding to nonspecific aspects of being treated. An approach to the diagnostic problem was found by Prusoff and colleagues (1979) who studied 35 ambulatory schizophrenics who had developed depressive symptoms. The findings suggest that depressive symptoms responded better in the group given amitriptyline plus perphenazine, but 75 per cent of those receiving combined treatment had an increase in blood-pressure and body-weight. Brockington's (1978b) study of 'schizo-depressives' suggested that chlorpromazine alone was as good as or better than combined treatment with amitriptyline. To complicate matters, Butterworth (1962) showed that extrapyramidal symptoms of 30 institutionalized patients improved significantly in 80 per cent of patients when imipramine was added. Patients with severe signs of Parkinsonism got worse. Such results emphasize the importance of distinguishing akinesia from true depression and show the risk of attempting diagnosis on the basis of specific response to treatment.

There are serious methodological problems in distinguishing between depression, akinesia, and the effects of institutionalism in chronic patients. Studies which separate these features and distinguish between specific and non-specific effects of treatment have not been carried out. In the meantime, good clinical practice will involve a trial and error approach to individual patients who have depressive symptoms, using one antidepressant at a time for a sufficient period to evaluate the effect of each.

Lithium for schizophrenic and schizo-affective psychosis

Analogous methodological difficulties concerning the value of lithium for schizophrenia or for schizo-affective disorders render any conclusion about their value premature. The effectiveness of lithium in schizophrenia has not been tested with adequate controls or sufficiently large samples, and any beneficial effect raises the question whether the sample included misdiagnosed atypical manic-depressives (Prien, 1979). Brockington and colleagues (1978a) suggested that chlorpromazine is more effective in the treatment of 'depressed schizo-affectives', while lithium is as good for 'manic schizo-affectives' if they are not grossly excited. However, the numbers in their study are small. In the absence of adequate studies it may be worthwhile adding lithium to the treatment regime on a trial and error basis when mood disorder is a disturbing and persisting feature.

Other physical treatments
Electroconvulsive treatment

Similar problems to those experienced in assessing the role of antidepressants beset an assessment of the use of ECT in schizophrenia or catatonic symptoms in association with schizophrenia. There is no doubt of the value of ECT in aborting catatonic stupor or excitement or bringing under control hypomanic excitement in schizo-affective patients. Treatment can be given daily or even twice daily in extreme cases where control of excitement presents an urgent problem. Amelioration of symptoms is usually seen after three or four treatments, if not sooner. Treatment gains should then be consolidated by the use of phenothiazines which are often given with ECT. Kalinowsky, Lothar and Hippius (1969) state that relapse rapidly follows if ECT is given alone unless followed

by further shocks, totalling 10 to 20 at decreasing intervals. Others who have reviewed the subject state that ECT has been undervalued in schizophrenia because it is incapable by itself of leading to sustained improvement (Weinstein & Fisher, 1971). Turek (1973) reviewed 12 studies, albeit mostly uncontrolled and methodologically unsound, although they included large numbers of patients. They suggest that, in combination with antipsychotic medication, ECT speeds the course of recovery in the early stages of treatment and lowers the patient's dose requirement for medication. Most of the more carefully controlled studies support this (Childers, 1961; Smith et al., 1967). Smith and colleagues (1967) randomly allocated 54 acute schizophrenics to ECT plus chlorpromazine (mean dose, 400 mg) or chlorpromazine only (mean dose, 655 mg). Although there was no important difference at the six-week and six-month follow-up on the IMPS and ward behaviour rating scales, the group receiving combined treatment improved more rapidly in a number of symptom areas and was discharged significantly earlier.

May and Tuma (1965) compared ECT alone with drugs, and controls with and without psychotherapy in acute schizophrenics with middle prognosis (worst and best prognosis excluded). The outcome for patients treated with ECT alone was intermediate between that of patients treated with drugs and that of patients given no physical treatment, though ECT by itself was not significantly better than controls. The main treatment effect was due to medication; the effect of drugs combined with ECT was not tested. Other authors have carried out well-controlled comparisons between ECT alone and conventional medication and have found that over a four- to eight-week period ECT was equal to but not better than phenothiazines given in adequate doses. Thus the weight of the evidence supports the view that, while ECT may offer the advantage of a more rapid recovery in the first few weeks when combined with medication, there is no advantage over neuroleptic medication after two or more months.

There are particular problems in assessing the role of ECT in schizophrenia. First, patients who respond best in many studies have affective symptoms. Given the widespread use in the USA in the past of ill-defined diagnostic criteria for schizophrenia and catatonia, many patients in earlier studies may have been suffering from a misdiagnosed affective illness. Second, patients who respond best are said to be those who have had an acute onset and are being treated in the first year of illness (Abrams & Taylor, 1977). But these are the patients who are most likely to have a spontaneous recovery and to have the most favourable long-term prognosis regardless of treatment. However, there is general clinical agreement.

A separate question is whether ECT is of therapeutic value in the absence of affective and catatonic symptoms. This question has not been adequately investigated in acute patients. The limited evidence available for *chronic* non-depressed schizophrenics shows that ECT is no better than anaesthesia without ECT (Brill *et al.*, 1959; Miller *et al.*, 1953).

Chemically induced convulsive treatment

Von Meduna introduced convulsive treatment for schizophrenic patients in 1934. He used camphor oil injected intramuscularly but soon changed to a soluble synthetic camphor preparation (pentylenetetranyl or Metrazole). Since 1957 the most popular chemical convulsive agent has been hexafluorodiethyl (fluethyl). It can be given intravenously but causes sclerosis of veins – inhalation is therefore the usual route of administration. The details of technique are summarized by Kalinowsky, Lotha and Hippius (1969) and the research on its clinical value is well reviewed by Small and Small (1972). Many studies including a double-blind evaluation in 100 patients, suggest that it is clinically as effective as ECT but no more. The evidence suggests that the essential therapeutic factor is whether seizures have been induced – a fact which is relevant to the issue whether the key factor in ECT is electricity or seizures. Disadvantages of fluethyl include difficulty of administration, occasional multiple seizures, plus other side-affects equivalent to ECT, except possibly fewer effects on memory. Its main advantage is as an alternative to ECT when there is a need to avoid electrical induction of seizures. Against occasional use of this sort is the fact that most psychiatrists today are unfamiliar with the technical aspects of its use.

Insulin coma treatment

This treatment, which has a reported mortality of 0.5 per cent, is mentioned for historical interest as it was the first biological treatment of importance to be used in schizophrenia. Experimenting with insulin subcoma in various psychiatric patients, Manfred Sakel noticed that some schizophrenics who developed coma as an unintended complication came out of it remarkably improved. He reported it as a treat-

ment for schizophrenia in 1933 and it rapidly became established, joined by ECT as the main treatment for schizophrenia until the advent of phenothiazines. The method is well reviewed by Kalinowsky Lothar and Hippius (1969). Although a respectable number of series have reported positive results, there are few controlled trials. Fink and colleagues (1958) randomly allocated patients to 50 insulin coma treatments or to chlorpromazine, 300–2000 mg per day, and found no difference in outcome on weekly observation over four months following completion of treatment.

Ackner, Harris and Oldham (1957, 1972) also failed to find a difference between insulin coma and barbiturate coma followed by amphetamines in a double-blind trial. These studies were limited in scope and cannot be regarded as decisive, but because the treatment is difficult, dangerous, uneconomic and has nothing to offer over standard chemotherapy, it has largely disappeared from use even in centres where it had the greatest support.

Psychosurgery

The problems of conducting controlled trials are most evident in relation to surgical techniques. There are no adequately controlled or randomized studies of psychosurgery for schizophrenia. Stengel (1950) reported that hallucinations were unchanged in 75 per cent of 154 cases and delusions undiminished in 72 per cent of 160 cases following leucotomy. The use of psychosurgery fell dramatically following the introduction of phenothiazines. General clinical opinion is that anxiety, tension, agitation, and depression form the main indications regardless of the underlying condition. Centres which specialize in psychosurgery do not regard schizophrenia as an indication but a few patients whose symptoms are very distressing and unresponsive to all other means of treatment are considered.

Special and experimental treatments

During the past ten years various treatments have been advocated and studies carried out using penicillamine, mega-vitamins, levo-dopa, serotonin precursors, nalorphine, thyrotropin releasing factor, and GABA, without impressive success. More recently renal dialysis, propranolol, and various endorphin molecules have been reported to have antipsychotic effects. None of these treatments has been sufficiently well examined in controlled trials to merit further comment. Their appearance reflects an understanding by psychiatrists that current treatments can ameliorate and control symptoms but not cure the disease. While we should be critical of premature enthusiastic advocation of new therapies, progress will depend on the willingness of clinicians, with due regard for safety, to give new treatments proper trial.

Side-effects of antipsychotic medication

A discussion of treatment is incomplete without mentioning side-effects. This is more so in psychiatry because, given that there are no differences between the antipsychotic effects of neuroleptics, indications for the use of a particular drug should be based on a knowledge of its other effects, wanted and unwanted.

Many side-effects are common and a few are serious but, over all, the wide difference between the therapeutic and the toxic doses of most neuroleptics places them among the safest groups of drugs used in acute medicine. Nevertheless side-effects can be psychologically distressing, physically painful, and rarely disabling or fatal. If detected early, most are reversible. It follows that the practitioner should be thoroughly familiar with their manifestations and management.

Unwanted neurological effects

Neurological side-effects can be classified by the system affected and by the time they develop after initiating treatment. The most common neurological symptoms are extrapyramidal.

Acute dyskinesia and dystonia

These are the most psychologically and physically distressing of the common side-effects. They generally occur within the first week of treatment and more frequently with potent low-dose neuroleptics such as trifluoperazine and haloperidol. One theory is that they are due to an initial compensatory overproduction of dopamine neurotransmitter in the nigrostriatum. Dramatic tonic contractions of the neck, mouth, tongue and postural muscles occur and may persist for hours or days if untreated. Opisthotonos, oculogyric crisis, torticollis, and involuntary movements of the tongue, face and neck may occur. Untrained doctors misdiagnose catatonia, hysteria, tetany or epileptic seizures and may wrongly give additional neuroleptics rather than decrease the dose. These side-effects rapidly respond to anticholinergic medication, which should be administered parenter-

ally at first; e.g. 10 mg of procyclidine or biperiden intravenously will abruptly terminate symptoms.

Parkinsonism

Drug-induced extrapyramidal side-effects including Parkinsonism are especially common in the first six months of treatment, but may appear at any time. Tolerance to the neuroleptic effects of medication develops with time and symptoms tend to come and go. The two most frequent manifestations of drug-induced Parkinsonism are akathisia and bradykinesis. Akathisia appears as motor restlessness, fidgeting, and a subjective need to pace; rocking movements may be a feature or be part of the underlying schizophrenia. It can be confused with anxiety and agitation, but the correct treatment is to reduce medication or to use anti-Parkinsonian medication. Bradykinesis or akinesia is treated in the same way but with less success. The syndrome is characterized by a reduction of the range, speed, and frequency of voluntary movements, including stillness of the face and staring. This can be a severe social handicap for patients because it gives them an odd and peculiar appearance. Festinating gait may be a feature. Klein and Davis (1969) were the first to identify a depressive akinetic syndrome which arises in conjunction with drug-induced Parkinsonism, including lack of drive, sadness, inactivity, and apathy. It has been said that the syndrome can be diagnosed rapidly by an immediate response to an intravenous injection of anticholinergic medication. Tremor, stiffness, and cogwheel rigidity are common; stooped posture, drolling, and other symptoms of Parkinsonism are uncommon. One should, of course, guard against overlooking a case of true Parkinson's disease, especially in the older population, in which case dopamine replacement with levo-Dopa or amantadine may be called for.

Tardive dyskinesia

This is the most serious and potentially disabling unwanted effect of treatment because it is irreversible in the majority of cases if not detected early. The commonest early signs are sucking, chewing, smacking, and lip-pursing movements and other signs of the bucco-linguo-masticatory syndrome, including protrusion of the tongue into the cheek in a darting 'fly-catching' manner, puffing of the cheeks, grimacing, and lateral movements of the tongue and jaw. The hands and fingers are frequently affected, as evidenced by complex, irregular movements. Choreo-athetoid jerking movements of the arms, legs, and feet occur, as well as flexor and extensor contractions of the neck and back and contractions of the respiratory musculature. Dysarthria, difficulty in swallowing, dyspnoea, and cyanosis may be late consequences. A striking and unexplained feature is the patient's lack of concern and apparent obliviousness of the disorder despite gross gyrations which cause marked social disability.

The relationship of tardive dyskinesia to dose and length of medication and other factors has been distorted by early reports intent on proving the existence of the disorder. These focused on large surveys of chronic hospitalized patients. Of 22 large-scale surveys, 14 showed a prevalence rate of about 10 per cent (Crane, 1978). More recently larval signs of tardive dyskinesia have been detected in as many as 43 per cent of 69 out-patients on neuroleptics for more than three months (Asni *et al.*, 1977). The symptoms are reversible if neuroleptics are reduced or withdrawn at an early stage, though improvement can take up to 16 weeks (Quitkin *et al.*, 1977). Crane states that the syndrome can be found among the elderly who have never had neuroleptics and that the prevalance increases markedly over the age of 55 among patients on neuroleptics. It can, however, occur at any age, even in children. An association with pre-existing brain damage has now been confirmed in seven or eight investigations reviewed (Crane, 1978). Though it is significantly more common in patients who have received more than 200 mg per day of chlorpromazine or its equivalent, and in younger age groups, patients who have had more than 1000 mg per day account only for 10 per cent of the variance.

Pathophysiology of extrapyramidal side-effects

Parkinsonism in general is attributed to an imbalance between cholinergic and dopaminergic systems in the basal ganglia with a relative excess of cholinergic over dopaminergic activity. In Parkinson's disease this is thought to arise from a deficiency of dopaminergic pre-synaptic neuron activity which can be ameliorated by giving supplementary levo-dopa or blocking cholinergic activity by giving centrally acting anticholinergics to restore the balance. In drug-induced Parkinsonism neuroleptics have blocked the dopamine neuroceptors so levo-dopa is relatively ineffective, but anticholinergics still work.

Tardive dyskinesia is thought to be due to an imbalance affecting a different part of the nigro-striatal system, because Parkinsonism may be present at the same time. Klawans has postulated that dopamine sensitivity, perhaps in the form of an increase in dopamine receptors, occurs as a compensatory mechanism in response to dopamine receptor blockade; hence the gradual tolerance which develops to Parkinsonian side-effects. Overcompensation leads to dopamine hypersensitivity relative to cholinergic activity and over-activity of post-synaptic neurons in part of the nigro-striatum. This explains why: (1) Parkinsonism precedes tardive dyskinesia: because dopamine blockade predominates at first; (2) anticholinergics are ineffective or exacerbate tardive dyskinesia: because they increase the dominance of dopaminergic activity over cholinergic; (3) tardive dyskinesia may be revealed or exacerbated when neuroleptics are stopped: because this allows dopaminergic function to increase when receptors have become more sensitive. It also explains the paradoxical observation that, in the short run, increasing the dose of neuroleptics decreases the dyskinesia. In fact, this is the only proven method of decreasing the severity of symptoms.

Every effort should be made to reduce neuroleptic medication if incipient signs of tardive dyskinesia appear. Drug 'holidays' have been advocated as a means of prevention, but their efficacy is unknown.

Other effects on the central nervous system

Most antipsychotic compounds are thought to decrease the epileptic threshold and they may induce epileptic convulsions in high dosage, but this is rare. Combinations with other drugs such as tricyclics or lithium could increase the risk of fits. Diazepam should provide rapid relief as an anticonvulsant; phenytoin can be used if necessary in conjunction with neuroleptics for longer-term use. The low-potency neuroleptics are more likely to cause convulsions at dose levels in the normal therapeutic range.

Sedation may be a problem, more so with the low-potency drugs. This is discussed with therapeutic effects above.

Toxic confusional states may occur at high dosage, but this is more likely with combined therapy as the anticholinergic activity of neuroleptics and anti-Parkinsonian drugs are additive. Loss of temperature control and hypothermia may result from chlorpromazine; other drugs less so. This could be dangerous for the elderly living in poorly heated conditions.

The anti-emetic effects of neuroleptics may be of value and can be mentioned here because they are believed to act on the chemoreceptor sensitive area of the brain stem which triggers vomiting.

Autonomic side-effects

At doses necessary to achieve equal antipsychotic effects, autonomic side-effects are more common in low-potency than high-potency antipsychotics. The anticholinergic effect of neuroleptics acts peripherally to cause such side-effects as blurred vision, dry mouth, difficulty in urinating, ejaculatory incompetence, constipation, and, rarely, paralytic ileus, which can be fatal.

The peripheral sympatholytic effects (due to α-adrenergic receptor blockade) of chlorpromazine and thioridazine, in combination with their anticholinergic effects, cause orthostatic hypotension and can lead to acute hypotensive crisis in the elderly. Autonomic side-effects are not uncommon with low-potency neuroleptics and are unlikely with the high-potency group, unless these are used in a very high dosage. Susceptibility is higher in the elderly and in patients with a specific vulnerability such as elderly males with prostatic hypertrophy who would be susceptible to urinary retention.

Metabolic and endocrine side-effects

Weight gain, increased appetite and decreased activity are common with prolonged use. Impairment of glucose tolerance and insulin release (chlorpromazine) have been described.

Galactorrhoea often accompanied by amenorrhoea is a frequent complaint of women given long-term treatment with low-potency neuroleptics. It is thought to be due to increased levels of circulating prolactin which is under the inhibitory control of dopamine neurons. Loss of libido is frequently reported in men and decreased growth hormone has been observed in children, as well as adults with chlorpromazine and haloperidol even with low doses.

Idiosyncratic, allergic, and toxic effects including those on the myocardium

Cholestatic jaundice which was commonly reported in the 1950s, usually in the first five weeks of treatment with chlorpromazine, is now rare. There is no established connection with high-potency neu-

roleptics. Agranulocytosis is also an early complication, but is extremely rare; nevertheless, it should always be considered in appropriate cases, since positive lupus erythematosis cells have been seen with chlorpromazine though not systemic lupus erythematosis.

A more serious problem is a toxic effect on the myocardium, which is most common with thioridazine in high doses. Abnormal tremor, prolonged ventricular repolarization, and ventricular tachycardia have been reported. Overdose with thioridazine is said to be frequently fatal, but unexplained sudden death has been reported with neuroleptics and probably results from their effect on the myocardium (Hollister, 1978).

Skin and eye lesions

Early in treatment a wide variety of skin eruptions can be seen and are of little consequence. A photosensitivity (sunburn) reaction commonly occurs with chlorpromazine but not with the high-potency neuroleptics in normal dosage or with the butyrophenones. Sun screens or avoidance of sunlight are prophylactic measures.

Blue-grey metabolic discolorations due to pigmentary granules which occur in areas of skin exposed to sunlight occur in patients having prolonged treatment and are more prominent when patients receive high doses. Similar deposits have been found in the viscera. More important are the granular deposits which occur in the anterior lens and posterior cornea seen on slit lamp examination. There is a statistical association between skin and lens changes, related to duration and total dose of treatment. Davis states that the majority have taken 1–3 kg of phenothiazine and he reports prevalence rates between 1 per cent and 30 per cent in state hospitals (Klein & Davis, 1969).

Treatment with thioridazine in doses over 800 mg is said to cause retinitis pigmentosa with substantial visual impairment or blindness which is irreversible but these serious complications have not been reported with other drugs.

Hollister (1978) reports that adults have survived single doses of chlorpromazine of 9.75 g and a one-year-old child survived 1.08 g. Severe overdose leads to central nervous system irritation and depression, coma, convulsions, slow low-voltage EEG, hypothermia, respiratory failure, shock, and cardiac arrest. Treatment consists of physostigmine as an antidote for anticholinergic effects, norepinephrine to counteract hypotension due to α-adrenergic blockade, diazepam for convulsion, and warmth for hypothermia.

Side-effects not related to dopaminergic blockade are more common in low-potency drugs where the milligramme dose is high and are rare in the potent low-dose group. Thioridazine which recommends itself because good sedation can be achieved without many extrapyramidal side-effects paradoxically carries the greatest risk of serious side-effects. Its use should therefore be limited to acute treatment under close supervision.

14

Rehabilitation and management of schizophrenia

J. K. WING

General principles

The general principles of psychiatric rehabilitation have been expounded in a recent publication from the Royal College of Psychiatrists (1981) which begins with the concept of 'social disablement'. This is the state of individuals who are unable to perform up to the standards expected by themselves, by people important to them, or by society in general. (Those who *choose* not to do so are not, of course, covered by the definition.) Three main types of cause – psychiatric symptoms or impairments, social disadvantages, and personal reactions to impairment or disadvantage – have been considered, in relation to the course of schizophrenia, in chapter 9. In this chapter, we shall be concerned with 'rehabilitation and management', i.e. with identifying and preventing or minimizing (over as long a period of time as necessary) the causal factors while, at the same time, helping the individual to develop and use his or her talents, and thus to acquire confidence and self-esteem through success in social roles. This general goal should not be translated into simple criteria, such as discharge from hospital or the attainment of full-time employment, which are then applied inflexibly whatever the disabilities and disadvantages of the patient. If the highest level attainable is a permanent settlement in a sheltered environment, achieving and maintaining this level is sign of success for that patient and not of failure.

The document sponsored by the Royal College

of Psychiatrists deals with the problems of formulating and updating a rehabilitation plan for each individual, and of trying to put it into practice. The headings used are: assessment, methods of rehabilitation and counselling, occupation and day environments, residential care, staff and training, and administration and coordination. General principles of rehabilitation are also considered in a forthcoming book by Bennett and Watts. This chapter will deal with the problems particularly likely to arise during the course of schizophrenia and with the achievement of 'the best level possible' in each individual case.

Prevention of clinical impairment

The work discussed in section 1 of this book does not suggest any effective means of primary prevention of schizophrenia. Measures taken to reduce physical abnormalities occurring during pregnancy and infancy may decrease vulnerability to some extent as will the avoidance of known precipitants such as amphetamine. There is no firm evidence that any particular kind of parental management during infancy or childhood will decrease the risk of schizophrenia developing later.

Social and psychological problems precipitating the onset of acute episodes can occasionally be prevented. Three kinds of factor were discussed in chapter 9. In the first place, it is important to be aware of possible iatrogenic factors. Florid symptoms can be reactivated when a patient is put under too much pressure in a rehabilitation unit, or in group therapy, or is discharged prematurely (Goldberg *et al.*, 1977; Stevens, 1973; Stone & Eldred, 1959; Wing, Bennett & Denham, 1964). Judging how much pressure to apply, particularly when a patient is reluctant to attempt to achieve a higher level of performance, is a skill that can only be acquired in clinical practice, since individuals vary a great deal, not only in degree of impairment but in personal reaction to it.

The second kind of precipitating factor consists of events in 'personal space' – including loss, separation, threat, or increased responsibility – that are experienced as disturbing by the patient. Most of these are everyday occurrences that are not preventable under ordinary circumstances of living. Most people experience them from time to time without having a severe or prolonged reaction but schizophrenic patients seem particularly sensitive. In a protected environment, such as a sheltered community, such events are less likely to occur and if they

do, may be less distressing because of the greater detachment from everyday life that institutionalism entails. The term 'asylum' or 'refuge' carries a connotation of escape from common stresses. Such relief may be helpful not only to people who need prolonged shelter but as a temporary measure. Part of the value of an admission to hospital is that it entails a period of 'retreat'; indeed, this is sometimes all that is required for recovery.

The third kind of factor arises from intrusive personal relationships, usually within a family setting. A degree of social withdrawal may then be protective to the patient by decreasing the amount of face-to-face contact and thus the exposure to overemotional or hostile interactions. Patients who go to work or who attend a day centre automatically spend less time at home. Some patients adopt apparently abnormal methods of reducing contact – walking the streets on their own, reading newspapers in public libraries, or even reversing the usual diurnal cycle by sleeping during the day and getting up when their relatives have gone to bed. Some patients learn for themselves that getting into arguments about sensitive topics, or entering into too emotional relationships with the opposite sex, brings back unpleasant symptoms (Wing, 1975).

Taking phenothiazine medication tends to reduce the risk of relapse when environmental circumstances are unfavourable and, conversely, it is less necessary when they are propitious (Brown, Birley & Wing, 1972; Vaughn & Leff, 1976).

Acute schizophrenic episodes tend to be associated with symptoms lower in the diagnostic hierarchy, such as depression, anxiety, worrying, muscular tension, and irritability. Such symptoms often occur by themselves in reaction to the difficulties and frustrations which all disabled people experience. It is just as much a mistake to assume that all psychiatric symptoms that occur in a patient who has experienced attacks of schizophrenia are part of 'schizophrenia' as it would be in chronically handicapping conditions such as multiple sclerosis or Parkinsonism.

The implications of these observations for long-term management and, in particular, for counselling the patient and family, will be considered later in the chapter. First it is necessary to consider the other type of clinical problem that commonly arises – the development of chronic affective and cognitive impairment. We have seen (chapter 7) that 'deterioration', in the sense of deficit relentlessly increasing with time, is not a common feature in schizophrenia. Nevertheless, social withdrawal and its concomitants (slowness, underactivity, lowered motivation, emotional flattening, self-neglect and poverty of verbal and non-verbal communication) commonly occur in some degree and may be severe.

This 'clinical poverty syndrome' is not immutable. It can be made worse by conditions of social isolation and understimulation such as can occur in the understaffed wards of large institutions, in group homes where disabled schizophrenic patients are left largely to their own devices, or in single bedsitters, hostels for the destitute, and conditions of 'sleeping rough' (Leach & Wing, 1980; Ryan, 1979). Fortunately, the extra deficit that accrues in such circumstances can be counteracted fairly rapidly if the social environment is made more stimulating (Wing & Brown, 1970). However, there are several qualifications to this general rule (Wing & Freudenberg, 1961). Improvement is proportional to the degree of understimulation that has caused the extra deficit – environmental changes cannot be expected to remove 'intrinsic' impairment. Further deterioration may occur if the environment later becomes understimulating again. There may be little 'transfer of training'; an improvement in one setting may not generalize to others. Providing a socially rich environment is not a mechanical exercise; it depends on the presence of people whom the patient can trust and who are emotionally supportive rather than intrusive. The patient needs to be able to keep a certain emotional distance from those he or she is living with.

It is quite difficult for staff to maintain a therapeutic approach to withdrawn and apparently apathetic patients, because effort seems likely to be unrewarded. For the same reason some relatives are critical of patients because of traits they call 'laziness' or 'unfriendliness', which they find difficult to explain in terms of illness. Critical comments by relatives are more often concerned with such traits than with florid manifestations such as delusions or hallucinations which are more evidently abnormal (Vaughn & Leff, 1976).

Even patients who are selected to go to an Employment Rehabilitation Centre because they appear to be only moderately disabled may appear, by contrast with physically handicapped people, to be slow, plodding, lacking in initiative, and unsociable (Wing, Bennett & Denham, 1964). Staff need special experience and training in order to maintain appropriate levels of stimulation.

Schizophrenic thought disorder is a further disabling factor. When severe, the patient finds it difficult, without intense and exhausting concentration, to keep to a purposeful line of thought, with consequences in speech and behaviour that are very puzzling to employers and relatives. One patient at a rehabilitation unit adamantly refused to put in all the screws necessary for an assembly, on the grounds that he was saving money by leaving some out. The effort required to maintain standards of self-care and general social performance, even when negative impairments and thought disorder are only moderate in severity, is difficult for normal people to appreciate, whether they be staff, employers, or relatives. A patient who manages to hold down an apparently simple, routine job may return to his lodging exhausted and have no energy left for shopping, managing a financial budget, preparing meals or keeping up appearances (Hewett, 1979; Hewett, Ryan & Wing, 1975).

The atmosphere of a workshop, in which a patient is expected to perform up to standards chosen because they are achievable by him or her, and in which the routine is structured and consistent but supervision is friendly as well as firm, provides an ideal balance between too much and too little stimulation. Moreover, companionship is available without being unduly intrusive. Unfortunately, the type of work available is often repetitive and boring and does not allow scope for the artistic and creative talents that some patients possess. Nor is there sufficient opportunity for non-manual types of work. Many patients, however, prefer the security of a well-established routine and do not seem to mind the monotony of the work. Acceptable occupation is one of the keys to a smooth course in schizophrenia and it is unfortunate that day centres are so rarely equipped to provide it. Unstructured group therapy is probably the least helpful form of activity.

Preventing social disadvantage

Measures which prevent social disadvantage due to poor educational or work opportunities, poverty, prejudice, or physical ill-health are likely, in general, to diminish the severity of disablement that follows the onset of any further illness. The relationship between unemployment and hospital admission rates is highly suggestive (Brenner, 1973; Dear, Clark & Clark, 1979). Most preventive efforts by the health and social services, however, will be concentrated on counteracting the effects of earlier disadvantages and trying to prevent new disadvantages from developing.

It is characteristic of the longer-term population of residential units such as hospitals, hostels, and group homes that the patients tend to have few occupational or social skills and to be living outside a family setting (Leach & Wing, 1980; Mann & Cree, 1976; Ryan, 1979). It has been pointed out in chapter 8 that a decline in level of social performance frequently occurs even before the first onset of florid schizophrenic symptoms and may be an early manifestation of the disease. However, some early advantages – particularly financial and social – are undoubtedly protective (Cooper, 1961) while some extraneous disadvantages make a poor social outcome more likely. It is therefore essential to ensure that opportunities are made available to correct earlier occupational and social disadvantages in so far as this is possible.

The social course of schizophrenia is undoubtedly affected by factors that occur following the onset. Up to the 1930s, the chance of patients given the diagnosis becoming long-stay residents was very high. In the years following the Second World War, a number of sociological studies, chiefly American, demonstrated that large institutions were often characterized by pauperism, social isolation, neglect, and stigmatization (Belknap, 1956; Dunham & Weinberg, 1960; Goffman, 1961; Scheff, 1964). The longer patients remained in such institutions the less likely they were to receive visitors, to be knowledgeable about conditions outside, or to practise everyday activities such as using public transport, shopping, and working, and the less able they became to undertake them. Although British hospitals, in general, provided rather more opportunities for exercising and maintaining social skills, particularly from the mid-1950s onwards (Bennett, 1975), a long tradition of environmental poverty had to be overcome. Measures of the social milieu and of patients' disabilities demonstrated that some hospitals provided particularly poor social conditions and that these were not necessarily dependent on the fact that patients were severely impaired (Wing, 1962; Wing & Brown, 1970). Patients with relatively mild disabilities were therefore exposed to extra social disadvantages which they might have avoided if discharged from hospital earlier.

These conditions are less often found in large hospitals nowadays but only because staff are aware of the necessity to prevent them and because public attitudes have become somewhat less stigmatizing and more caring. It is still possible to find a bleak institutional atmosphere in parts of some hospitals and in other places where disadvantaged schizophrenic patients tend to accumulate, such as casual wards and reception centres (Leach & Wing, 1980; Wing & Olsen, 1979).

Fostering self-confidence

Chronic disabilities of every kind cause distress and even despair to the sufferer. Schizophrenia is no exception; indeed, the 'invisible' nature of the impairments and the stigma that is still attached to the concept of severe mental illness make a loss of self-esteem and self-confidence almost inevitable. It can be detected even in patients who 'lack insight' into the fact that they are disabled.

Hewitt (1949) studied the life-style of unemployed physically disabled men and found that there was a general tendency to do nothing but walk the streets and read newspapers in public libraries. They frequently developed attitudes of resentment against society at large. These traits, in people with schizophrenia, are too frequently regarded as 'part of the illness'. Hewitt's conclusion, that 'the attitude of mind of the disabled men is the largest single factor in determining the prospects of future employment', contains a germ of truth for schizophrenia. One of the most important aims of rehabilitation and management is to avoid, as far as possible, the development of self-attitudes that are unnecessarily disparaging and hopeless, thus increasing the degree of dependency and disablement. In part, this can only be achieved by changing the attitudes of people who are important to the patient including relatives, employers, and medical, nursing, and social workers.

The development of adverse self-attitudes that increase social disablement is particularly obvious in 'institutionalism' – a condition of gradually increasing dependence on a protected environment, the institutional way of life eventually replacing and precluding any active participation in the general community, so that, finally, the patient no longer wishes to leave. This condition can develop in people who are not severely disabled (although a mild degree of schizophrenic impairment probably acts as a predisposing factor), and in settings which are socially pleasant to almost the same extent as in those that are characterized by pauperism and neglect (Wing, 1962; Wing & Brown, 1970). Techniques of correcting this tendency were developed during the 1950s (Barton, 1959; Bennett, 1975; Freudenberg, 1967).

Very few patients now stay for long periods in hospital and those who do are likely to be severely impaired (Mann & Cree, 1976; Wykes, 1982). But a similar process may take place in all the alternative environments in which moderately disabled people accumulate unless staff are aware of the need to weigh self-attitudes against potential capacity and to provide appropriate help and encouragement to those who can achieve a more independent life (Edwards & Carter, 1979; Hewett, Ryan & Wing, 1975; Leach & Wing, 1980; Ryan, 1979; Wing, L. *et al.*, 1972).

Assessment

Rehabilitation and management, to be successful (i.e. to achieve the optimum level of social functioning for each individual patient), must be based on systematic and regular assessment in order to determine the nature and severity of the clinical symptoms and impairments, the presence of talents that might be developed, the harmful or protective features of the social setting in which the patient is living, and the nature and mutability of his or her self-attitudes. Upon this assessment is based a plan of professional and self-help in which the family must be included, and the prescription of services which will ensure that the appropriate help is available when and where it is needed. Repeated assessment is required because progress is rarely uniform and circumstances are constantly changing (Wing & Morris, 1981).

Techniques of rehabilitation and management

Rehabilitation in schizophrenia consists of a long series of small steps, each depending on the success of the previous stage, but often with long periods in between during which little progress appears to be made. Benign social pressures need to be kept up throughout because they prevent progress from being lost; success is often measured by the fact that social disablement is not getting more marked.

Techniques include: medication (the dose being varied to allow for the interplay between social factors and the illness), occupation, education and training, individual counselling, family counselling, behavioural modification, physiotherapy, and small-group living and working programmes. Exploratory psychotherapy is very rarely helpful.

Such techniques should be used as part of a continuous process. Target problems are selected in order of priority, realistic goals are set in collaboration with patient, relatives and other people concerned, and new goals adopted as necessary. The over-all aim is a gradual reduction in dependence but only to the point where further pressure would begin to have harmful effects. The ladder model of rehabilitation described by Early (1965) requires the provision of resting places for those who cannot make steady progress to the top, and allows for the fact that progress may be uneven in different areas of social functioning. A satisfactory outcome is reached when the patient's potential assets are realized as fully as possible, even if this falls short of full independence. This optimum condition should then be maintained by attention to factors that might lead to deterioration or relapse.

Hemsley (1978) provides a useful discussion of chronic cognitive impairments in schizophrenia and of behaviours which can be understood as an attempt to adapt to or cope with these impairments. He emphasizes that operant procedures applied to patients without understanding their basic impairments may either fail or actually result in making symptoms worse. Gwynne Jones (1978) discusses the advantages and limitations of token economies.

Family problems

Very few schizophrenic patients now stay for long periods in hospital. On discharge, the majority live for most of the time at home with relatives: 40 per cent with parents, 37 per cent with a spouse, 8 per cent with some other relative, and only 15 per cent in lodgings or residential jobs. Parents tend to be elderly: 40 per cent over the age of 70. There is a high divorce and separation rate, particularly among men (Brown *et al.*, 1966).

The social problems experienced by parents and spouses are somewhat different. It is fairly socially acceptable for a mother to explain that her son is handicapped or ill in order to account for his strange behaviour, but much more difficult for a husband or wife, particularly if the couple have children. Patients do leave parental homes, partly because of the death or illness of parents or because of a normal process of gaining independence. Parents, often rightly, fear that patients will not be able to cope by themselves, but people with schizophrenia are motivated by the same wish to be free of parental dominance as other youngsters and have to learn by experience what their capabilities are.

As time goes on, if relative and patient stay together, they tend to acquire a tolerance which neither might have had earlier. There is often, however, a turbulent phase first, which can be lengthy and profoundly distressing for all concerned. It is during this phase that the family needs most help. One of the central problems concerns the admission to hospital of someone who is clearly unable to make rational judgements but who lacks insight into the fact. Relatives have to take the initiative and are frequently blamed for it by the patient. Doctors and social workers need to appreciate the relatives', as well as the patients', difficulties.

Other problems arising in family life are much the same as occur in a hospital ward where schizophrenic patients are living. Relatives, like nurses, acquire a good deal of experience in handling difficult behaviour. Unlike nurses, they have no training and no professional ethos to sustain them, they are 'on duty' all the time, and their normal emotional involvement with the patient makes it very difficult to adopt a neutral caring role. Nevertheless, many relatives do manage to find the most helpful ways of responding to the patient. They learn to accept the validity of schizophrenic experiences and to understand what lies behind odd speech and behaviour. They do not argue about the content of delusions but lay down clear limits as to behaviour which they are not prepared to tolerate. They discover how far they can expect the patient to respond to pressure to perform up to ordinary standards and at what point further stimulation is likely to lead to negative results. More than half the relatives interviewed in recent surveys were judged to have a tolerant, supportive, and non-critical attitude towards the patient (Brown, Birley & Wing, 1972; Vaughn & Leff, 1976).

It is hardly surprising that some relatives do not learn to cope as well as this. They may try to argue patients out of their delusional convictions, may not accept that schizophrenic experiences are real rather than imaginary, and, above all, fail to appreciate that slowness and lack of motivation may be disabilities rather than traits such as 'laziness' and that social withdrawal can be protective. It is from such relatives that the theory of 'schizophrenogenesis' has arisen.

Professional helpers should be aware of the real problems that arise in the family (Creer & Wing, 1974) and try to foster the healthy elements that are always present. Organizations such as the National Schizophrenia Fellowship, which has branches or groups in most parts of the country (NSF, 1979) deserve full professional support. Group meetings, at which inexperienced families can learn from experienced ones, are particularly helpful. The prescription of the right services at the right times is essential.

In the long run, even in families where there has been a long history of turbulence, if the patient remains at home or returns there, a routine develops which is fairly successful. Often the parents of unmarried or separated patients are elderly widows who are glad to have some companionship and help with household chores and are not too worried by not being able to live a life of their own. This is another kind of institutionalism, less expensive and less demanding of the patient than a good hospital with workshops, leisure activities, and socialization programmes would be and sometimes a good deal more restricting on the activities and interests of relatives. Few, however, complain. The major problem for them is worry over the patient's future. One father called this the 'when I am gone' syndrome.

Services and their prescription

At various points during the course of schizophrenia a wide variety of services, both statutory and voluntary, may be needed. These include admission to hospital during acute episodes which cannot be managed at home, day and occupation units, residential units such as hostels and group homes, and leisure time facilities such as dinner and social clubs. Counselling is needed concerning the use of these services, medication, work opportunities, family problems, welfare arrangements, and the day-to-day problems of 'living with schizophrenia'. Many kinds of professional people become involved: general practitioners, psychiatrists, community physicians, hospital and community nurses, social workers and social care staff, occupational therapists, occupational supervisors, resettlement officers, clinical psychologists, physiotherapists, probation officers, police, clergy, workers in voluntary organizations.

Some relatives and patients manage to obtain the best from the services available but many do not receive optimum advice and care, not only because the full range of services is not available but because there is no single agency committed to long-term management. Suggestions concerning the co-ordination of services for psychiatrically disabled people are made in 'Psychiatric Rehabilitation in the 1980s' (Royal College of Psychiatrists, 1981). Key recommendations are that there should be a consultant psychiatrist in every health district who accepts special responsibility for planning, co-ordination, management, and training, that each district should have a multidisciplinary rehabilitation committee, and that there should be a review system by which individual assessments are regularly updated and needs matched to services. Above all, each patient and family unit needs an individual counsellor who should be able to make appropriate care or advice available, whatever the agency involved. In order to allow this, the agreement of all the agencies concerned has to be obtained to the concept of a single service providing rehabilitation in its most appropriate form for each individual.

Information concerning occupational rehabilitation for chronically disabled people generally, including those with schizophrenia, is given by Bennett (1975) and Wansbrough and Cooper (1980). Information on various forms of residential care is given by Hewett (1979), Ryan and Wing (1979), Wing (1975) and Wykes (1982).

Counselling patients and relatives

The concept of rehabilitation has tended to be unduly restricted in the past to the theories appropriate to some one professional group (group or individual psychotherapy, behaviour modification, occupational or domestic training, medication, etc.) rather than to embrace all the multifarious problems that arise during the course of a condition such as chronic schizophrenia. The best use will not be made of services, and the stimulus to improve the often inadequate services now provided will not be consistently forthcoming, unless more attention is given to the need for good long-term counselling.

Attitudes to medication provide a specific example. Three highly intelligent professional people who contributed to a volume of essays on experiences of schizophrenia each said that they found medication dampening and depressing although they were grateful for the relief it brought from acute symptoms (Wing, 1975). Up to one-third of patients with schizophrenia do not persist with medication (Hirsch et al., 1973). Serious attention given to explanations about the drugs available, the use of other drugs to minimize side-effects, the circumstances under which the dose may need to be varied, and the effects of discontinuing medication under different conditions of stress, may prove very helpful, particularly if the patient's own experience is used in illustration.

Some patients learn eventually to recognize situations which make them feel worse and which might trigger off episodes of relapse. One said: 'There is a sensitivity in myself and I have to try to harden my emotions and cut myself off from potentially dangerous situations. . . . When I get worked up I often experience a slight recurrence of delusional thoughts.' He avoided arguments on topics that made him emotionally upset. Another found that sometimes, when sitting in a subway train, he noticed the eyes of another passenger begin 'to radiate'. Then he would deliberately turn his attention to something else; in fact, he had evolved a relaxation technique in order to deal with such occasions. Another experienced hallucinatory voices only last thing at night, when his attention began to wander before he went to sleep, but he knew that he would not act on them and quite enjoyed them. A very bright girl chose her men friends among people who were not her intellectual equals because she did not get so involved with them and found she could control the situation better.

Social withdrawal is a technique that can be consciously manipulated by patients and used in a specific way to avoid situations they find painful. It is important that they know the dangers of going too far, since understimulation carries its own risk of increasing morbidity. A degree of external social stimulation is necessary for ordinary social functioning. Nevertheless, being withdrawn is often found preferable to being forced into unwanted social interaction.

Equivalent problems arise when counselling relatives. The role of relatives as caring agents is often not understood by professionals, who thereby fail to learn from the expertise of those who cope well (and who may have learned to do so by trial and error in default of useful advice being available). The traditional patient–doctor or client–social worker relationship may also prevent professionals from accepting opportunities for useful collaboration with relatives in the care of patients. When most people with schizophrenia tended to become long-term in-patients relatives were relieved of their responsibility. Now they need all the help they can get. Nurses often prove the most sympathetic helpers since they themselves take over the responsibility for patients from relatives from time to time and are in a position to understand the problems of management that can arise from day to day.

One of the commonest complaints of relatives is that they do not receive practical advice on how to react to deluded or withdrawn patients, what to do when a patient refuses to claim benefits or to take the medication prescribed, or even how to deal with the patient's jealousy of a normal sibling (a problem quite frequently met with in the case of chronic physical disability). The counselling expertise that has long been available to the families of people with diabetes or multiple sclerosis rests, of course, on a securer foundation of knowledge about the nature of the disabilities involved, but there is now quite a substantial body of knowledge about schizophrenia which is not always applied (Creer, 1978; Priestley, 1979; Wing, 1977). Making the fullest use of the services available, and raising the standard of advice to that already made available by some professional helpers, would be a major factor in improving the social course of schizophrenia and ensuring a better quality of life for patient and relatives.

PART II
Affective psychoses

Section 4

CHAPTERS 15–20

Clinical

15
Manic-depressive psychoses: mania

JAMES L. GIBBONS

In this group of functional psychoses, often also called affective psychoses, the primary change appears to be in the patient's mood, which is either elevated (mania) or lowered (depression). In either case other symptoms can be intuitively understood as consonant with the mood change.

The term manic-depressive psychosis was coined by Kraepelin and included all periodic and circular psychoses, all manias and most depressions, together with affective personality disorders and some cases previously classified as amentia (delirious states). He based this synthesis, one of his greatest achievements, on similarities in symptoms, on the good prognosis for the individual episode of illness, and on the family history.

Recently, as a result of family studies, manic-depressive psychoses have been divided into bipolar and unipolar disorders. The concept originated with Leonhard (1961), who used the term 'monopolar', and was developed independently by Angst (1966) in Switzerland and by Perris (1966), who introduced the term 'unipolar' in the interests of etymological purity, in Sweden. For these European workers 'bipolar' referred to patients who had had attacks of both mania and of depressive psychosis, 'unipolar' to patients who had recurrent attacks of mania alone or of depressive psychosis alone. All three investigators found an increased morbid risk for bipolar disorder in the first-degree relatives of bipolar, but not of unipolar, patients. Following family studies carried out by Winokur and his colleagues (Winokur, Cadoret, Dorzab & Baker, 1971; Winokur, Clayton & Reich, 1969) American workers apply the term 'bipolar' to patients who have had an attack of mania, whether or not they have ever been depressed: 'unipolar' is restricted to patients who have had episodes of primary depressive illness (not necessarily the same as the European concept of depressive psychosis) but no episodes of mania. Winokur appears to prefer the terms 'manic-depressive disease' and 'depressive disease'. An excellent summary of these and other family studies of affective disorder is provided by Kay (1978).

A further modification has been introduced by Fieve and Dunner (1975): 'bipolar I' includes any patient who has been admitted to hospital for mania; 'bipolar II' comprises patients who have been admitted to hospital for depression and have had one or more episodes of mania (referred to as hypomania) which did not require admission; 'bipolar other' includes patients with a history of both depressive and manic episodes that have not required admission.

Another dichotomy, introduced by the St Louis group and of much influence in the United States, is between primary and secondary affective disorder. Primary affective disorder occurs in patients with no previous history of psychiatric disorder other than depression or mania. Secondary affective disorder, almost always depression, follows some other psychiatric disorder (including alcoholism and sociopathic personality disorder) or is associated with an incapacitating or life-threatening physical illness. This last qualification, however, is no longer used by the St Louis group (Spitzer, Endicott & Robins, 1978).

Manic syndromes

Mania is characterized by elevation of mood, pressure of talk, over-activity, and expansiveness or grandiosity. Kraepelin's account in the eighth edition of his textbook (Kraepelin, 1913) is available in English (Kraepelin, 1921) and remains worth reading. The most detailed recent account of the symptoms of mania is by Winokur and colleagues (1969). Other recent series are referred to in table 15.1.

Mood

Mood is elevated. The patient is cheerful and displays an infectious hilarity or jollity. He looks happy, smiling with frequent peals of laughter. 'I'm high, in great spirits, on top of the world.' The observer is often moved to smile, or even laugh, with the patient. However, sustained euphoria is unusual, except in mild cases. Most patients are also irritable: frustration, even of a trivial kind, leads to anger and even hostility and aggressiveness. In more severe cases, although euphoria still occurs at times, the mood is labile and capricious. Episodes of depressed mood, tearfulness and sadness, replacing elation and lasting from a few minutes to a few hours, were seen in two-thirds of the patients of Winokur and colleagues (1969): some patients expressed suicidal thoughts and fleeting depressive delusions. Other recent observers, using nurses' ratings of the patients' entire waking day, have also been impressed by the frequency of depressive moods and of depressive symptoms generally in manic patients (Loudon, Blackburn & Ashworth, 1977; Murphy & Beigel, 1974; Kotin & Goodwin, 1972). In general, depressive symptoms are more frequent and more intense in more severe episodes of mania. Murphy and Beigel (1974) conclude: 'mania appears to be not as well characterized by elation but rather by a state of heightened overall activation with enhanced affective expression together with lability of affect.' Loudon and colleagues (1977) noted minor non-specific symptoms of anxiety and tension, as well as definite symptoms of depression, in many of their manic patients. They comment, 'It seems probable that elation in pure culture is rather rare and that the majority of patients diagnosed as manic show signs of a mixture of mood states.' Certainly many, but not all, patients report after recovery that their excitement was unpleasant.

Speech and thought

Manic patients talk excessively, sometimes almost incessantly, and show pressure of speech. Many patients appear to feel a great need to seek out other people and to talk to them at length. Speech is often rapid and the voice unnecessarily loud. In milder cases it is easy to follow the direction of the patient's thoughts, in spite of circumstantiality and distractibility. In more severe cases flight of ideas occurs: the patient's thinking leaps from topic to topic with changes of direction determined by puns or rhymes or by chance distractions from the environment (a cough outside the door, the noise of a car in the street, a sudden gust of wind, the colour of the doctor's tie). Although the aim is lost, the shifting direction of thought and the connection between successive topics can usually be understood by an observer. Some patients describe a subjective aspect of flight of ideas, the feeling of thoughts racing through their minds, idea generating idea at a great

Table 15.1. *Percentage frequency of manic symptoms in recent series*

	Winokur *et al.* (1969)	Carlson & Goodwin (1973)	Taylor & Abrams (1973)[a]	Leff *et al.* (1976)	Loudon *et al.* (1977)[b]
No. of patients	100	20	52	63	16
Euphoria	98	90	31[c]	97	69
Lability	95	90	29	–	38
Irritability	85	100	81	–	56
Hostility	83	75	48	–	38
Depression	68	55	29	–	44
Over-activity	100	100	100	81	63
Over-talkativeness	99	100	100	86	88
Flight of Ideas	93	75	77	49	25
Distractibility	100	70	–	16	56
Grandiosity	86	100	–	–	63
Delusions	48	70	60	67	38
Hallucinations:					
Auditory	21	40	48	–	13
Visual	9		27	–	
Extravagance	69	–	–	32	–
Insomnia	90	–	–	63	63
Hypersexuality	55	80	–	27	25

[a] Criteria for mania probably less strict than in other series.
[b] Based on ratings at first interview only.
[c] 'Expansive' mood in 66 per cent.
A dash indicates that the frequency of the symptom was not stated.

rate (subjective ideomotor pressure). Other patients demonstrate such pressure by voluminous writings.

In very severe mania, flight of ideas may degenerate into incoherent and unintelligible speech (Carlson & Goodwin, 1973).

The content of thought is expansive and indicates enhanced self-esteem. The patient has never felt so well, he is at the height of his powers, his opportunities are limitless. Religion and wealth are common themes. Many patients express frank delusions. They may be evanescent or expressed in a half-joking way, but sometimes they are persistent. The majority of delusions are grandiose and they can be classified according to the scheme used by Leff, Fischer and Bertelsen (1976):

(1) Delusions of special abilities: the patient is an inventor, he can cure all sick people, he has a greater talent than Shakespeare. One manic mathematician was convinced that he could completely alter the basis of arithmetic by his brilliant reasoning.

(2) Delusions of grandiose identity: the patient is of royal blood, the most important statesman in history, an archangel, a reincarnation of Moses. One patient asserted that she was a close blood-relative of both the Queen and the Pope.

(3) Delusions of wealth: the patient is a millionaire, he has a fleet of ships anchored every two miles across the Atlantic, he owns more oil wells than all the Arab nations put together.

(4) Delusions of a special mission: he is to bring peace to Northern Ireland, to solve the problems of poverty in the third world, to unite all the great religions under his spiritual leadership.

Non-grandiose delusions are sometimes expressed, especially delusions of persecution and reference. Often these seem metaphorical or exaggerated expressions of the patient's frustrations. Some American authors (e.g. Winokur *et al.*, 1969; Taylor & Abrams, 1973) claim that delusions of control and other first-rank symptoms of schizophrenia occur in a sizeable minority (10–20 per cent) of manic patients (see chapter 19). Fleeting depressive delusions, including hypochondriacal ones, may be expressed during spells of depressed mood during the manic episode.

Occasional patients report hallucinations, auditory or visual. They are fleeting and inconstant and usually consonant with mood. Examples from Carlson and Goodwin (1973) are: 'hearing the Hallelujah Chorus from Messiah', 'seeing a box open with beautiful flowers', 'seeing a kaleidoscope of colours running together'.

Activity and behaviour

Over-activity is characteristic of mania. Very often, largely because of distractibility, the over-activity is unproductive, the patient never completing one task before embarking upon another. One patient rose early, completed her housework in chaotic fashion by 7 a.m., and then called on several of her neighbours to offer her services to them. Other patients stay up all night, constantly changing their activities, allowing no sleep to anyone in the household. In hospital patients are constantly on the go, repeatedly visit the nurses' station, get out of bed moments after being put into it, perhaps engage in singing and dancing. Simple acts like dressing or eating are complicated by inappropriate movements, by cries, by bursts of laughter.

Winokur and colleagues (1969) point out that many patients are over-active for only part of the time, with periods of quiescence and normal behaviour. In general over-activity tends to decline if environmental stimuli diminish.

In the severest cases patients engage in a constant frenzy of activity, rushing about, perhaps screaming and shouting, attacking and destroying furniture, bedding and clothing, sometimes attacking other patients or staff. Such extreme over-activity, persisting for days with little or no sleep or food, can lead to exhaustion.

The combination of pressure of activity, expansiveness, grandiosity, and disinhibition (also characteristic of mania) easily leads to extravagant behaviour, of which overspending is the most characteristic. Patients give lavish parties to which they invite casual acquaintances. They buy lots of expensive clothes, order large new cars. One patient, employed in a sweet shop, gave away the entire stock to passers by in two hours. Another, actually on his way to a psychiatric clinic, ordered several thousand pounds' worth of furniture and carpets in a Regent Street store. Other patients are full of schemes for making money or plan a series of ambitious business ventures, sometimes persuading their friends to invest in them. The effects on the patients and their families may be disastrous, all savings spent and large debts accumulated in just a few weeks. One patient, seen recently just after recovery from a brief manic episode said, 'I'm just waiting for all my bounced cheques and all my credit card accounts to come in. If the bank manager is sympathetic, I could be solvent again in a couple of years.'

Extravagant behaviour can take many other forms. Patients often dress in outlandish style, perhaps bedecking themselves with garish ornaments. Sexual drive is often increased and this may lead to sexually provocative behaviour, to foolish proposals, to unfortunate liaisons, to promiscuity. In the series of Winokur and colleagues (1969), however, most of the patients' increased sexual activity was of a socially approved kind and only 11 per cent were promiscuous.

Excessive drinking is common during a manic episode. Although the drinking is usually in company in pubs and bars and is rarely solitary, it can still be a serious drain on the patient's financial resources. By causing even more disinhibition alcohol can lead to even greater social problems for the manic patient. One patient, in the course of a two-month manic episode, had himself barred from all six pubs in his neighborhood, was arrested for being drunk and disorderly, and lost his driving licence for driving with too high a blood-alcohol concentration.

In the community the manic patient's extravagance can lead to ruin. In hospital some of the patient's outrageous behaviour is suggestive of a game, of playing to the audience. As Ey (1954) remarked, the patient manipulates reality, amuses himself with people about him, at times is acting a part; unfortunately it is all bad theatre!

Cognitive function

Patients are usually correctly oriented for time and place, except at the height of the illness. Formal psychometric testing is very difficult with excited and over-active patients, but Henry, Weingartner and Murphy (1971) have produced evidence that manic patients show a reversible defect of recent memory processes, particularly retrieval of information. This contrasts with the traditional view that hypermnesia, the ability to recall precise details of all sorts of past events, characterizes some manic patients.

Physical symptoms

Insomnia is a cardinal symptom of mania. Decreased duration of sleep is often the first symptom noted by the patient or relatives. One patient was always aware that a manic episode was imminent when it took him an hour to get off to sleep instead of his usual two to three minutes; this was also always noticed by his wife, who would persuade him to take a neuroleptic drug even before he consulted his doctor next day. Insomnia is often also the last symptom to disappear. The sleep disturbance has been studied clinically by Winokur and colleagues (1969) and by Weckers and Meyer (1977). The duration of sleep is reduced, because of initial insomnia or early waking or both disorders. Characteristically the insomnia is not associated with fatigue and the patients wake refreshed, even those who in health are slow to reach full alertness in the morning. EEG studies confirm the diminution of sleep time and also show a reduction in delta sleep (Hartmann, 1968; Mendels & Hawkins, 1971).

Appetite is usually good and most manic patients enjoy their meals, although a few patients neglect food because of distraction from other interests. Nevertheless, because of over-activity, moderate weight loss is quite common.

Insight

Manic patients often refuse to admit that they are ill and resent being admitted to hospital. Yet they are sometimes aware of the effect of their behaviour on others and may be able to restrain themselves and even pass as normal during a brief clinical interview. Of the patients of Winokur and colleagues (1969) almost a third had insight (i.e. the ability to understand that admission had occurred because of psychiatric illness) all the time, a third part of the time and a third none of the time during the first 24 hours in hospital.

Classification of mania

Kraepelin described four forms of mania: hypomania (the mildest form with predominant euphoria, over-activity, disinhibition); acute mania (more severe, with transient grandiose delusions, a more labile mood, and at times incoherent talk); delusional mania (with less excitement but with more persistent grandiose delusions and occasional hallucinations); delirious mania (with disorientation for time and place, vivid visual and other hallucinations, variable delusions, a very labile mood ranging from excitement to despair to panic, and frenzied over-activity). The most severe forms of mania are rarely seen now, presumably because of neuroleptic drug treatment. Carlson and Goodwin (1973) analysed the records of patients on a research ward where drugs were withheld and described three stages during the course of mania; they resembled the hypomania, acute mania and delirious mania described by Kraepelin.

Murphy and Beigel (1974) have proposed the division of manic patients into two categories, 'elated grandiose' (the majority) and 'paranoid destructive'. Loudon and colleagues (1977), using a similar rating scale, found no clear distinction between the two categories.

Most authors have regarded mania as a unitary disorder. There have been none of the disputes which have raged over the classification of depression. However some earlier French and German authors described 'reactive mania', a short-lived episode closely following a severe traumatic experience (Ey, 1954). Recently Krauthammer and Klerman (1978) have drawn attention to secondary mania, where a manic syndrome is associated with an antecedent physical illness (such as metabolic disturbance, influenza, encephalitis, or celebral neoplasm) or drug treatment (steroids, isoniazid, levodopa). The patients were usually over forty and had no family history of bipolar affective disorder.

Finally, there used to be a condition, in the days before effective treatment was available, of 'chronic mania'. In this condition, the mood of elation became less pronounced although many of the other symptoms remained present. A similar picture may occasionally be seen nowadays when the affective disturbance is suppressed by medication, leaving many of the other symptoms in isolation.

16
Depressive syndromes
JAMES L. GIBBONS

This chapter is concerned with depressive illness, a primary disorder of mood with a variable number of associated symptoms such as insomnia, anorexia, weight loss, poor concentration, and so on. The description that follows is of 'depressive psychosis' or 'endogenous' depression – the meaning of these terms is considered later in the section on classification – and symptoms of other varieties of depression are only briefly referred to. The classic account in English of depressive symptoms was written by Lewis (1934), and this paper is still very much worth reading. In the subsequent 45 years very severe depressions have become less frequent in psychiatric practice and what was commonplace then (for example, nihilistic delusions) is now rare. Nevertheless many patients suffering from the 'endogenous' depressive syndrome still seek treatment and milder forms of the disorder, for which Taylor (1979) suggested the term hypomelancholia, are not always recognized.

Mood
Mood is lowered. Patients describe themselves as low in spirits, depressed, sad, miserable, unhappy, unable to stop crying. 'There's nothing to live for.' Depression is like a black cloud which envelops the patient. When severe it is all pervading. The mood is often described in physical terms – a heavy weight on the head, oppression in the chest, a feeling of pain. Mild depression may be likened to ennui, a lack of

zest, but severe depression is an intensely unpleasant mood, a psychic pain less bearable than even the severest physical pain previously experienced. Some patients ascribe a 'distinct quality' to their depressed mood: it is not just ordinary unhappiness multiplied, but rather a feeling of a quite different kind. Many patients complain of the mood change; others describe their gloomy sadness when asked about it although their primary complaint is of some associated symptom, most often in physical terms: a few seem unable to express their melancholy in words and admit only to associated symptoms.

Most patients look sad, with drooping posture and lack-lustre eyes and perhaps tears. In general, tears, however profuse, bring little or no relief. Some patients complain rather of the inability to cry, their expressions being of dry-eyed misery. Patients with milder depression, however, may not look in any way distressed, or only an intimate friend may notice a lack of sparkle.

The depressed mood is often described as unchanging from day to day, uninfluenced by the environment. The patient is just as wretched alone or in the company of dearest friends. Neither good news nor bad news affects his melancholy. As Winokur, Clayton and Reich (1969) remark, if the sadness and pessimism do fluctuate, neither the patient nor his family has any control over them. However, a lightening of mood later in the day, with symptoms at their worst in the morning ('diurnal variation') is well recognized and regarded as characteristic of the endogenous syndrome. One patient, a bipolar depressive, was so filled with gloom early in the day that he could scarcely dress and wash, yet he was able to do two or three hours of useful work if he went to his office in the late afternoon, only to wake in a state of wretched despondency early next morning.

The depression colours, or rather darkens, the patient's perception of the world. Everything looks black, the future is hopeless, the patient is helpless. Even in mild cases interests are lost, the woman skilled at embroidery can scarcely pick up a needle, the avid reader listlessly looks at the same page for minutes at a time, the musician gets no enjoyment from his piano. In severe cases the anhedonia is complete: there is no source of pleasure, no reward, no joy. This is the setting in which suicidal ideas are only too prone to arise, particularly when guilt and self-reproach are prominent.

Most depressed patients are anxious; in Lewis' apt phrase, they experience an unpleasant state with expectation, but not certainty, of something unpleasant happening. Physical symptoms of anxiety and tension are also common and frank anxiety attacks are by no means unusual. Some patients are also irritable, becoming angry when disturbed or frustrated. The combination of inexplicable gloom and uncharacteristic irritability and hostility is often particularly difficult for relatives and friends to bear.

Speech and thought

The most typical change is a reduction in the amount and rate of speech, in retarded patients. The voice becomes more monotonous, there is a pause before questions are answered, the voice may die away before the sentence is completed. Many such patients complain that their thinking is slower and less clear than usual, although others report a ceaseless round of repetitive, unpleasant thoughts. In the agitated patient, however, there is a great deal of talk, often with much circumstantiality and expostulation although with only a limited range of topics. In milder cases no abnormality of speech may be detectable.

The content of thought in depression comprises one or more of three main themes, guilt, hypochondriasis, and poverty. The degree of the disorder ranges from anxious preoccupation to full delusional conviction. In pathological guilt the patient blames himself unreasonably, feels that the illness is somehow his fault, that he has let down his family. Often attention is concentrated on some minor peccadillo from the past. One patient was severely troubled by the memory of finding and keeping sixpence several years previously. Another reproached herself for having been a month late in purchasing her television licence. Other patients feel themselves somehow to blame for any misfortune that befalls friends or relatives. In all of these instances the patient will agree that the guilt is excessive, but he is unable to banish the feeling. Delusions of guilt, however, are held with full conviction. The patient has brought shame and disgrace on his relatives, he has committed an unforgivable sin, he is damned and rightly so, his punishment will be terrible but he deserves it. Some delusions of guilt are grandiose: 'All the trouble in the world today is my fault. If it wasn't for me there would be peace in the Middle East and everywhere else.'

Similarly some patients are preoccupied with bodily functions, wonder if some physical disease might be responsible for their symptoms. Other patients express frank hypochondriacal delusions: they have widespread cancer, their bowels are blocked, they have an incurable disease and will die soon.

Nihilistic delusions (syndrome of Cotard) may take a hypochondriacal form: the patient's skull is empty, he has no stomach, no internal organs. In extreme cases patients may be convinced that they are dead, all their relatives are dead, perhaps even the whole world has ceased to exist. Here again the grandiose quality of some depressive delusions is evident.

Preoccupation with money is a common symptom. The patient may worry unnecessarily or may exaggerate minor financial difficulties. One patient was preoccupied by the rate of inflation, another worried about an impending bill for alterations to his house, even though he agreed he had enough money to pay for it. Delusions of poverty may develop, in which the patient is convinced that he is ruined, that his debts are unpayable, that all his possessions will have to be sold. Occasionally such delusions are expressed so plausibly that the doctor may at first be deceived and consider the depression understandable in one so unfortunate.

Delusions of persecution are not uncommon in depressive psychosis. The patient is being followed, he is watched by the police, he is going to be taken to prison and hanged. It is usually stated that depressed patients regard any such persecution as justified, but this is not always so, as Lewis (1934) pointed out. However, the delusional conviction disappears as the depressed mood lightens.

Auditory hallucinations are uncommon but well-recognized. Typically, the patient occasionally hears a voice which speaks directly to him in a derogatory way. Usually few words are spoken.

Activity and behaviour

Even in mild depression patients describe a subjective slowing up. Energy and efficiency are reduced, work output is less, the housewife does her housework less well, the student does unexpectedly poorly in his examinations. However, the inadequacy is often exaggerated by the patient.

In terms of motility patients may be retarded or agitated. Retardation is a decrease in purposive movement and in speech. The patient is slow in all his actions, slow to obey commands or to answer questions. Gait is slow and laboured. The rare extreme form of retardation is depressive stupor, in

which the patient is mute and almost immobile and fails to react to external stimuli. Some patients may need to be fed, but incontinence is rare and the depth of stupor is not as great as in catatonic stupor. In agitation there is purposeless motor restlessness, sometimes amounting to ceaseless but pointless activity. Patients pace up and down, wring their hands, rock back and forwards. Speech is usually repetitive, expressing distress, anguish or despair. Although retardation and agitation are often regarded as polar opposites, they can coexist (Lader & Wing, 1969). Retardation is characteristic of bipolar depression (Blackburn, 1975) and agitated depression is almost always unipolar (Himmelhoch, Coble, Kupfer & Ingenito, 1976).

Suicide

Suicide, an ever-present risk in depressive psychosis, is discussed in chapter 22. The suicidal act is sometimes preceded by the murder of relatives, especially young children. The motive is to save them from disgrace and ruin (Batt, 1948). Less serious criminal offences associated with depression (perhaps more often depressive neurosis than psychosis) include shoplifting and exhibitionism. A few depressed patients drink to excess during their illness and recent alcohol abuse is occasionally the presenting feature. More often patients report that alcohol fails to relieve their misery, which may even be accentuated after a bout of drinking.

Other psychiatric syndromes

These may appear for the first time or become more severe during a depressive episode. Obsessional symptoms were prominent in a fifth of Lewis's cases and in almost a third of patients with depressive psychosis reviewed in a case-note study by Gittleson (1966a). Kendell and Discipio (1970) found them at interview in 20 of 92 patients. They also found that the frequency of obsessions increased with the severity of the depression. Some patients had obsessional symptoms, usually less severe, before the onset of the depression, but other patients, especially those with depressive psychosis, had not. Occasionally pre-existing obsessions disappear when a depression develops. Kendell and Discipio, as well as Gittleson (1966b), confirmed the clinical impression of earlier writers that the content of depressive obsessions is almost always aggressive, with thoughts of killing or harming oneself or others. During a depressive illness there may be a transition from an obsession to a delusion: a fear of contamination may become a conviction of infestation.

Depersonalization

Depersonalization, discussed in the next chapter, occurs in about a fifth of psychotic depressives (Gittleson, 1967). Patients' guilt may be accentuated by their lack of feeling for their loved ones. A much less common occurrence during a depressive psychosis is the emergence of morbid jealousy, usually in a patient who has always been jealous of his or her spouse (Shepherd, 1961).

Cognitive function

Depressed patients are usually correctly orientated and can give a full history if the interviewer is patient enough. Any apparent defect in memory or grasp is usually attributed to impaired concentration, itself often due to preoccupation with depressive ideas. Several investigators have found reversible impairment of memory by means of psychological tests (e.g. Strömgren, 1977). Cutting (1979) found both verbal memory and pattern recognition to be impaired and suggests that memory defect may be intrinsic to depressive illness. In occasional patients, usually but not always elderly and usually of below average intelligence, disorientation and memory defect may be severe enough to resemble senile or presenile dementia. This 'depressive pseudodementia' disappears with recovery from the depression (Post, 1966).

Physical symptoms

These always occur in depressive psychosis and are often the presenting complaints. *Sleep* is reduced and less refreshing. The characteristic, but by no means invariable, complaint is of waking earlier than usual, perhaps by an hour or two, without any particular difficulty in falling asleep (Kiloh & Garside, 1963). Several other studies, but not all, have supported the diagnostic importance of early waking in 'endogenous' depression. A study of psychiatric outpatients suggested that anxiety was associated with initial insomnia and broken sleep, sadness with some delay in falling asleep and with early waking. 'Endogenous' depressives reported both delay in falling asleep and early waking, while 'neurotic' depressives woke just as early but took almost twice as long to get to sleep (Stonehill, Crisp & Koval, 1976). Polygraphic studies in sleep laboratories have shown that depressives as a group take longer to fall asleep, sleep less and less deeply and wake earlier than normal subjects. (For references see Chen, 1979.) Differences between 'endogenous' and 'reactive' or 'psychotic' and 'neurotic' patients have not yet been established and there is much disagreement about how the various EEG stages of sleep are affected by depression. Current and also recent use of both hypnotics and antidepressants may affect the patients' experience of sleep and the EEG findings.

A group of American workers has claimed that bipolar depressives experience increased sleep rather than insomnia, at least when they are not taking medication (Detre *et al.*, 1972). This report runs counter to reports of a series of patients (Winokur *et al.*, 1969) and to clinical experience: two of my bipolar patients, neither taking medication, constantly reported waking at 5 a.m. rather than 7 a.m. during depressive episodes. Mendels and Chernik (1975) did not find hypersomnia in their bipolar patients, although those patients had generally less severe sleep disturbance than unipolar patients. Increased duration of sleep does, of course, occur in some depressed patients, more usually in 'neurotic' depressives.

Appetite is decreased in depressive psychosis, but may be increased in younger 'neurotic' depressives (Paykel, 1977). Many patients lose several kg in weight. This may be due to a loss of appetite, to retardation, to guilt about consuming food in a hungry world, even to delusions of being poisoned. Increase in appetite and in weight does occur in some depressives: in Paykel's experience this is confined to women with milder 'neurotic' depression. Antidepressant drugs, of course, can increase appetite (and weight) even though they do not alleviate the depression.

Other physical symptoms include constipation (which may also be due to antidepressant medication) and loss of sexual drive and interest. Impotence in the male and failure to achieve orgasm in the female may be both the result of depression and the cause of marital acrimony. Increased sexual desire, perhaps leading to uncharacteristic promiscuity, has been attributed to 'atypical' depression, but is extremely rare, if not unknown, in the 'endogenous' syndrome.

The depressives' lack of energy and sense of fatigue have already been mentioned. These may be presenting symptoms which suggest physical disease. Numerous other physical symptoms, particularly complaints of pain, pressure, or heaviness in various parts of the body (including the vertex, shoulders, chest, abdomen, and back), are reported by depressed patients. Antidepressant drugs, so freely prescribed now, may also cause symptoms resembling those of depressive illness, such as constipation, dry mouth, tachycardia, tremor, and so on.

Insight

To assert that 'neurotic' depressives have insight and that 'psychotic' depressives lack insight is, as Lewis (1934) remarked, 'an extreme, almost extravagant assertion'. A patient suffering from typical depressive neurosis may attribute all symptoms to some supposed physical illness, whereas a 'psychotic' depressive may be afraid that he is going mad. Most of the depressed patients seen by psychiatrists nowadays are seeking help for distress, whether they perceive it in physical or psychological terms, whether or not they have depressive delusions. Lewis's quotation from Lange (1928) remains apposite: 'A more or less obscure awareness of illness is rarely absent even in severe melancholia; indeed it can coexist with pronounced delusions; in that case, however, it nearly always refers to the bodily state only, while the possibility of there being any mental disorder is repudiated'.

Classification of depression

In this section only the better-known classificatory systems can be mentioned. The reader should consult the admirable comprehensive review by Kendell (1976), with its apt title of 'a review of contemporary confusion'. In the British literature there has been a prolonged if intermittent controversy about the relationship between 'endogenous' and 'reactive' depression, whether they represent two separate (if symptomatically overlapping) categories or the two extremes of a continuum. The classical concept of endogenous depression includes three criteria which do not necessarily coexist: the clinical syndrome (pervasive and unresponsive depression, early waking, diurnal variation of mood, depressive ideation, disturbance of motility, marked physical symptoms, etc.); the lack of an obvious precipitant; a stable premorbid personality (Rosenthal & Klerman, 1966). In the case of reactive depression the classical criteria are: the clinical syndrome (a more fluctuating depression, responsive to environmental change, self-pity rather than self-blame, and so on); a clear precipitant; a vulnerable personality.

Recent work suggests that patients with the endogenous syndrome are just as likely to have experienced a major threatening event in the months before the onset of the illness as patients with the reactive syndrome (Brown & Harris, 1978).

To avoid the conceptual difficulty of reactive endogenous depression, Klein (1974) coined the term 'endogenomorphic' to describe the clinical syndrome. In British and European literature 'depressive psychosis' is more or less synonymous with the endogenous syndrome. In American usage, however, 'psychotic depression' applies only to those depressed patients with 'psychotic' features such as delusions, hallucinations, or stupor. Some American workers have suggested that psychotic depression should be considered a separate disorder from the endogenous syndrome without psychotic features because, they claim, the former does not respond to tricyclic antidepressants. In my experience, some clearly deluded depressives do respond to imipramine or amitriptyline. For references, see Nelson and Bowers (1978). Depressive neurosis generally corresponds to the 'reactive' clinical syndrome.

The use of multivariate statistical techniques has not resolved the controversy. Discriminant function analysis and similar techniques, which assign weights to different items of mental state or history in order to achieve the best possible separation between the two groups of patients, have sometimes suggested that 'endogenous' and 'neurotic' depressions are distinct categories (Carney, Roth & Garside, 1965), sometimes that they merge imperceptibly to form a continuum (Kendell & Gourlay, 1970; Bhrolcháin, Brown & Harris, 1979). In any case there is no doubt that significant clinical overlap is found. In these studies the external criterion is the clinical diagnosis, which may be deficient in both reliability and validity. An alternative approach is to use some form of cluster analysis. Paykel (1971) derived four clusters from 165 depressed patients: one corresponded to the endogenous syndrome, the other three to different groups of neurotic depressives – an older anxious group, and two younger groups characterized in one case by hostility, in the other by personality disorder. Several other authors (for references see Kendell, 1976) have found a cluster of depressives corresponding to the endogenous syndrome, but none found a single cluster of depressive neurosis. The formulation of Kiloh, Andrews, Neilson and Bianchi (1972) may be quoted here. They suggest that there is a category of 'endogenous' depression; some of the patients respond to the illness by developing neurotic symptoms as well. Neurotic depression is 'a diffuse entity encompassing some of the ways in which the patient utilises his defence mechanisms to cope with his own neuroticism and concurrent environmental stress'. Bhrolcháin and colleagues (1979) remind us that those neurotic depressives who reach the psychiatric services are probably a selected sample anyway. Wing and his colleagues have compared the affective disorders found in in-patients, out-patients, and a sample of the general population (Wing *et al.*, 1978). They suggested that a hierarchical model incorporating both dimensional (severity) and categorical (symptom type) elements would be theoretically and practically useful and deserved further investigation.

The distinction between bipolar and unipolar depression, referred to in the preceding chapter, is now generally accepted and it is usually assumed that the clinical picture of bipolar depression is the endogenous syndrome. This conforms with my own experience and with the clinical description of bipolar depressives by Winokur, Clayton and Reich (1969).

In the United States there has been widespread acceptance of the distinction between primary and secondary depressive disorders, originally put forward by the St Louis group in order to avoid the endogenous-reactive and psychotic–neurotic dimensions. As mentioned in the previous chapter, depression is secondary when it has been preceded by another psychiatric disorder. Clear research diagnostic criteria are available (Spitzer, Endicott & Robins, 1978). As Kendell (1976) comments, the primary–secondary distinction is a useful strategy. However, it does not solve the endogenous—neurotic problem, it merely ignores it. A depression arising against a background of obsessional or anxiety neurosis may well be different from a primary depression, but it is hard to see why a depression arising at 50 in a woman who had an episode of phobic anxiety at 20 should necessarily be different. The research diagnostic criteria distinguish between major and minor depressive disorders; the latter has fewer symptoms and no 'psychotic' features. Cases of the endogenous syndrome and of the neurotic syndrome (of at least moderate severity) would both be diagnosed as major depressive disorder. There are, incidentally, criteria for endogenous major depressive disorder.

Winokur (1973) has suggested the subdivision of unipolar depressive disorder into depressive spectrum disease (characteristically affecting a young woman with depressed female relatives and alcoholic or sociopathic male relatives) and pure depressive disease (characteristically affecting an older man with a relatively low but equal risk of depression in male and female relatives). Originally the distinction depended on whether the first attack of depression occurred before the age of 40, a relatively straightforward criterion. More recently he has suggested that family history (a much less reliable datum) be used as follows: pure depressive disease where there is a history of depression but not of alcoholism or sociopathy in first-degree relatives; depressive spectrum disease where there is a history of alcoholism or sociopathy in a first-degree relative; sporadic depressive disease where there is no family history of alcoholism, sociopathy or depression (Winokur, Behar, VanValkenberg & Lowry, 1978). These are stimulating if over-simplifying ideas, but their clinical or therapeutic significance remains to be demonstrated.

17
Mixed affective states and other syndromes

JAMES L. GIBBONS

This chapter is concerned with 'mixtures' of mania and depression (mixed affective states) and of schizophrenia and affective psychoses (schizo-affective psychoses), with involutional melancholia and with two syndromes (depersonalization, hypochondriasis) that are often, but by no means always, associated with a depressive syndrome.

Mixed affective states

Kraepelin postulated that mood, activity, and thought sometimes varied independently during the transition from depression to mania or vice versa, producing 'mixed states' (*Mischzustände*). There are six possible permutations which he described as follows:

(1) depressive or anxious mania (flight of ideas, over-activity, anxiety)
(2) excited (agitated) depression (inhibition of thought, over-activity, depressed mood)
(3) unproductive mania (inhibition of thought, over-activity, elation)
(4) manic stupor (flight of ideas, gross motor retardation, elation)
(5) depression with flight of ideas (flight of ideas, motor retardation, depression)
(6) inhibited mania (inhibition of thought, motor retardation, elation)

These states were usually transitional, occasionally persistent. Kraepelin also pointed out that an otherwise typical manic episode might be briefly interrupted by depressive symptoms and vice versa. Elated patients sometimes reiterated hypochondriacal delusions, while depressive delusions sometimes had a grandiose quality.

We have already seen, in the chapter on mania (chapter 15), that modern authors have noted that depressive symptoms are common in mania. Loudon, Blackburn and Ashworth (1977) doubted the usefulness of the concept of mixed states because of this. American authors speak of mixed states when patients satisfy criteria for the diagnosis of mania and depression during a single episode of illness. Himmelhoch, Mulla and Neil (1976) reported that the first episode of affective illness was mixed in this sense in 31 per cent of 84 bipolar patients. Winokur, Clayton and Reich (1969) observed mixed episodes in 10 to 61 bipolar patients. In general the patients showed 'manic' speech and activity, but 'depressive' vegetative symptoms. Delusions were more often depressive than manic, but mood fluctuated remarkably from ecstasy to despair.

Clinical experience supports the conclusion drawn from the reports mentioned above, that Kraepelinian mixed states with *sustained* mood change are now very rare. Agitated depression, far from being a mixed state, appears to be almost confined to unipolar patients (Beigel & Murphy, 1971; Himmelhoch *et al.*, 1976). However mixed states with variable mood do occur and may be very difficult to diagnose if they are persistent rather than transitional phases. A history of previous discrete episodes of frank mania or depression or of depressive symptoms immediately prior to the mixed episode was the rule in the cases of Winokur and colleagues: and this observation should prove helpful in diagnosis.

Schizo-affective psychoses

This term was coined by Kasanin (1933), who described nine cases of psychosis of sudden onset and relatively short duration (a few months) with fantastic delusions and sometimes hallucinations in young people in the face of recent or persistent stress. He used the term because he considered that the patients showed both schizophrenic and affective symptoms. In subsequent years the diagnosis has been applied to a variable group of patients showing features of both schizophrenia and affective psychosis during the same episode. According to the criteria of Spitzer, Endicott and Robins (1978), for

example, such patients must meet the criteria for either mania or depression and exhibit at least one characteristic feature of schizophrenia (such as delusions of control). The topic has recently been reviewed by Procci (1976).

Some workers, on the evidence of follow-up and family studies, have concluded that schizo-affective psychosis is a form of affective psychosis (Clayton, Rodin & Winokur, 1968). Others, using similar methods of investigation but different diagnostic criteria, regard the disorder as a form of schizophrenia with a marked tendency to become chronic and disabling (Welner, Welner & Fishman, 1979). A third view is to regard these patients as a mixed group of as yet undiagnosed schizophrenics and affective psychotics. Thus Tsuang (1979) concluded from a twin study that schizo-affective psychosis with an onset before 30 is most often genetically related to schizophrenia; when the onset occurs after 40, the disorder is genetically related to affective psychosis. Finally some workers contend that there is a form of psychosis, with a benign if sometimes relapsing course, that is intermediate between schizophrenia and affective psychosis but nosologically distinct from both. The most recent example of this view is Perris's (1974) concept of 'cycloid psychosis', based on an earlier formulation by Leonhard (1961).

An explanation of this confusion and disagreement is provided by Brockington and Leff (1979), who applied eight sets of criteria for the diagnosis of schizo-affective psychosis to 119 newly admitted psychotic patients under the age of 65. The number of patients satisfying the various criteria ranged from 1 to 17 and the concordance among the various sets of criteria was low, much lower than in similar studies of schizophrenia and mania. It is clear that there is little agreement about which patients should be included in the schizo-affective group.

It is thus impossible at present to judge among the four different concepts mentioned above. Yet the problem is an important one because the number of these patients is considerable. Indeed Brockington and Leff argue that the incidence of schizo-affective psychosis is comparable to that of mania. The problem of defining schizophrenic symptoms and of detecting them in excited patients is considered in chapter 19. It must also be remembered that some schizophrenic patients become depressed as a result of their schizophrenic experiences; it would be wrong to regard such patients as schizo-affective.

Involutional melancholia

This term was applied by Kraepelin to a form of depression that he considered nosologically distinct from manic-depressive psychosis, although he later changed this view. It referred to agitated depression, especially with hypochondriacal and nihilistic delusions, occurring for the first time in late middle life and likely to last for three to four years. In the 1930s a number of American authors described series of such patients, stressing their pre-morbid obsessional personalities. With the advent of electroconvulsive treatment, fully developed typical cases were seen less frequently. Stenstedt (1959) argued from a family study that involutional melancholia was a mixture of cases of manic-depressive psychosis and of neurotic depression. Later Kendell (1968) concluded from multivariate analysis of clinical data that the disorder could not be distinguished from psychotic depression. The whole topic has been well reviewed by Rosenthal (1968). It now seems that classical involutional melancholia was merely untreated unipolar depression occurring in later life.

Depersonalization

This is a feeling of change in the self, experienced as one of strangeness or unreality. Derealization, which is often associated with depersonalization, is a similar feeling about the outside world. The experience is unpleasant and the subject has insight into the 'as if' quality of the experience, which is not elaborated in a delusional way. A complaint of inability to feel, a loss of affective response, is usual (Ackner, 1954). The experience is very difficult to put into words. Typical expressions include: 'I feel dead.' 'I'm detached from everything, distant, remote.' 'It's like a curtain between me and everything else.' 'The world looks as if it's made of cardboard.' 'Nothing looks real any longer. It's all two-dimensional.' 'Everything's changed. It's all grey.'

Other symptoms, not always present, include distortion of the body image ('my fingers feel huge', 'my body is too light'), metamorphopsia, physical symptoms ('pressure on the head'), the experience of seeing oneself as if from outside the body, slowing in the subjective sense of time, even olfactory hallucinations. At the most severe, the patient may complain of having no head, no face, no shadow, being 'like a living ghost'.

Depersonalization occurs in otherwise normal subjects: in at least 40 per cent of groups of students investigated by questionnaires. The experience has been recorded in fatigue, after alcohol consumption, after sleep deprivation, in febrile illness, during hallucinogenic drug use, all conditions possibly associated with minor alterations of consciousness (for references, see Sedman, 1966). The experience is also a well-known symptom in several psychiatric and neurological disorders. The latter include temporal lobe epilepsy and cerebral tumour, although depersonalization is rare in gross organic psychosyndromes. It occurs in anxiety states, particularly in phobic anxiety (Roth, 1960), when it may be chronic or recurrent but fleeting. Depersonalization is well known in schizophrenia: in one study it was detected in 11 per cent of 54 consecutive admissions (Sedman & Kenna, 1963). Unfortunately, one well-known writer used the term 'depersonalization' to mean delusions of control (Langfeldt, 1960). This usage should not be imitated. Its occurrence in depressive states has been the subject of controversy. Lewis (1934) observed depersonalization in 31 per cent and derealization in 34 per cent of his series, while Gittleson (1967) found depersonalization recorded in the case notes of almost 20 per cent of a large series of depressive psychosis. Roth (1960) has contended that depersonalization is rare in 'endogenous depression'. The discrepancy is explained by Sedman and Reed (1963), who found depersonalization in 30 per cent of depressed patients ('psychotic' and 'neurotic') with insecure personalities, but in only 4 per cent of 'psychotic' depressives with normal personalities.

Occasional patients present with depersonalization as the primary symptom, with any affective disturbance clearly secondary. This disorder, like depersonalization generally, is commoner in women and characteristically begins suddenly in adolescence or early adult life: it may persist for years, sometimes with remissions (Shorvon, 1946; Davison, 1964).

The occurrence of depersonalization at the height of phobic anxiety and in response to life-threatening danger (Noyes & Kletti, 1977) suggests that it may sometimes be a protective mechanism. Consideration of the various theories of depersonalization is beyond the scope of this chapter; the reader should consult the excellent review by Sedman (1970).

Hypochondriasis

This brief section can do no more than touch on the complex problem of hypochondriasis. For more detailed consideration and references to the literature the reader is referred to the review by Kenyon (1976) and to volume 4, chapter 8.

Hypochondriasis is a morbid preoccupation with one's state of health: the subject is excessively and unpleasantly worried about his health and is unable to control his worry. Minor physical symptoms, often due to perception of physiological changes, are exceedingly common in the general population (Wadsworth, Butterfield & Blaney, 1971). In certain individuals, particularly of anxious or obsessional personality, the experience of illness in themselves or others or some other influence makes the symptoms the object of morbid scrutiny that leads to medical consultation. At this stage the doctor, by giving specific reassurance, may relieve the symptoms, but he may perpetuate them if he is unaware of the nature of the complaint (Mayou, 1976).

In psychiatric practice hypochondriasis is most often associated with, and considered to be secondary to, depression. (This may be due to selection and may not be the case in general medical clinics, as Mayou (1976) points out.) Hypochondriasis is more usually associated with neurotic depression and is often listed as a symptom that helps to distinguish between endogenous and neurotic syndromes (Kendell, 1968). Hypochondriacal delusions, however, are characteristic of the endogenous syndrome. Delusions of bodily change or disease are also, of course, seen in schizophrenia and sometimes appear as 'monosymptomatic' psychoses (Riding & Munro, 1975). Examples of the latter, which sometimes occur in a setting of depression, are patients who believe that they emit an odour or believe that some part of their body (e.g. nose, mouth or ears) is too large, too small, or in some way disfigured. When depressive symptoms are present it may be difficult to decide whether they are primary or secondary. (See also chapter 5.)

There remains a small but important group of patients, sometimes said to be suffering from primary hypochondriasis, who have chronic and disabling physical complaints, usually of pain, for which no physical cause is found despite intensive investigation. Spontaneous psychological complaints are few. These patients tend to be referred to psychiatrists as a last resort, much to the patients' annoyance. The St. Louis group have described a form of this disorder, said to occur only in women and regarded as a manifestation of hysteria, which they call Briquet's syndrome. Characteristic features include recurrent pains, conversion symptoms, nervousness, sexual and marital discord, repeated admissions to hospital, and repeated surgical operations (Guze & Perley, 1963). Kendell (1974), in an interesting paper, suggests that 'primary hypochondriacs' are best regarded as people who derive benefit from the sick role and he suggests an appropriate therapeutic approach. However, Kreitman, Sainsbury, Pearce and Costain (1965) claim that a proportion of such patients are suffering from a depressive illness – they do not look depressed or complain of depression, but give much the same answers to questions about mood and associated symptoms as depressives generally – and respond to antidepressant treatment. Symptoms of depressive illness should therefore always be sought in patients with apparently primary hypochondriasis.

18
Affective psychosis in adolescence

PHILIP GRAHAM

Prevalence

It is well recognized that psychotic disorders of affective type do occur during adolescence, although the experience of those running adolescent units (Sands, 1956; Warren, 1965) suggests that they are uncommon and that bipolar illness is rarely observed. More controversial is the issue whether such psychoses can occur before puberty. Most authorities consider that they do, but again with extreme rarity, and when such pre-pubertal disorders do occur it is usually in the year or two before external secondary sexual characteristics appear. As endocrine changes in the body precede the appearance of such characteristics by a couple of years, and as, in most case reports, the description of the stage of pubescence which the patient has reached is usually not provided, the issue remains uncertain. Depression occurring in children is discussed in volume 4, chapter 5, and the meagre genetic literature in chapter 36 of the present volume.

Causation

The question whether pre-pubertal affective psychosis occurs is by no means an academic one, but crucial to a consideration of causation, for if the condition does not occur before puberty, the physiological and/or psychological changes associated with sexual maturation must be of vital importance for the condition to appear. As in older patients suffering from these conditions, the frequency of first-degree relatives being affected suggests that genetic factors are of importance. A history of early deprivation or early loss is not uncommon as a background feature. Precipitating factors include environmental stress and febrile illness. The condition occurs too rarely in adolescence for any of these factors to have been systematically examined in this age period.

Clinical picture

Most adolescents with this condition present classically with features of hypomanic or depressive illness similar to those occurring in adulthood (Anthony & Scott, 1960). In general, adolescents tend to show rather more florid symptomatology with antisocial behaviour prominent in hypomanic episodes, and to be somewhat more responsive to environmental change such as admission to hospital. However, this is by no means invariable. A number of authors have suggested that manic-depressive psychosis can present in childhood and early adolescence with an entirely different clinical picture. Davis (1979) suggests that the condition should be diagnosed when outbursts of severe loss of emotional control are accompanied by hyperactivity and disturbed interpersonal relationships in children with a strong family history of manic-depressive disorder. Clearly caution is required before assuming that an over-active child with severe tantrums is showing a form of affective psychosis, but where the problem appears severe and atypical, and occurs in the presence of a family history, it would certainly be reasonable to consider the use of treatment usually reserved for more classically presenting affective psychoses. In differential diagnosis in pre-pubertal children, the possible presence of the much more commonly occurring conduct or emotional disorders should always be taken into account. In adolescence, purely depressive disorders may be confused with anorexia nervosa and, where thought disorder, delusions, and hallucinations are present, an early form of schizophrenia will be an alternative diagnosis.

Management

Disabling affective symptoms are usually an indication for a period of in-patient assessment and treatment. In early adolescence, it is certainly helpful to be able to admit to an adolescent or child psychiatric unit partly because such units are generally more geared to the family approach necessary with disorders occurring in the dependent young, and partly because they contain educational provision. Older adolescents may be satisfactorily nursed on adult wards, although many feel that here, too, the adolescent or young people's unit provides a more satisfactory alternative. In appraising the problem, interviews with the whole family may be a helpful supplement to individual sessions with the patient and parents.

In treatment, attention to stressful factors and supportive psychotherapy will usually need to be supplemented by medication, especially antidepressants and tranquillizing agents (see chapter 26). Except in early adolescence, when dosage should be adjusted to body weight, levels prescribed can be similar to those used in adulthood. The use of lithium carbonate in children and adolescents has been helpfully reviewed by Youngerman and Canino (1978) who suggest that the proven effectiveness of this agent in young people is limited to those with a history of affective disorder in a first-degree relative, although the drug may be prophylactic in other situations. ECT is rarely indicated in adolescence.

Prognosis

Although it is sometimes suggested that disorders in adolescence are of less ominous significance because of the fact that adolescence is normally a turbulent period, the evidence for this view is lacking. Certainly some adolescents do suffer from isolated episodes but the appearance of an affective psychosis in adolescence may also be a prelude to recurrent episodes of disabling disorder.

19
Differential diagnosis of affective psychoses

JAMES L. GIBBONS

Mania

The main problem is to distinguish mania from schizophrenia (or from what some investigators call the manic form of schizo-affective psychosis). The hypothesis put forward in this volume is that schizophrenia and mania are related in an hierarchical manner, so that definite and persistent schizophrenic symptoms indicate a diagnosis of schizophrenia, even though the patient shows other features that would support a diagnosis of mania. Such schizophrenic symptoms include, as well as first-rank symptoms, persistent non-affective hallucinations and delusions. Thought disorder is often put forward as a diagnostic feature of schizophrenia and contrasted with flight of ideas. However, the speech of an acutely excited manic patient may become as incoherent as that of a schizophrenic with 'loosened associations'. Indeed formal tests for schizophrenic thought disorder failed to discriminate between schizophrenics and manics (Breakey & Goodell, 1972). At the height of a severe manic state it may be impossible to perform an accurate mental state examination or to decide whether a patient's account of an apparent first-rank symptom is a direct account of experience or has an 'as if' quality. Too much attention should not therefore be paid to apparent schizophrenic symptoms in very severe mania: these may disappear as the extreme excitement begins to subside (Carlson & Goodwin, 1973). Other features besides the mental state must be taken into account in doubtful cases: a stable and extravert previous personality, a history of depressive symptoms immediately before the current episode of illness, a history of a previous attack of typical mania or depression with full recovery, and a family history of mania would all support a diagnosis of mania.

The hierarchical principle has therapeutic as well as theoretical implications. The acute schizophrenic symptoms are treated first, with the expectations that any 'secondary' affective symptoms or anxiety (which are very common) will subside as the schizophrenic symptoms disappear. Of course if the latter do not respond to treatment, the affective symptoms are treated in their own right (see chapter 20).

Until recently many American psychiatrists diagnosed schizophrenia in patients whom British psychiatrists regarded as manic. This situation has changed and several American workers seem to have concluded that mania is hierarchically 'superior' to schizophrenia, so that a patient fulfilling diagnostic criteria for mania should be diagnosed as manic even if he displays first-rank symptoms, non-affective delusions and hallucinations, and so on (Pope & Lipinski, 1978). In a series of papers Abrams and Taylor (1976) have claimed that patients who meet their criteria for mania (over-activity; rapid or pressured speech; euphoric, expansive, or irritable mood; flight of ideas or grandiosity; no recent drug abuse) and who also show 'schizophrenic' symptoms resemble typical manics in pre-morbid personality, outcome, response to lithium, and family history. This claim must be taken seriously and confirmed or refuted by other investigators. One possible cause of error is how rigorously first-rank symptoms are defined and detected. Wing and Nixon (1975) studied cases in the International Pilot Study of Schizophrenia where there was a clinical diagnosis of mania in spite of the recorded presence of first-rank symptoms. In several instances the examples given by the clinician suggested that a first-rank symptom had been recorded when it was not in fact present, as when a patient whose thoughts were 'so great they came from God' was incorrectly said to have thought-insertion. (See also chapter 6.)

There may be occasional diagnostic confusion between mania and organic psychoses. In acute mania, disorientation, apparently purposeless over-activity, and incoherent speech may suggest delir-ium. Symptoms resembling hypomania may be prominent in subacute delirious states and in chronic organic psychoses such as neurosyphilis. Here clouding of consciousness and/or recent memory defect should enable the distinction to be made.

Depressive psychosis

The same hierarchical principle applies in the distinction between depressive psychosis and schizophrenia (see also chapter 6). Persistent non-affective delusions or hallucinations, and even depressive auditory hallucinations that are continuous rather than occasional, suggest a diagnosis of schizophrenia. Where the nature of the hallucinations or delusions is uncertain, their temporal relationship to the mood change is important. If they first become apparent after the onset of the depression, and if they decline as the intensity of the depression lessens, they can be regarded as probable depressive symptoms. Schizophrenic patients, of course, do get depressed because of their bewildering and terrifying experiences, and the development of a depressed mood after the onset of psychotic symptoms can often be understood in this way. It is also well known that schizophrenic patients, whether or not treated with long-acting neuroleptics, may develop an endogenous depressive syndrome shortly after the remission of an acute schizophrenic episode (for references see Sheldrick, Jablensky, Sartorius & Shepherd, 1977).

In the elderly depressed and paranoid patient it is sometimes difficult to distinguish depressive psychosis from *late paraphrenia*. A diagnosis of depression is almost certainly correct when there are only a few persecutory symptoms with depressive colouring. When the paranoid symptoms are more extensive and the depression is marked, it may be wisest not to make a firm initial diagnosis but rather to decide whether the first line of treatment should be directed against depression or paraphrenia (Post, 1976).

A much commoner problem is to distinguish between depression and dementia, because depressive illness can closely mimic a chronic organic psychosyndrome (depressive pseudodementia). This occurs more often in the elderly, but is well documented in middle-aged patients, in whom pre-senile dementia may erroneously be diagnosed (Kiloh, 1961). More immediately obvious than the depressive features may be disorientation, impaired recent memory, and a poor knowledge of current events.

Personal habits may deteriorate and the patient may have difficulty in performing simple tasks. Occasional patients give ridiculously incorrect answers, suggesting the operation of hysterical mechanisms (Post, 1976).

Clues to the correct diagnosis include the presence, when sought for, of depressive symptoms (which may have preceded the 'organic' symptoms), a short history with a relatively acute onset, and a history of a previous episode of 'endogenous' depression with full recovery (Kiloh, 1961). Routine psychometric tests may fail to distinguish between depression and dementia, but a specialized test battery, recently revised, is reported to discriminate well (Kendrick, Gibson & Moyes, 1979). The EEG may be helpful and Kiloh (1961) has remarked that a normal EEG with well-developed alpha rhythm in any 'demented' patient should lead to careful consideration of the possibility of depressive pseudodementia.

In the elderly, as Post (1976) has pointed out, a severe depressive illness of rapid onset may be mistaken for an acute psycho-organic syndrome. Here misdiagnosis is less serious, because the diagnosis of depressive psychosis is likely to have become clear by the time physical investigations have been completed.

The distinction between endogenous (or psychotic) depression and neurotic (or reactive) depression has been mentioned in chapter 16. Typical examples of either disorder are readily recognized, but there is considerable clinical overlap. One well-known device to discriminate between the two syndromes is the Newcastle Diagnostic Index, whereby a score is calculated from the presence or absence of a number of clinical and historical features as follows: adequate personality, +1; no adequate psychogenesis, +2; distinct quality of depressive mood, +1; weight loss, +2; previous episode, +1; depressive psychomotor activity, +2; anxiety, −1; nihilistic delusions, +2; blames others, −1; guilt, +1. A score of six or more indicates 'endogenous', a score of five or less, 'neurotic' depression (Carney, Roth & Garside, 1965). Definitions of these items are given in the original paper.

The controversy over the possibility of drawing a sharp distinction between depression and anxiety is mainly concerned with 'neurotic' depression (for references see Tyrer, 1979). Patients with 'endogenous' depression usually admit to symptoms of anxiety on direct questioning; occasionally their presenting complaints are physical or, less often, psychological manifestations of anxiety. Occasionally a depressed patient may complain of dread, on first waking, of what the day holds for him. At its most severe, this symptom can develop into delusions of catastrophe. Any apparently anxious patient should be asked about depressive symptoms. This is particularly so when the patient is over 40 and is experiencing his or her first episode of psychiatric disorder. It should be recalled that severe anxiety states can be accompanied by 'secondary' depression, particularly the chronic phobias.

'Endogenous' depression is often misdiagnosed as physical disease when the patient's presenting complaint is one of the many physical symptoms of depression, such as loss of weight, constipation, occipital headache, pressure on the chest, and so on. A careful history will usually indicate the depressive origin of all these complaints. Nevertheless, since the endogenous syndrome is more likely to occur after forty, when physical disease is also more common, appropriate physical investigations should accompany treatment of the depression if there is doubt about the significance of any of the physical symptoms. Clinical experience suggests that the depression accompanying physical disease is most likely to resemble 'neurotic' depression. Therefore, if a patient has both physical and depressive symptoms, it seems likely that the more typical his psychiatric symptoms are of the 'endogenous' syndrome, the more likely are both groups of symptoms to be due to depression and to respond to antidepressant treatment. This view, although plausible, lacks experimental evidence at present.

The distinction between 'normal' grief and clinically significant depression mainly concerns the 'neurotic' syndrome. Studies by the St Louis group showed that depression, sleep disturbance, and crying are very frequent after bereavement. Retardation and the fear of going insane were not seen. Most subjects improved within two to three months. A small proportion had more persistent symptoms, but rarely sought psychiatric help (Clayton, Halikas & Maurice, 1972). It is well-known, of course, that a typical episode of 'endogenous' depression may follow bereavement, often after a symptom-free interval.

The distinction between clinically significant depression and normal sadness generally is also chiefly concerned with 'neurotic' depression. A diagnosis of depression is usually considered to be justified when depressed mood is accompanied by symptoms such as anorexia, insomnia, loss of libido, etc., or when the depression is itself a burden on the patient. However the case of bipolar patients shows that minor 'endogenous' episodes, readily recognized by the patient, occur. One such patient said that he would have regarded his earlier waking (at 6 a.m. instead of 7), his drowsiness in the mornings, his diminished libido and his mildly impaired concentration as a normal variant if it had not been for his previous experience of similar but much more severe symptoms in an episode of frank depression. In the absence of a previous history of mania or of endogenous depression, the significance of such minor symptoms is a matter of clinical judgement. Sometimes a trial of antidepressant medication may be thought worthwhile, although any subsequent improvement may be a placebo response rather than a pharmacological effect.

20

The course and prognosis of affective psychoses

PAUL E. BEBBINGTON

Methodological problems

Kraepelin's early opinion that the course of a psychiatric disease should be one of the criteria for its diagnosis has cast a long shadow over studies of outcome in the psychoses. It explains why some authors regard a case of manic-depressive psychosis with a poor outcome as something to be explained away whatever the cost (Astrup et al., 1959). Kraepelin (1920) later withdrew from this extreme and logically untenable position. Other authorities have always held that the syndrome complex rather than the course must be the basis of disease theories in psychiatry (Hoch, 1912).

The adoption of a syndromal approach allows an open-minded review of similarities and differences in outcome. This means that we can become interested in, rather than embarrassed by, those cases which show unequivocal symptoms of affective disorder but later develop episodes with schizophrenic symptoms or pursue a chronic course characterized by persecutory delusions or by the negative symptoms which are often seen in chronic schizophrenia.

A further difficulty is left over from the Kraepelinian insistence that course is a necessary part of the disease definition. If someone displays schizophrenic symptoms, is he then classed as schizophrenic for all time? Are subsequent non-schizophrenic psychiatric symptoms to be taken as incipient or partial schizophrenic relapse? It is more logical and informative to classify relapses in their own symptomatic right as the hierarchical approach would suggest (see chapter 7). This approach has only recently been adopted (McGlashan & Carpenter, 1976; Sheldrick *et al.*, 1977) but it holds out the possibility of a more complete account of the course of the functional disorders, freed from *a priori* assumptions.

Dissatisfaction with categorical classification in psychiatry (Kendell, 1976) has led to an increased interest in the hierarchical grouping of psychiatric disorder (Foulds & Bedford, 1975; Wing, 1978b; Wing *et al.*, 1978). These groupings are based upon certain key symptoms which predict but are not predicted by lower-order symptoms. Any such grouping is arbitrary unless it can be shown to specify other aspects of the disease concepts involved. Perhaps the best justification for a hierarchical classification would arise if at least some of these aspects were themselves arranged hierarchically. The course of affective psychoses provides one such opportunity to test their position in the symptomatic hierarchy.

The hierarchy of psychiatric disorders has been expounded by Wing (1978b). Organic symptoms take precedence over those of functional psychoses and neuroses which in turn are of higher order than the 'lesser psychiatric disorders' – non-specific syndromes for which no disease theory has been convincingly put forward. Within the functional disorders, schizophrenia pre-empts other psychoses, which in turn take precedence over depressive neuroses and the anxiety states. At the base of the hierarchy are the minor non-specific neuroses.

Any attempt at comparing prognostic studies makes it immediately apparent that authors use different concepts and definitions of the affective disorders and that the distinction between depressive psychosis and neurosis is particularly poorly standardized. Most studies have hitherto been carried out on series of in-patients or out-patients (Zis & Goodwin, 1979; Nyström, 1979), thus imposing a degree of limitation on the range of severity. Even so, series based on University clinics or on specialist units (for instance, those particularly interested in lithium therapy) must restrict the generalizability of the findings. Recent studies of general population samples, however, have markedly extended the range of severity (Weissman & Myers, 1978; Wing *et al.*, 1978).

The policies and practicalities of service use are important in the assessment of course, as in the determination of cases (Perris, 1968). They determine the duration of the attack before admission and the way eligibility for discharge is governed by mental state. Where the length of admission defines duration of attack and discharge is taken to indicate recovery, an artificially better prognosis for the individual episode will arise within community-orientated services.

From an early stage, a distinction was made between the *Streckenprognose*, the prognosis for the attack, and the *Richtungsprognose*, the long term outcome, of affective psychosis. These two issues demand different resources of investigation; the immediate prognosis is more easily made. However, after discharge the patient may remain well, or relapse and be readmitted, or relapse and seek treatment elsewhere. He may have minor relapses or mood disturbances without seeking help from a physician. He may suffer some social disadvantage as a result of his diathesis which does not come to medical notice. The patient's disabilities may involve his family who may react to it, suffer from it, and cover it up. The longer the follow-up period and the more information, other than re-admission, available, the less optimistic the prognosis.

Early workers used medical records as a means for both case designation and follow-up (e.g. Swift, 1907; MacDonald, 1918). These were usually of one hospital, although Pollock (1931) had access to New York State records, and Passkind (1930) reported only on the out-patients seen by one private psychiatrist.

Such studies are obviously but to an unknowable degree dependent upon the quality of the hospital records. As follow-up information derives from the subjects' readmission to hospital only those of poor prognosis are truly followed up and an unknown number even of readmitted cases may be given a good prognosis because they have been admitted elsewhere without the author's knowledge. Such studies may not state the actual length of follow-up. Studies based on a cohort of patients for follow-up by interview with patient or relative carry the possibility of more extended criteria of outcome, including information about intervening episodes and mental and social state at follow-up, supplemented by data from other sources. Most weight must be placed upon such research. Some studies have the additional virtue of providing individual case histories (e.g. Lewis, 1936).

Duration of the attack

The problems of chronicity and incidental death are avoided by using an actuarial method: plotting the probability of recovery against duration of the attack. Only Norris (1959) has done this (fig. 20.1).

Studies which give information about the length of episode are listed in table 20.1 and the factors which modify this are given in table 20.2. It is not easy to arrive at a consensus about duration. Studies pre-dating effective treatment include those showing the longest duration. This is not due to the inclusion of chronic cases, which were specifically excluded by Steen (1933). Huston and Locher (1948) were able to show shorter illnesses after the introduction of ECT. However, Rennie (1942) recorded quite short attacks before this. It may well be that varying service traditions distort the picture. Bratfos and Haug (1968), Shobe and Brion (1971) and Angst and colleagues (1973) are the only authors who date onset from the start of symptoms. The importance of this has recently been underlined by Winokur (1976) in whose study 22 per cent of manics, 54 per cent of bipolar depressives and 54 per cent of unipolar depressives had been ill for six months before admission. The short duration reported by Angst and colleagues (1973) may be accounted for by inclusion of non-treated and out-patient cases. Passkind (1930) showed that attacks treated on an out-patient basis were indeed briefer.

Angst and colleagues (1973) and Pollock (1931) failed to demonstrate any tendency for episodes to become longer in individual patients, although Rennie (1942) claimed that later manic attacks were longer than earlier ones. Constancy of episode length agrees with the negative findings of Steen (1933) and Bratfos and Haug (1968) regarding the effect of prior attacks (table 20.2). The most robust (and most tested) result in table 20.2 is that episodes of manic-depressive psychosis in later life last longer. There is soft evidence that this distinction has been reduced by the introduction of ECT. It can be assumed that sex, family history of affective disorder, and severity have no effect upon duration. Data concerning personality and physique are suspect and are not included in the table.

In the absence of an actuarial approach, a full account of the immediate prognosis requires that we complement information about duration with the probability of recovery. Findings from the literature are presented in table 20.3. The issue of the nature of the chronic effects of manic-depressive illness will be dealt with later. It may be mentioned here that these figures, albeit in reasonable agreement, often involve assumptions concerning mental state at and after discharge. Recently Paykel and colleagues (1974) and Weissman and Klerman (1977) have revealed that persistent minor disablement can occur in a significant proportion even of those who are less severely affected.

Likelihood of relapse

The likelihood of relapse (table 20.4) presents further difficulties of definition and procedure (Perris, 1968). If length of hospital stay is the criterion of episode, liberal policies tend to show more episodes of shorter duration. Episodes undoubtedly occur which do not lead to admission: Bratfos and Haug (1968) reckon readmissions accounted for only 70 per cent of subsequent episodes in their series. If these are to be counted, problems of reliability of definition and of reporting immediately arise. This issue becomes more significant in the light of the follow-up studies of Kiloh and colleagues (1960), Kessel and Holt (1966), and Bratfos and Haug (1968), which reveal high rates of minor relapse during short term follow-up. These reports are also of interest in terms of the actuarial study of Fleiss and colleagues (1978) which suggests that relapse probability may have short- and long-term components.

Relapse rate is also dependent upon patient selection; if only first attenders are included in a given period of selection, a lower relapse rate will result

Fig. 20.1. Manic-depressive reaction. Weekly discharge rates per 1000 exposures (From Norris, 1959, p. 149).

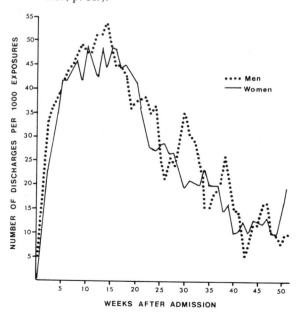

Table 20.1. *Duration of attack*

Study	N	Duration	Notes
Panse (1924)	205	7 months mean	All attacks. Only cases first admitted age: 40–65
Malzberg (1929)	11393	9 months mean	1st admissions
Wertham (1929)	2000	8½ months mean	Mania only
Pollock (1931)	424	1.1 years mean	1st attack
Steen (1933)	493	1.5 years mean	All admissions. Chronic cases excluded
Fuller (1935)	327	6 months mean	All admissions
Rennie (1942)	208	3½ months mean: mania 6½ months mean: depression	1st admissions
Lundquist (1945)	319	6 months mean (age < 30) 8½ months mean (age > 30)	No difference between manic and depressive attacks
Huston & Locher (1948)	80 (no ECT)	1.75 years mean 1.25 years median	1st attacks
	74 (ECT)	12½ months mean 9 months median	
Kinkelin (1954)	146	6 months mean: mania 7½ months mean: depression	1st admissions
Taschev (1965)	372	6 months mean: males 4½ months mean: females	All admissions
Bratfos & Haug (1968)	176	13 months mean 7 months median	Attacks dated from beginning to end of symptoms. Mean hospital stay 9 weeks
Shobe & Brion (1971)	111	8 months mean 6 months median	Attacks dated from onset of symptoms; private practice. Out-patients
Angst et al. (1973)	1027	3 months mean	All attacks, including those untreated; dated from onset of symptoms

than if all attenders are eligible. In the latter case, relapsers will have a greater chance of selection than those remaining well.

The rate of relapse is obviously dependent upon the duration of follow-up. Angst and colleagues (1973) argue that if cases are followed long enough, virtually all relapse. Oltman and Friedman (1962) who studied completed life histories give figures which support this. After my correction for chronic cases (table 20.4), 92 per cent relapsed. The definition of relapse is related to that of the interval between attacks. Like duration of attack, and for similar reasons, these two aspects of prognosis are therefore best dealt with jointly in an actuarial manner, by the computation of relapse probability during given time periods. A crude attempt at this was made in the admirable early study of Lundquist (1945). A sophisticated use of this approach is the study of the effects of lithium prophylaxis on relapse by Fleiss and colleagues (1978).

A large majority of studies from Kraepelin's (1920) onwards show a decreasing interval between attacks. These surveys are based upon *mean* intervals. Lewis (1936) felt that the study of individual cases gave scant evidence for this. Slater (1938) pointed out that a case with three illnesses in a set follow-up period could not have intervals of as great potential length as a case with only two illnesses and thus all second intervals arrived at in such a way must be shorter on average. This in fact applies whether

Table 20.2 *Factors which modify the duration of episode*

Study	N	Sex	Family history	Prior attacks	Slow onset	Bipolarity	Mania	Severity	Hallucinations	Delusions	Confusion	Monotony	Stupor	Late onset
Wertham (1929)	2000													+
Pollock (1931)	8438	0												+
Steen (1933)	493			0	+				-	+			-	0
Rennie (1942)	208		0					0						+
Lundquist (1945)	319	0		0	+[b]		0		? -	+[a]	-	+		+
Huston & Locher (1948)	154	0		0	0			0						+[c]
Kinkelin (1954)	146													+
Bratfos & Haug (1968)	176	0		0			-							0
Shobe & Brion (1971)	111						0	0						
Angst et al. (1973)	1027					-								+

[a] In the younger group only.
[b] In the older group only.
[c] In the non-ECT group only.

Explanation + = positive association with long duration; 0 = no association; - = negative association otherwise variables are not reported.

Table 20.3. *Probability of recovery from first episode*

Study	N	Follow-up in years	% recovered	Notes
Steen (1933)	493	3–12	*81*	
Fuller (1935)	327	10	*72*	
Lewis (1936)	57	7–8	*88*	
Rennie (1942)	208	*c.* 20	*79*	recovered and improved group, plus some who recovered post-discharge
Lundquist (1945)	319	<10–30	*92* mania *80* depression	
Huston & Locher (1948)	80	1–12	*79*	
Astrup *et al.* (1959)	70	>5	*70*	highly selected 'typical cases'
Norris (1959)	2298	2–5	*81*	includes 10 per cent self-discharges against advice
Bratfos & Haug (1968)	218	1–12	*79*	
Shobe & Brion (1971)	151	14–20	*80*	
D'Elia *et al.* (1974)	72	10, average	*92*	'non-psychotic'

the follow-up period is set or randomly variable. Slater (1938) studied 116 of Kraepelin's own patients and using analysis of variance was unable in the individual patient to show a declining interval.

Very few authorities seem aware of 'Slater's fallacy'. Bratfos and Haug (1968) were, but it is not clear that they avoided it although they did not find decreasing duration of subsequent intervals. It should also be noted that in their large series, Angst and colleagues (1973) do claim to show a decreasing interval in the individual patient.

When we turn to the factors which are associated with likelihood of relapse, we must share Lewis's (1936) pessimism. Severity of first episode (Brodwall, 1947; Shobe & Brion, 1971) and sex (Pollock, 1931; Perris, 1968) do not seem associated. There is suggestive evidence that the relationship between age of onset and relapse is U-shaped, with a higher probability in the youngest and oldest age groups (Swift, 1907; Pollock, 1931; Rennie, 1942) which makes it strange that Carlson and colleagues (1977) should compare these groups in order to test the idea that early onset manic-depressive psychosis has a poor prognosis. Winokur (1975) suggests that whatever the

age of onset, attacks tend to occur in flurries and the process 'burns out'. The really robust finding is that unipolar depression has a lower likelihood of relapse than circular, alternating or manic illnesses.

Norris (1959) showed that the distribution of readmissions differs from that expected from the Poisson distribution. More single episodes and more high-frequency relapses occurred than expected. These results suggest a tendency towards two separate patterns but Norris did not analyze the data in terms of polarity.

Chronicity

Manic-depressive psychosis may become 'chronic' by virtue of social impairment, continuation of affective symptoms, or a change in symptomatology. It seems likely that social impairment in this condition is largely due to the influence of persistent affective symptoms which may however be trivial in themselves. Indeed Weissman and Paykel (1974) claimed some social impairment in their unipolar depressed women even when euthymic. Holmboe and colleagues (1968) report stable working capacity in less than half of their series of 45 manic-depres-

Table 20.4. *Likelihood of relapse*

Study	N	Follow-up period	Probability of relapse %	(See note below)	Notes
MacDonald (1918)	451	not stated	65	A	1st admissions
Pollock (1931)	8438	? 10–20 yrs	40–50	A	1st admissions. High proportion of mania
Fuller (1935)	327	10 yr mean	63	B	1st admissions
Rennie (1942)	208	? 20 yrs	79	A	
Lundquist (1945)	319	<10–30 yrs	39 depression	A	
			45 mania	A	
Poort (1945)	141	10–15 yrs	70	A	
Brodwall (1947)	110	9–15 yrs	38	–	Poor response rate Postal survey
Huston &	80	1–12 yrs	63	B	Pre-ECT
Locher (1948)	74	2 mo–4 yrs	51	B	Post-ECT
Stenstedt (1952)	288	0–3 yrs	42 depression	A	
			68 mania	A	
Kinkelin (1954)	146	½–72 yrs	84	A	
Forssman & Janssen (1960)	240	5 yrs exactly	72 at least some symptoms	–	1st admissions
			45 marked relapse		
	239	10 yrs exactly	76 at least some symptoms	–	
			52 marked relapse		
Oltman & Friedman (1962)	187	Whole life	79	A	
Carlson *et al.* (1974)	47	½–9 yrs	43	–	

Note: Relapse rates are very often given in different ways. It is frequently not recorded whether chronic cases become chronic at first attack. Relapse rates are often indicated in the form '*x* per cent had only 1 attack'. Where this percentage includes subjects who became chronic at first admission these obviously have to be removed from both numerator and denominator which means that the probability of relapse is higher than the percentage of those having more than 1 attack (studies marked 'A' above). As an example the figure given by Oltman and Friedman (79 per cent) becomes 92 per cent. In studies marked 'B' above, the relapse rate is in the form '*x* per cent were not readmitted'. Chronic cases then only have to be removed from the denominator.

sives; 38 per cent had 'low' working capacity. Bratfos and Haug have reviewed this topic and noted marked social decline in 28 per cent of patients who were chronic. In their study of early onset cases, Carlson and colleagues (1977) reported that 20 per cent were socially impaired even after exclusion of the chronic cases. Dunner and colleagues (1978) and MacVane and colleagues (1978) do not report poor social function-ing in their euthymic manic depressives but both groups studied lithium clinic attenders who may be a low-risk group. Nyström (1979) records an unfavourable work prognosis in 17 per cent of his depressives followed up for 10 years.

Table 20.5 lists findings on chronicity in manic-depressive psychosis, related partly to length of stay in hospital and partly to persistence of affective

Table 20.5. *Chronicity in manic-depressive psychosis*

Study	N	Follow-up in years	% Chronic	Notes
Rennie (1942)	208	? 20	*c. 8*	Refers to chronic at 1st attack
Poort (1945)	141	10–15	*c. 33*	*c.* 20 per cent chronic and in hospital
Brodwall (1947)	110	10	6	
Huston & Locher (1948)	80	6–10	*c. 8*	Chronic and in hospital
Norris (1959)	2298	2–5	10	Readmissions much more likely to be chronic
Forssman & Janssen (1960)	479	5 & 10	9	
Bratfos & Haug (1968)	176	6	28	Chronic affective symptoms throughout follow-up period
Shobe & Brion (1971)	111	14–20	20	Private patients. 6 per cent had been in hospital for at least 2 years
Carlson *et al.* (1974)	53	½–9	36	Persistent affective symptoms
Nyström (1979)	83	10	5	Unrelieved depression following index admission
Taschev (1974)	122	Whole life	8	'Cyclothymic depression'
	134	Whole life	16	'Recurrent depression'
	335	Whole life	22	'Involutional depression'
	23	Whole life	4	'Reactive depression'
	38	Whole life	13	'Recurrent mania'
	652	Whole life	17	All types

symptoms. Intensive study reveals a high probability that affective symptoms will persist (Bratfos & Haug, 1968; Shobe & Brion, 1971; Carlson *et al.*, 1977). These symptoms may be relatively minor and fluctuating but cases showing continuous severe symptoms for many years have been documented (e.g. Wertham, 1929). Norris (1959) underlines the very low likelihood of discharge following an admission lasting as long as two years.

Finally, chronicity may take a non-affective form. Many studies record a small percentage of cases which have a schizophrenic symptomatology at outcome. Astrup and colleagues (1959) give case histories of 13 patients (out of 96) who, they thought, were schizophrenic at follow-up. In the writer's opinion 3 of these showed no features allowing an initial diagnosis of schizophrenia but ended up with a defect state, similar to that of schizophrenia. Four similar cases are reported by Lewis (1936) and Lundquist

(1945). A further 3, of whom 2 were euthymic, had entered a chronic paranoid state.

Further light on the tendency for manic-depressive psychosis to become chronic under present-day conditions of treatment is shed by the study of Mann and Cree (1976) on the 'new long-stay' patients (patients who had been in hospital between one and three years). Affective psychosis was the second most common diagnosis in this group, accounting for 15.8 per cent compared with 44.4 per cent for schizophrenia.

Subclassification

There have always been authors who regarded Kraepelin's synthesis of manic-depressive psychosis as unwise (e.g. Hoch, 1910). The recent differentiation of the unipolar and bipolar subtypes, notably by Leonhard, Perris, Angst, and Winokur, confirms these reservations. We have seen that bipolarity in virtually all studies indicates a poorer prognosis. There is a higher likelihood of an early onset, of relapse (although some of this is tautological) and of chronicity in bipolar illness. The methodological problems of follow-up do not damage this conclusion. The likelihood that a subject who has had one depressive episode will develop a bipolar course is probably between 4 per cent and 6 per cent (Lundquist, 1945; Winokur & Morrison, 1973; Dunner *et al.*, 1976). In the study by Dunner and colleagues (1976), all patients who later developed full-blown manic episodes had had detectable minor hypomanic symptoms beforehand.

Other subclassifications include the distinction between pure (unipolar) depressive disease and depressive spectrum disease (Winokur *et al.*, 1975). Winokur (1979) feels that depressive spectrum disease, although lying symptomatically with the depressions, partakes more of the nature of personality disorders. The implications of this for prognosis are not fully clarified; depressive spectrum disease may be more likely to be episodic, pure depressive disease to be chronic (Winokur, 1974).

Conclusions

What may be extracted from this profusion of studies of differing sophistication? We may conclude tentatively:

(1) Episodes leading to hospital admission are likely to have a total duration of several months. Much of the episode will precede admission. Episodes which do not lead to hospital admission occur but are shorter and milder.

(2) Episodes of mania may possibly be of more rapid onset and of shorter duration than episodes of depression.

(3) Most people will either recover completely or nearly so from the first attack (70–92 per cent). Some of this group will have a fairly rapid recurrence of minor affective symptoms. Episodes occurring later in life last longer and may be more likely to be chronic. It is not clear that this tendency has been modified by ECT. Sex and family history of affective disorder does not influence duration but slow onset may indicate slow recovery.

(4) A majority of those who recover will relapse.

There may be a subpopulation of non-relapsers who are much more likely to be depressive than manic. Some have claimed that the chance of recovery becomes less with succeeding episodes but the literature as a whole does not provide conclusive evidence for this.

(5) A substantial minority develop a chronic disability which may follow the first episode. The proportion of chronic cases increases with intensity of follow-up. Between 5 per cent and 10 per cent may be long-term hospital in-patients and an additional 25 per cent may have persistent affective symptoms which are to some degree incapacitating. There is considerable social impairment in this group.

(6) Chronicity may take a non-affective form. A small proportion of patients develop schizophrenia, a few cases develop a chronic defect state having never had schizophrenic symptoms, and a few change to a chronic paranoid state.

(7) The attempt to incorporate prognosis into a hierarchical organization of psychiatric disorders survives this review in a statistical, but not a logical, form. All the possible outcomes of schizophrenia may also be seen in manic-depressive psychosis. Unfavourable outcomes are, however, considerably rarer in manic-depressive psychosis.

(8) All the studies reviewed in this chapter are in some way methodologically unsound. The analysis of prognostic factors is often naive. The most informative presentation for prognosis is actuarial: Norris (1959) uses this technique but her data refer only to hospital admission. A full account of the prognosis of affective psychosis has therefore yet to be rendered. This should ideally be part of an account of functional disorders as a whole. The recent specification of the questions to be asked (e.g. bipolarity versus unipolarity) does represent an advance. This review emphasizes once again the serious prognostic import of manic-depressive psychosis; a concern which has been expressed by many over the years since the condition was recognized (Swift, 1907; Poort, 1945; Norris, 1959; Welner *et al.*, 1977).

Acknowledgement
My thanks are due to Dr Thomas Herzog for help with German translation.

Section 5

CHAPTERS 21–25

Aetiology and pathology

21
Epidemiology of affective psychoses

K. RAWNSLEY

Introduction

The fundamental statistic of epidemiology, frequency of a defined condition in a defined population, is hard to capture with precision and assurance in the field of affective illness. Even where the numerator of the fraction is confined to hospital-treated cases, the controversial issue of diagnosis remains and figures will depend upon the particular classification adopted and the conceptual standpoint of clinicians.

In general, this review will be concerned with the epidemiology of the most severe affective disorders – mania, manic-depressive psychosis, and severe depression. However, there are real problems in discriminating between these groups and the milder affective disorders. It will be necessary, therefore, to include many studies which have not made a clear distinction between them. Reference should also be made to comprehensive reviews (Bebbington, 1978; Rawnsley, 1968; Silverman, 1968).

Frequency

Hospital admission rates for affective disorders are principally an index of availability of hospital resources, coupled with attitudes of patients and of referring agencies. Thus the rise in first-admission rates for manic-depressive disorders in England and Wales from 1952 (males 16.1 per 100 000; females, 26.0 per 100 000) to 1960 (28.8 and 49.3 respectively) gives little information about secular trends in the general population. A further example is the decline in English first-admission rates of 'depressive psychoses' between 1970 and 1976 (from 10 to 8 per 100 000 for males and from 18 to 14 per 100 000 for females).

Scandinavian psychiatrists have been preeminent in endeavouring to calculate the 'lifetime morbid risk' for affective disorders. The excellent population registers available in these countries greatly facilitate this work (Table 21.1). The 'biographical' method of Klemperer (1933) has been used in Bornholm (Fremming, 1951) and in Iceland (Helgason, 1964); morbid risk figures for a rural population in Sweden were based on retrospective scrutiny of psychiatric hospital admissions and of parish records (Larsson & Sjögren, 1954). Estimates of lifetime risk from first admissions to mental hospitals have been made for Norway (Ødegård, 1961) and, for her London material by Norris (1959). In 1947 Essen Möller and his colleagues made a painstaking survey by direct interview of the mental health, past and present, of the entire population of two adjacent parishes in Southern Sweden (Essen Möller, 1956). The lifetime morbid risk for affective disorders was estimated as: male 17 per 1000, female 28 per 1000. In 1957 the population of the same parishes was reexamined by Hagnell. Using the data available from this survey Essen Möller and Hagnell (1961) made an estimate of the lifetime morbid risk by Weinberg's method yielding 85 per 1000 for males and 177 per 1000 for females. These high figures may result, in part, from the closer scrutiny inherent in the prospective method and in the inclusion of relatively mild cases. However it is interesting to compare this finding with the material reported by Watts (1966), a general practitioner who has kept a careful account of psychiatric disorders in his practice for many years. Watts has seen 1127 patients with depressive illness in the course of 19 years' observation, approximately 1 in 10 of the population at risk. This figure is of the same order as that quoted by Essen Möller & Hagnell for the lifetime risk calculated from the decade incidence.

Regarding the period of risk for affective illness, Slater (1935) found 60 per cent of the total morbidity for women and 56 per cent for men to have passed by the age of 50. Norris (1959) also using mental hospital data found 79 per cent of the morbid risk for women and 69 per cent for men to have passed by the age of 65.

Table 21.1. *Expectation through life of affective disorder*

		Per 1000 births	
		Male	Female
Bornholm	(Fremming, 1951)	10.2	22.4
Sweden	(Larsson & Sjögren, 1954)	9.0	12.0
Norway	(Ødegård, 1961)	4.2	6.2
Iceland	(Helgason, 1964)	18.0	24.6
London	(Norris, 1959)	8.0	14.4

Essen Möller and Hagnell's work quoted above is an example of a survey endeavouring to escape from the shackles of 'treated' prevalence. Many attempts have now been made to measure the prevalence of 'depression' in whole populations or in representative samples thereof. A useful and critical discussion of the many difficulties of method and of interpretation has been made by Bebbington (1978).

The problem essentially is to find a way of distinguishing individuals with affective disorders from among the myriad subjects who report themselves as feeling 'depressed' in response to questions. Hare and Shaw (1965) compared representative samples of the population of a new housing estate and of an old-established area in Croydon, England. Four per cent of men and 11.8 per cent of women from the newer areas and 4 per cent of men and 8.7 per cent of women from the old area claimed to be currently 'depressed'. Even higher rates were reported by Comstock and Helsing (1976) in samples from Kansas City, Missouri, and from Washington County, Maryland. The Centre for Epidemiological Studies Depression Scale was used to assess depressive symptoms and the results are summarized in Table 21.2.

Application of the Present State Examination (PSE) (Wing, Cooper & Sartorius, 1974) to community surveys introduces a form of assessment which is of proven clinical relevance. Global diagnoses based on the PSE used in the Camberwell, England, survey reported by Brown and Harris (1978), in two samples of women age 18–65, yielded 14.8 per cent of subjects with depressive disorder. A similar method in the Hebridean island of North Uist yielded a prevalence of 8.4 per cent for depressive disorder among women (Brown *et al.*, 1977). Wing and his colleagues have devised a method for distinguishing between defi-

Table 21.2. *Percentage of population with CES – D scores of 16 or more*

| | Kansas City | | Washington County |
	Blacks	Whites	Whites
Male	22.2	15.7	11.9
Female	29.6	22.4	20.7

nite threshold and below-threshold conditions, by applying a set of clinical rules incorporated in a computer program to PSE profiles (Wing *et al.*, 1978).

Socio-demographic correlates

One of the few consistent positive associations is between affective disorder and female sex. Whether this connection depends upon biological susceptibility or upon social conditioning is critically reviewed by Weissman and Klerman (1977). Less clear-cut is the link between affective illness and age. Some enquiries indicate a decline in prevalence with age (Comstock & Helsing, 1976; Uhlenhuth, Lipmann, Balter & Stern, 1974); others an increase (Hare & Shaw, 1965; Brown, Bhrolcháin & Harris, 1975). In general, rates of depressive illness among the married are lower than rates among the single in both sexes (Grad de Alarcon, Sainsbury & Costain, 1975; Adelstein *et al.*, 1968), although teen-age marriages seem to carry a higher risk.

Enquiries into the association between affective disorders and social class have yielded conflicting results due perhaps in part to variations in the source of case material and in part to differences in definition of social class. The first-admission rates and the rates for second and subsequent admissions to psychiatric hospitals in England and Wales for males age 20 and over with manic-depressive reaction show a clear peak for social class V (unskilled workers) (Registrar General, 1960). First admissions to Norwegian mental hospitals show highest rates for affective psychosis among seamen, farm labourers, and domestic servants (Ødegård, 1961). By contrast, the study by Sundby and Nyhus (1963) of male admissions to psychiatric wards mostly attached to general hospitals in Oslo yields a relatively high incidence of affective disorder among the inhabitants of the western suburban areas. These are the most well-to-do parts of the town and contain mainly professional and business men. Among sixteen selected occupational groups the highest rate for affective psychoses was among seamen officers followed by university men. Bagley (1973) reviews the issue and, from his own work, suggests a link between higher social class and the limited category of circular manic-depressive psychosis. At the level of community surveys which do not depend upon 'treated' prevalence little association has been found between depressive phenomena and social class (Warheit, Holzer & Schwab, 1973, Uhlenhuth *et al.*, 1974, Brown *et al.*, 1975, Taylor & Chave, 1964; Hare & Shaw, 1965).

When the epidemiological focus is upon race and culture, problems of method and interpretation loom large. Marsella (1978) pin-points the issue firstly for 'treated' prevalence by underlining the enormous variability in motivation between cultures to seek help. Identification of 'untreated' cases is affected by variations in definition of depression and in the particular manifestations of depression among different ethno-cultural groups. Fernando (1966) points out that the older German literature considered manic-depressive illness as a typically Jewish psychosis. He draws attention to contrasts between the findings of studies of affective disorders in Jews living in the USA and in Jews resident in Israel. Thus Malzberg (1962) found a significant higher rate for admissions to New York City hospitals of Jews with manic-depressive psychosis than of Christians. Studies in Palestine (Halpern, 1938) and in Israel (Hes, 1960) do not indicate an unusually high prevalence among Jews. In New Zealand, striking differences are found between Maoris and the population of European origin (Foster, 1962). Although the crude rate of admission for manic-depressive illness was more than twice as high in Europeans than in Maoris, manic and circular states were commoner in Maoris.

The early literature on African populations indicated a relatively low proportion of affective illness among all psychiatric attenders in Eastern and Southern Africa compared with that in Western areas (Table 21.3). These figures must be subject to all the reservations attending 'treated' prevalence findings more particularly in cross-cultural comparisons.

Frequencies obtained from studies of African random samples using case-finding techniques which have also been employed in British settings support the view that depressive ailments are very common in Africa. Thus Orley and Wing (1979) using the Present State Examination found 9.3 per cent of Camberwell, London, women to have depressive disor-

Table 21.3. *Proportion of affective disorder in patients attending for psychiatric treatment*

		%
Kenya	(Carothers, 1947)	*1.6* 'depressives'
South Africa	(Laubscher, 1937)	*3.8* manic-depressive
Ghana	(Tooth, 1950)	$\begin{cases} 19.6 \text{ manic-depressive} \\ 2.3 \text{ depressive} \end{cases}$
Ghana	(Weinberg, 1965)	*23.5* manic-depressive
Nigeria	(Leighton, *et al.*, 1963)	*16.9* depression main symptom

der of at least 'threshold' severity as against 22.6 per cent of women from two small Ugandan villages. The nine-centre International Pilot Study of Schizophrenia found severe manic and depressive disorders to occur in all the areas investigated (WHO, 1973).

Precise comparison of such disparate populations is rendered difficult by a cross-cultural gulf in the conceptualization of depression and cognate emotional states and by the language available (Leff, 1973; Bebbington, 1978).

Among Western societies, Ødegård (1961) has drawn attention to two populations which appear to be at opposite extremes of the scale: the Hutterites (an anabaptist religious sect living in the North American West) and rural communities of North Sweden. Eaton and Weil (1955) found a ratio of schizophrenia to affective disorder of 0.23:1 among Hutterites. Böök's (1953) finding for North Swedish rural parishes established a ratio of 46.0:1. The 'life-time morbidity risk' for all psychoses was similar in the Hutterite and Swedish communities. A sociological explanation of the relatively high frequency of affective disorder among the Hutterites is preferred by Eaton and Weil. There is a strong tradition of communal co-operation with emphasis upon duty both to God and to society. Aggression is frowned upon. Responsibility rests heavily upon the individual who must accept guilt within himself rather than project it on to others. In the semi-arctic North Swedish community conditions are very different. Most of the inhabitants live in isolated farmsteads. Social cohesiveness in the Hutterite sense is not a prominent feature. Böök, however, points out that differential migration into and out of his northern Swedish area, together with a high frequency of first-

cousin marriages, provides the basis for a genetic explanation.

The link between 'life-events' and depression is discussed in chapter 23 and in Volume 4, chapters 1 and 5.

Seasonal correlates

In a study of seasonal patterns of suicide, depression and electroconvulsive therapy, Eastwood and Peacocke (1976) found the three phenomena to be positively related and to show peaks of frequency in the Ontario spring and autumn. Symonds and Williams (1976) found a peak for the admission of female manic patients in August–September for England and Wales, but not for males. However, Myers and Davies (1978) found the highest rate of admission of manic patients (of both sexes) to occur in summer with a trough in winter. (See chapter 22 for a fuller discussion of the epidemiology of suicide).

The question of a link between season of birth and affective illness has been examined and a useful review of the literature is by Videbech, Week and Dupont (1974). From their own Danish material these authors found no association between season of birth and affective illness whereas there was a surplus of schizophrenic patients born in the first trimester. This finding for schizophrenia has been supported by several other studies but the pattern for affective illness varies in different materials. Thus Sauvage Nolting (1955), Dalén (1968), Koehler and Jacoby (1976), and Danneel and Faust (1979) found no association. Lang (1931), Petersen (1935), and Huntington (1938) found a trend towards positive association with birth in the first trimester. Hare (1978) showed a significant association between affective illness and birth in the last quarter of the year.

Conclusion

It seems that affective disorder, like schizophrenia, has a world-wide distribution. 'Treated' prevalence rates are powerfully influenced by availability of therapeutic resources and by a variety of nosocomial factors. The 'iceberg effect' is very striking as case-finding is carried to greater depths and the lifetime morbid risk is of the order of 10 per cent.

Although many socio-demographic factors have been shown to have association with affective illness in individual studies the only consistent positive link is with female sex. The pathoplastic influence of culture in determining the content of affective disorders is clear. Although for this and other reasons the manifestations of depressive illness vary considerably between different populations, Bebbington (1978) concludes: 'There seems to be a consistent depressive core of loss of sleep, libido and appetite with a tendency to somatic complaints.'

22
Suicide: epidemiology and relationship to depression

PETER SAINSBURY

Epidemiology of suicide

The national mortality statistics allow us to identify not only the characteristics of those most at risk but also the social conditions and events that predispose to the act. Though it is evident that depressive and other mental disorders conduce to suicide, illnesses of this kind are common occurrences, whereas suicide is comparatively rare. They are therefore not, in themselves, sufficient causes; other factors besides the psychological ones need to be taken into account, in particular the effects of the social environment and of psychosocial stresses such as bereavement, if the occurrence of suicide is to be understood.

Age and sex

Suicide statistics reveal very consistent differences in rates of suicide between demographic groups, between nations and over time. Women, for example, invariably commit suicide less than men do, despite their being more prone to depression. In the last two decades, however, the ratio of male to female suicide has been falling in all European countries, largely due to the rising incidence in women: an observation not without implications regarding the changing status and roles of the sexes.

Though suicide also rises steeply with age in Western cultures – depressive disorders too are commoner in later life – it is among the four most frequent causes of death at ages 15–34. Moreover, throughout Europe suicide has recently been increasing in the youngest age groups, particularly among men. The increase in women, on the other hand, has been more apparent in middle and late life. Thus, the suicide rate of women aged 65–74 rose in 16 out of 18 European countries in the decade 1963–73, England and Greece being the only exceptions (WHO, 1968, 1973, 1976).

Nations and their trends

Countries also maintain their characteristic incidence of suicide over long periods. In Europe during 1972–4 suicide rates ranged from a mean of 3.4 per 100 000 per year in Ireland to 38.2 in Hungary. England and Wales has a low rate (7.8), the rate having fallen by a third since 1963, whereas in all other European countries except Scotland and Greece rates have been increasing during this period. Explanations of the surprising decline in Britain have been sought in terms of social changes, loss of availability of the preferred means because of the reduction in the carbon monoxide content of domestic gas (Kreitman, 1976), and to improved psychiatric services, of which the first has so far proved the best predictor of whether a country's suicide rate will change. Using multivariate analysis, a composite of 15 social variables correctly allocated 18 countries into those with increasing and those with decreasing suicide rates. Variables depicting changes in the role of women were the best predictors; next were the indices of affluence and of social isolation (Sainsbury, Baert & Jenkins, 1978).

The social environment

Marital status also relates to suicide in a uniform way: married people with children have the lowest rate followed in increasing order by the unmarried, the divorced, and the separated. In general, it would seem that belonging to a closely knit group, such as the family, protects against suicide; by the same token suicide tends to be lower in rural than in urban communities; it is also lower among poorer classes than among more affluent ones.

The consistency with which national trends change with political and economic events also suggests that the social milieu has substantial effects on suicide: in 22 countries suicide increased during the depression in 1930–33, while it decreased in both world wars. A less well understood but remarkable statistical regularity is for the incidence of suicide to reach a peak in spring or early summer. The ten-dency for any country to maintain a low or high suicide rate relative to other countries led Durkheim (1897) to propose that the predisposition to suicide is socially determined. More specifically, his theory claims that suicide varies with the extent of the individuals' ties with their domestic, occupational, religious or neighbourhood groups. He termed the suicide of those who become socially isolated 'egoistic'. Many of the observations already quoted support this view; while others also show that those who live alone, immigrants, the separated, the unemployed, and those without religious affiliations, commit suicide more often than do those without these characteristics (Sainsbury, 1973). Furthermore, suicides occur more often in socially disorganized city districts where social pathology such as homicide, child neglect, delinquency, and so on is rife, i.e. where the community's social control of its members is lacking. Suicide occurring in these conditions Durkheim refers to as 'anomic'.

Most other social theories of suicide are variations on Durkheim's theme; but the transactional school, typified by Douglas (1967), rejects all suicide statistics and epidemiological findings derived from them, because methods of ascertainment and the definition of suicide varies from place to place. This view has been widely canvassed. However, when the differences between ascertaining officials and procedures are allowed for, the distinctive suicide rates of populations persist. For example, immigrants to the USA and to Australia from countries with a high rate still have higher rates than immigrants from low rate areas. Similarly, differences in suicide between the county boroughs of England persist despite changes in the coroner (Sainsbury & Barraclough, 1968). Further, when national differences in reporting and defining suicide are obviated by adding open verdicts and certain categories of accidental death to reported suicides, and a new 'combined' rate is calculated for each nation, the rank orders remain virtually identical (Barraclough, 1973). Epidemiological studies using official mortality statistics can therefore validly describe differences between populations and elucidate predisposing causes.

Psychosocial stresses

Consideration of life-events and crises as precipitants of suicide also emphasizes the interplay between social and psychological factors. When the risk of suicide is compared in people who have and have not experienced particular events it is apparent that certain adversities increase the risk; notably, recent bereavements, separations, moving house, and, to a lesser extent, some terminal and chronic illnesses (Sainsbury, 1975; Whitlock, 1978).

Methods
Hanging is still the means suicides use most; and since domestic gas is no longer lethal, drugs and poisons come next and are increasingly used everywhere. Otherwise, men prefer firearms and women prefer drowning. The barbiturates still easily head the list of drugs, though other hypnotic and psychotropic medications (notably tricyclics) are assuming greater importance (WHO, 1968). The question whether the easy availability of a means of suicide, such as drugs, can increase the incidence of suicide rather than simply the proportion of people using the method is important for preventive action: the epidemiological evidence points to the latter (Sainsbury, Baert & Jenkins, 1978).

Attempted suicide
In general, people who attempt suicide differ from those completing the act – in many respects they are opposites (Kreitman, 1977; Bancroft et al., 1975). Thus attempts are mostly made by women and the young. They also differ from suicides in being common in the lower socio-economic groups and, allowing for age, among the married; moreover, the most frequent precipitants are domestic and marital conflicts. And unlike suicide the incidence of self-poisoning in Britain has been rising sharply over the last two decades. As many as one per cent of all women aged 15–24 make an attempt each year and these acts now account for some 30 per cent of all medical emergencies. The questions these observations pose as to the social predicament and needs of young people are pressing (see volume 4, chapters 5, 6, and 8, and volume 5).

Though fewer attempters have a mental illness than do suicides, more have disordered personalities (Pallis & Birtchnell, 1977). Nevertheless, the two populations overlap in an important practical respect. Some 8 per cent of those attempting will eventually die by suicide and in perhaps a fifth the intent to die is serious (Stengel, 1972).

Relationship to depression
The association between suicide and depression is more than a matter of clinical interest; it has considerable practical significance. Research in recent years has established not only that the majority of suicides suffered from an unequivocal and treatable depressive illness, but that most also contacted their doctors during the period immediately preceding their death. These observations have important implications for suicide prevention. The evidence that a high proportion of suicides have a primary depressive illness derives from three sources: follow-up studies, interviews with relatives, and comparison between suicide and attempted suicide.

Follow-up studies
First, when patients with manic-depressive illnesses are followed up a consistent finding is that about 1 in 6 of them will die by suicide (see Table 22.1). More recently Miles (1977) reviewed 30 follow-up studies of patients with a primary depressive illness in which he included 7 cohorts of 'neurotic depressives'. He also reached the conclusion that 15 per cent of depressives, whether classified as endogenous or neurotic, will ultimately die by suicide.

Prevalence surveys give a lifetime morbidity risk for depressions severe enough to be referred to a psychiatrist which varied between about 2 per cent and 4 per cent. If the lower figure is taken, there should be about 10^6 depressives in England and Wales; and if the life span of depressives is 66 years (Oltman & Friedman, 1962) the expected annual number of depressed suicides will be $15/100 \times 10^6/66 = 2273$. As on the average 5000 suicides a year were reported in 1960–69, the proportion occurring in depressives would be 45 per cent which is similar to the 64 per cent found by Barraclough, Bunch, Nelson and Sainsbury (1974) in a clinically assessed sample of suicides.

Of particular value are surveys in which the mortality of a population has been recorded over long periods. Helgason (1964), for instance, followed a cohort of 5395 born in Iceland in 1895–7 through 60–62 years. From national records he ascertained that nearly 2 per cent (103) of the probands developed a manic-depressive illness of whom 34 were dead by 1960, 18 from suicide. Over half of their deaths therefore were by suicide and 17 per cent of the manic-depressives in the cohort committed suicide. Similarly, he identified 139 neurotic depressives of whom 15 died, but only 1 by suicide (7 per cent of the deaths). In a more recent survey Hagnell and Rorsman (1978) followed a cohort of over 3500 residents of Lundby through 25 years, 28 died by suicide. They

Table 22.1. *Death by suicide in affective disorder*[a]

	Cases N	Follow-up in years	Dead N	Suicide N	Death due to suicide %
Langeluddecke	341	40	268	41	15.3
Slater	138	30	59	9	15.3
Lunquist	319	20	119	17	14.3
Schulz	2,004	5	492	66	13.4
Stenstedt	216	10	42	6	14.3
Pitts & Winokur	56	Death	56	9	16.0

[a] Adapted from Eli Robins *et al.* (1959).

established a diagnosis of endogenous depression in half the suicides.

As manics often become depressed their mortality is also of interest. When Tsuang and Woolson (1978) followed 100 manics through four decades they found 9.3 per cent of the deceased committed suicide – most of them in the first decade.

Interviews with relatives

Eli Robins and colleagues (1959) in St Louis were the first to use diagnostic interviews with suicides' relatives. They concluded that 94 per cent of 134 suicides were mentally ill and that 45 per cent suffered from a manic-depressive illness. Dorpat and Ripley (1960) similarly diagnosed 30 per cent of suicides in Seattle as having a depressive disorder.

In England, Barraclough and colleagues (1974) obtained standardized social as well as clinical data by interviewing the relatives and friends of 100 consecutive suicides and 150 controls from the general population (matched for age, sex and whether ever married) in two county districts. In addition, the suicide's general practitioner provided information on any medical care given. The sample was representative in so far as the demographic characteristics of the suicides did not differ from the national figure.

The diagnoses were made by an independent panel of three consultant psychiatrists. The panel agreed that 93 per cent had an identifiable mental disorder and that 64 per cent had an uncomplicated primary depressive illness – this figure increased to 77 per cent if those suicides whose principal diagnosis was alcoholism, but who also had a severe depressive illness, were included.

Clinically most of the 64 depressions were of the endogenous type, but 17 per cent of subjects had also suffered manic episodes. In order to see how the suicidal depressives differed from living ones, a comparison was made with a random sample of 128 endogenous depressives (matched on age and sex) drawn from the same population as the suicides (Barraclough & Pallis, 1975). The rank order of the frequency of 15 leading depressive symptoms was the same for both groups; though severity was rated higher in the suicides. They differed significantly on only three items: persistent insomnia, self-neglect, and impaired memory. Insomnia is important not only because Rosen (1970) and Farberow and McEvoy (1966) have also claimed it to be characteristic of the suicidal depressive, but because many suicides are prescribed barbiturates over a long period and then use this hypnotic as their means of suicide (Barraclough *et al.*, 1971). Self-neglect and impaired memory were not associated with organic cerebral disease, but may well be the effects of a severe depressive illness on cognitive function and morale.

Others (McDowall *et al.*, 1968; Farberow & McEvoy, 1966; Flood & Seager, 1968) have compared depressives who committed suicide and diagnostically matched controls. The suicides, however, were selected (psychiatric admissions) and the sources of data lacked uniformity (case notes). McDowall and colleagues (1968) assessed the suicides as more severely depressed but less hypochondriacal than the controls; while Farberow and McEvoy's anxiety-depressions were more agitated, depressed and anxious. In all three controlled comparisons the suicides had made significantly more previous attempts (41 per cent v. 4 per cent in Barraclough & Pallis). It is also apparent (Pokorney, 1964; Temoche, Pugh &

MacMahon, 1964; Copas, Freeman-Browne & Robin, 1971) that depressives have a much higher risk of suicide immediately following discharge from hospital, a third or more occurring within six months. On the other hand, the duration of the suicides' illness tends to be longer than that of the controls (Barraclough & Pallis, 1975) and their deaths are more likely at the start and end of an episode of an illness (Copas *et al.*, 1971). Other predisposing factors distinguish the depressed suicides: they are more often male, older, separated, recently bereaved (Bunch *et al.*, 1971) and socially isolated.

The two groups did not differ on number of previous episodes of illness – about 40 per cent in both – nor on family history of mental illness: about 20 per cent of the first-degree relatives of both groups had had an affective disorder and 6 per cent had committed suicide. These figures are similar to those that genetic studies report for depressive psychoses (Perris, 1966). The depressive groups also resembled each other closely on predisposing social factors; but with one very conspicuous difference: 42 per cent of the suicides had lived alone, whereas only 7 per cent of the living depressives did.

The close resemblance between the suicides with depression and a series of depressives with a confirmed diagnosis of endogenous depression supports the validity of the suicides' diagnoses retrospectively determined. The salient considerations, however, are that more than half of the suicides have been shown to have a readily identifiable and treatable illness and that their depression has some distinctive clinical features denoting a suicide risk. Considerable scope for preventive action therefore exists.

Relation to attempted suicide

Some recent findings on attempted suicides have contributed to an understanding of the relation of depression both to suicide and to its prevention. On the one hand, Bagley (1973), Henderson and colleagues (1977), and Kiev (1976) have used principal components and cluster analysis to identify categories of attempted suicide. These investigations are consistent in differentiating a psychotically or severely depressed group of patients who made a serious attempt in circumstances which made discovery unlikely. And on the other, the consensus of ten clinical projects is that the variables most positively associated with the seriousness of intent to die are a diagnosis of manic-depressive or primary depressive

illness and a high score on a depression scale (Pallis, 1977). Pallis inferred that patients making a serious attempt resemble suicides rather than attempted suicides in general, and indeed, more patients whose attempts are rated as serious subsequently commit suicide than do the less serious attempters, e.g. Rosen (1970), Pallis (1977).

Pallis (1977) and Pallis and Sainsbury (1976) clinically assessed 151 consecutive suicide attempts admitted to the Emergency Department for the Chichester district. Pallis scored each of them on Beck's Intent Scales and on a Suicide-risk Scale, and also obtained an independent rating of the medical seriousness of the attempt. Intent to die not only correlated significantly with both suicide-risk and medical seriousness, but also with the number and severity of depressive symptoms. The depressive features that distinguished (1 per cent level) high from low intent were insomnia, pessimism, and impaired concentration. The high and low intent groups also differed significantly on those social variables which we have already seen to be strongly associated with consummated suicide: male sex, younger age, being single or separated, and living alone. The depressive and other features of the serious suicide attempt are therefore very similar to those ascertained by interviewing relatives of completed suicides.

Personality

Pallis and Birtchnell (1977) also looked at personality and the seriousness of attempts by comparing the MMPI scores of non-suicidal patients, attempts rated serious and non-serious, and patients who later died by suicide. The samples were drawn from the N.E. Scotland Psychiatric Case Register.

The personality profiles of the suicides and serious attempts were similar and differed from the much more deviant non-serious group; but they did not differ from the non-serious on the MMPI depression scale despite more being diagnosed depressive. High introversion was the only distinctive feature of the suicides (Pallis, 1977).

Other possible causative factors

So far we have established that suicides commonly suffered from a primary depression, and that attempted suicides in whom intent to die is serious have a high incidence of severe depression and subsequent suicide. Clearly diagnosing depression is a priority in assessing the risk of suicide. Nevertheless, the clinical similarities between depressed suicides and living depressives are more apparent than the differences. Accordingly, other interacting factors need to be taken into account in order to explain the depressives' vulnerability to suicide and to predict those who will die by suicide. These other components include the socio-cultural milieu (there is a higher incidence of suicide and depression in more affluent social classes and in those who live alone), psychosocial stresses and adverse events (bereavements in the preceeding two years, moving house, and loss of employment precipitate both suicide and depression, see Sainsbury, 1973), and personality attributes, such as introversion.

In order to elucidate the interdependence of some of these factors and to pursue the hypothesis that the more closely the individual attempting suicide resembles the completed suicide the greater the risk of his subsequently killing himself, Pallis (1977) compared samples of suicides whose relatives were interviewed with attempted suicides assessed on 55 clinical and social items from the standardized interview schedule that both groups had received. A stepwise discriminant function analysis identified the best discriminators and enabled 92 per cent of the combined sample of suicides and attempted suicides to be correctly allocated to their respective groups.

The suicides were characterized by the familiar clinical and demographic attributes of the manic-depressive. On the basis of these findings Pallis constructed and validated a risk scale of 18 items with a short form of 6 items for screening use by casualty officers. The practical implications of these studies are that intent and risk scales not only point to the severely depressed, whether categorized as endogenous or neurotic, as being highly vulnerable, but that they can also efficiently predict the short-term risk of suicide; hence they have practical value in quickly assessing the management of attempted suicides and in prevention. Indeed, the feasibility of suicide prevention largely depends on the ability of the primary care services to recognize the risk characteristics of depressed patients, provide effective treatment, and organize efficient after-care. The ways in which the suicidally depressed are identified and managed by services can be quoted to bolster these claims.

Barraclough and colleagues (1974) inquired about warnings by suicides. Thirty-three per cent of the 64 uncomplicated depressives made an unequivocal threat of suicide in the month before death, and nearly half of the alcoholic ones did so. Of greater preventive relevance was that 62 per cent of the depressives contacted a general practitioner and-or psychiatrist in the previous month and 42 per cent did so in the previous seven days. A high proportion of depressed suicide attempters are also reported as having seen their doctors just prior to the act (Bancroft *et al.*, 1977). It is apparent that with the majority of suicidal depressives there are ample opportunities for intervention, provided the doctor has the required skills.

It is of interest, therefore, to see how the GPs managed the suicidal depressives and hence whether prevention is a practicable proposition. Eighty-one per cent had been prescribed hypnotics and tranquillizers, so their doctors at least recognized that they were distressed. Nevertheless, in only 1 of the 19 given antidepressants was the dosage and type appropriate. Furthermore, over half had been prescribed barbiturates, and half of the depressives dying from barbiturates had received the tablets in the previous week, all but 2 using the prescribed tablets to commit suicide (Barraclough *et al.*, 1974, 1971).

Clearly in 1966, there was scope for more expertise in the primary care of suicidal depressives but we have reason to believe that recognition and management may have improved with the rapid extension of postgraduate education.

While seeking explanations for the decline in suicide in England, one of the possibilities we entertained was that it could be ascribed to improved mental health services, especially primary care. Jenkins therefore compared the consultation rates and diagnoses recorded in two surveys of general practice in England: one in 1955–6 (Logan & Cushion, 1958) and the other in 1970–71 (Office of Population Censuses & Surveys, 1974). He found that whereas consultation rates for *all* conditions fell, those for psychiatric disorder increased by 60 per cent. The general practitioners' diagnoses in the more recent period were more in accordance with psychiatric conventions and the number of patients being recognized as suffering from disorders with a high suicide risk, especially depressive disorders, had greatly increased (Sainsbury, Baert & Jenkins, 1978). We tentatively inferred that general practitioners' attitudes to the depressive patient are changing in a direction that could curtail suicide.

The practicability of applying advances in the treatment of depression to suicide prevention can be illustrated by considering the potential benefits of lithium clinics. Using the criteria of recurrence and the success rate that Coppen and colleagues (1971) reported in a controlled trial of the prophylactic value of lithium in recurrent depression, Barraclough (1972) identified 21 recurrent depressives in his sample of suicides who would have qualified for the trial. He then calculated that had these depressives been treated with lithium as successfully as had been the trial patients, a fifth of the suicides would have been prevented; and extrapolating to the country as a whole there would have been 750 fewer suicides.

The psychiatric management of the depressive is equally in need of reappraisal: too many depressives in psychiatric treatment commit suicide. We know that the quickest and surest way of removing the suicidal depressive from danger is still by admission to hospital and giving ECT (Greenblatt, 1977; Medical Research Council, 1965); despite this, suicides not only received less ECT than other depressives and spent less time in hospital, they also antagonized the staff more (Farberow & McEvoy, 1966; Flood & Seager, 1968; Robin, Brooke & Freeman-Browne, 1968). These problems of management led Pallis (1977) to ask general practitioners, psychiatrists, nurses and Samaritans about their knowledge of suicide risks and attitudes to the suicidal. Only the psychiatrists considered a primary responsibility for preventing suicide lay with them and, though most respondents knew that depression increases the risk of suicide, they were largely ignorant of other risk factors.

Further, the suicide rates of resident psychiatric patients in England and elsewhere (Sainsbury *et al.*, 1978) show a disturbing increase, and one which coincides with the introduction of more liberal regimes; whether the present preference for early discharge and for treating depressives in the community places the suicidal patient at greater risk has yet to be decided. Nevertheless we have sufficient facts to plan preventive management. We know that the danger of suicide relates to the onset of a depression and to its duration; it also increases in the weeks following discharge from active treatment: the importance of systematic after-care in the community is evident.

Walk (1967) has given grounds for claiming that a well-organized community psychiatric service might in fact be able to reduce the suicide rate. He compared the suicide rates of all patients in contact with a psychiatrist during the five years before and after the introduction of the Chichester Community Psychiatric Service in which 86 per cent of all referrals were treated extramurally. He found a significant decrease in the suicide rate of elderly psychiatric patients. Since it was the aged depressed patients who had benefited most, and whose level of referral had increased most after starting community care, there is a likelihood that the new services were responsible.

Summary

The available facts on the relation of suicide to depression, on the characteristics of the suicidal depressive, and on new opportunities that we have for providing effective treatment are such that suicide must now be considered a preventable disorder, at least to the extent that it should be mandatory for health services to implement preventive measures for the affectively disordered.

23
Social and psychological causes of affective disorders

E. S. PAYKEL

The possible causes of affective disorder discussed in this chapter include social factors such as recent life-events, longer-term environmental difficulties and problems occurring during childhood and psychological factors which have been studied empirically. The psycho-dynamic literature, which has been well reviewed by Mendelson (1974), will not be considered. In the first part of the chapter no distinction will be made between 'psychotic' and 'neurotic' forms of depression but consideration will be given to the problem of classification in later sections.

Recent life-events
Controlled studies of depressed patients
The last fifteen years have seen a large volume of research into the relationship between life-events and depression, reviewed in detail elsewhere (Andrews & Tennant, 1978; Paykel, 1982). Careful interview techniques have been needed to solve methodological difficulties. Retrospective recall of events is subject to distortions, magnified in the depressed patient by the 'effort of meaning', and by guilt and pessimism. Psychiatric illness may produce new events which are consequences rather than causes of illness. One precaution is to confine attention to time periods preceding symptomatic onset. A second is to concentrate attention on 'independent' events which, because of their specific circum-

stances, appear highly unlikely to have been brought about by the patient (Brown & Harris, 1978).

Two large studies have compared events reported by depressed patients with those reported by general population controls. Paykel and his colleagues (1969) found that depressives reported almost three times as many events in the six months before onset. Brown and Harris (1978) found the rate elevated only in the three weeks before onset, but for events rated as markedly threatening it was elevated over the entire 48 weeks studied. Studies comparing depressives with medical patient controls have found smaller differences, perhaps because events may cluster before medical illness or admission. Epidemiological studies also show that events precede and accompany the minor psychiatric disorders, mostly depressive, that occur in the community.

A highly specific hypothesis would suggest that certain events produce depression, and only depression. However, there is clear evidence that similar events also precede other psychiatric disorders including schizophrenia, suicide attempts and mixed neuroses. Effects for depression appear greater than for schizophrenia, but about the same as for mixed neuroses. There are greater patient–control differences for those who attempt suicide, particularly during the month before the attempt (Paykel, 1978).

Types of event

Depression has usually been regarded as related to certain types of events, particularly losses. The psycho-analytic concept of loss is broad, including not only deaths and other separations from key interpersonal figures, but also loss of limbs and other bodily parts, loss of self-esteem and of narcissistic self-gratification. These are better considered separately.

Deaths and interpersonal separations have received most study. In nine studies reporting separations, six found raised rates in depression. One study found 'exit' events related to depression while entrance events were not (Paykel *et al.*, 1969). Marital separations and arguments appear particularly important.

However, the relation between recent separation and depression is far from specific. A substantial proportion of the depressives do not report recent separations, and all studies of other types of events have also found some to be commoner in depressives.

A second group of events emphasized in the psychological and psycho-analytic literature comprises threats to self-esteem and failures. They have not been distinguished separately in recent empirical studies but do seem evident in the type of events reported.

One kind of event which does not emerge in empirical studies is the success event. Nevertheless, clinical observation suggests that a small proportion of depressions follow promotion, an unexpected economic windfall, or the achievement of a long-desired goal. These may contain disguised threats, such as great increases in responsibilities and disruptions of life routine.

The strongest associations have been reported in studies where a broad concept of stress has been used to categorize events. Brown and Harris (1978) found a high relationship with events rated as markedly threatening in relation to their context; Paykel and his colleagues (1969) with events categorized as undesirable. The general picture appears to be of a somewhat non-specific model of stress. Certain events, most notably separations, appear particularly related to depression. However, the range of events is too wide to be usefully included in any single specific formulation, including that of loss.

Magnitude of effect and predisposing factors

It has often been pointed out that the events reported by depressives are frequently experienced without depression occurring, so that their true contribution to causation is questionable. Most of the events reported in research studies are common concomitants of the life cycle, rather than rare catastrophes, so that the criticism has some validity.

In order to quantify the causative effect Brown and Harris (1978) derived an index of 'brought forward time', an estimate of the average time by which a hypothetical spontaneous onset was advanced by life events. They obtained a figure of 10 weeks for schizophrenia, regarded as only 'triggering', but about two years for depression, regarded as 'formative' in effect. Paykel (1978) used a modification of an epidemiological concept, the relative risk. This is the ratio of the rate of the disease among those exposed to a causative factor to the rate among those not exposed. Applying this to the data from his own work and other studies, he obtained figures of around 6 for the risk of developing depression in the six months after the more stressful classes of events, and considerably lower figures for schizophrenia. Risk fell off rapidly with time.

These figures indicate that a large part in determining whether an event is followed by depression must be attributed to interaction with other factors. These fall under the general rubric of predisposition or vulnerability.

In a seminal study, described in more detail in volume 4, chapters 1 and 5 of this Handbook, Brown and Harris (1978) found development of depression in women after a life-event or severe chronic difficulty more common where there were presence in the home of several young children, absence of a confidant with whom the subject could discuss worries, lack of full-time or part-time employment, and loss of mother by death or separation before the age of 11.

Brown's vulnerability factors are mainly additional social supports and stressors. There are many other possible predisposing elements, which have been little studied in interaction with life-events. Some personalities may be vulnerable to events in general; others to specific events such as loss. Such vulnerabilities might be genetic in origin, or environmental. In addition there must be vulnerabilities to specific disorders, psychiatric or somatic. For affective disorder these might involve habitual psychological defence mechanisms and reaction patterns, cyclical changes in function, variations in metabolic pools of transmitter substances. The psychological effects of events must have neurophysiological substrates, where they interact with other neurochemical, physiological, and pharmacological aspects of CNS function, and so influence the pathways regulating mood and causing depression.

Such considerations indicate markedly multifactorial aetiology in which many factors converge on the final state, even in a single case. Jaspers (1962) proposed for a psychiatric reaction that there should be a meaningful connection between content of the experience and that of the abnormal reaction; that the precipitant should appear adequate and be close in time to the reaction; and that the reaction should come to an end when the cause is removed. These criteria are less relevant to an additive model. In any case, the last is usually untestable, the first seems irrelevant, and the second may ask too much in a multifactorially determined condition.

Chronic stressful situations

There has been less research into effects of current stressful situations which are persistent rather than new events or changes. These might include such problems as a chronically bad marriage, physical invalidism, poverty. Brown and Harris (1978) rated presence of existing difficulties in addition to new events. Difficulties which were rated as threatening and had lasted two years were associated with increased depression. The effect was found in absence of severe events, but added little where an event was also present. However, most of their 'vulnerability' factors, which did not increase depression by themselves but only after an event or difficulty, were also chronic stresses. Tennant and Bebbington (1978), in a re-analysis, suggested that these had an independent effect in producing disorder.

Epidemiological studies, reviewed in chapters 21 and 22, also throw light on stressful situations which may predispose to depression. Rates are higher in females (Weissman & Klerman, 1977; Paykel & Rowan, 1979). Possible explanations include sex-linked genes, hormonal effects, and culturally determined modes of acknowledging distress, but perhaps the most plausible is in terms of social stress (Paykel & Rowan, 1979). There is evidence of high rates of depression in mothers of young children (Hare & Shaw, 1965). In case-register studies young married women show high rates of neurotic depression, while rates in single women and men rise with age (Grad de Alarcon *et al.*, 1975). The excess is not limited to the post-partum period. The most likely cause would appear to lie in the social situation of young wives and mothers lacking adequate support from husbands and extended families. Some epidemiological studies of life-events suggest occurrence of more stressful life-events in women. However, the majority show no differences in life-event occurrence, but greater symptom levels at the same life-event stress level. The findings of Brown and Harris (1978), although limited to women, also point to the dependence of young wives on social support.

The relation between affective disorders and social class is less clear-cut. Bagley (1973) reviewed the literature and concluded that there was some relation between higher social class and severe depression. Part might be due to diagnostic bias, part to vulnerability to depression of some personalities such as the ambitious, obsessional, or hypomanic; part to the stress of upward social mobility. On the other hand some recent community surveys have found higher rates in working class subjects. It may be that the neurotic depression and subclinical depression so identified, show a pattern different from affective psychoses.

Early environment

Studies of early environment have mainly concerned loss of a parent in childhood. Such studies require careful controls and matching. Rates of early parent death have declined progressively through this century, and divorce rates have risen. Childhood bereavement is more common in lower social classes and in conditions associated with greater parental age. Findings could also indicate genetic association with suicide in affectively disordered parents, or with patterns of behaviour conducive to early death, marital separation and divorce.

Granville-Grossman (1968) reviewed controlled studies of childhood loss, and several more have since been published. Findings are equivocal. For loss by death, eleven studies have now compared depressives with actuarial norms, general population subjects, or medical/surgical controls (Paykel, 1982). Five found excess in depressives, and six failed to do so. Two studies found greater parental death in depressed than in non-depressed psychiatric patient controls, but seven failed to do so.

Other studies have examined losses not due to death or have not reported type of loss. Three found greater loss in depressives than in general population or medical controls; five failed to do so. Only one of five comparisons with other psychiatric patients showed higher rates for early loss in depressives. Suicide attempters appear to show consistently higher rates; they are best regarded as a separate group from depressives.

The studies of depressives do not agree as to which sex of parent is most important. They do suggest that female children are more vulnerable to loss of a parent than are males.

Granville-Grossman (1968) reviewed other studies of family pattern. Most studies of birth rank have shown no particular relationship to affective disorder. Some studies have found selective firstborn, last-born, and other sibship positions, but they are inconsistent. Studies of parental age have not shown consistent deviations from the expected.

A review of the relevant literature by Tennant and colleagues (1980a) suggested a number of factors that might confound the relationship between early loss by death and depression. After controlling for these factors, the same authors were unable to find any association between early loss by death and subsequent minor neurotic disorder in a population sample. Early loss or separation also showed no asso-ciation with likelihood of disorder. However, if disorder was present, early loss by separation was associated with whether the individual contacted a psychiatrist or not (Tennant *et al.*, 1980b).

Social stress and affective psychoses
Endogenous and psychotic depressions

So far this chapter has made no distinction between depressive neuroses and psychoses. How relevant are findings to the latter? Many of the studies make no separation.

In hospital practice depressions are encountered which appear unrelated to any life stress. In one study of a representative sample, 15 per cent of episodes were judged endogenous (Paykel, 1974). In most depressions there are some psychological elements, although these are often incomplete as full causes.

The endogenous – reactive and psychotic – neurotic distinctions are conceptually separate, but have become partly fused (see chapter 15). In addition to absence of precipitating events, endogenous depressives are regarded as showing a specific symptom pattern with severe depression, psychomotor retardation, more somatic disturbances, morning worsening, early morning wakening, and absence of fluctuations with concurrent environmental change. A third element concerns pre-morbid personality, which is variously characterized in endogenous depressives as non-neurotic, obsessional, or stable.

A number of factor-analytic studies of classification have included precipitant stress. Unfortunately this has usually been recorded in a simple yes–no judgment, unreliable and prone to bias since the situation is often one in which an event has occurred but is not sufficiently overwhelming to be a sole cause of the depression.

Some studies have approached the problem more critically. Thomson and Hendrie (1972), using weighted stress scores, found diagnosed endogenous depressives to have experienced as much stress as reactive depressives. Paykel (1974) employed separate raters for symptoms and life-events to avoid interviewer bias, and also weighted life-events to form a quantitative score. This correlated with presence of an endogenous symptom pattern, but only very weakly. Both these studies reported unimodal distributions of stress scores. Brown and colleagues (1978; 1979) also found only relatively weak relationships between life stress and the distinction between psychotic and neurotic depression based on symptoms.

The relationship between stress and symptom picture is therefore at best relatively weak. The distinction rests more on symptom features, and the term endogenous thus appears unsatisfactory to describe such depressions.

A few studies have examined early loss in relation to symptoms. Brown and Harris (1978) found early loss by death to be associated with psychotic depression; early loss in other ways with neurotic depression. It was suggested that the more severe and irredeemable loss led to a greater lowering of feelings of mastery and self-esteem. Birtchnell (1970), also found more early parental death in severely depressed patients than in moderately depressed ones. Other studies have been inconsistent.

Bipolar affective disorder

The distinction between bipolar and unipolar affective psychoses has received relatively little attention in the life-event literature. Most studies have been in predominantly unipolar samples. A small prospective study of bipolars found no excess of events prior to affective episodes, except for employment difficulties, possibly illness consequences (Hall *et al.*, 1977).

In mania, Ambelas (1979) found independent life-events more common in the four weeks preceding admission, particularly for first attacks, than in surgical controls. Leff and colleagues (1976) reported an uncontrolled finding that 28 per cent of patients experienced an independent event in the month before onset of mania.

Perris (1966) found no differences between unipolars and bipolars regarding childhood bereavement and recent precipitating factors, but there was a higher incidence of unfavourable home conditions in bipolars. Woodruff and colleagues (1971) found that male bipolars reached higher educational and occupational levels than unipolars. The same applied to their brothers, suggesting some familial social advantage.

Psychological studies
Aggression and ambition
Although the psycho-analytic literature is outside the scope of this chapter, some of its themes have featured in empirical studies. Kendell (1970) reviewed

empirical evidence relating depression to internally-directed hostility. He put forward a hypothesis that depression, both as mood and as syndrome, is caused by inhibition of aggressive responses to frustration. Cochrane and Neilson (1977), using measures of drive and aggression, found evidence supporting inhibition of aggression. However, hostile behaviour is increased rather than decreased in some depressions (Weissman & Paykel, 1974).

Price (1968) suggested that depressive behaviour performed an evolutionary adaptive function in primates during a fall in position in a dominance hierarchy. Others have suggested an adaptive function of energy conservation and withdrawal for the infant separated from its mother (Schmale, 1973).

A series of investigations reviewed more fully elsewhere (Weissman & Paykel, 1974) derive from a psycho-analytic study by Mabel Cohen suggesting that manic-depressives come from families striving to improve their status, with much envy and competition. The individual who subsequently develops depression is chosen as the vehicle of the ambition, and develops a pattern of striving, with guilt, a tendency to undersell himself, and inability to achieve interpersonal intimacy. One small study comparing manic-depressives with schizophrenics confirmed this family background. Two other studies failed to to find any increased achievement motivation in manic-depressives.

Behavioural approaches
In recent years theories of depression have been put forward by behavioural psychologists. Seligman (1975) proposed a model of learned helplessness based on animal experiments. Dogs exposed to electric shocks from which they cannot escape develop a severe subsequent aversive learning deficit, remaining immobile instead of escaping shock by jumping a barrier after a signal. The crucial feature appears to be the uncontrollable nature of the aversive stimulus. Additional behavioural and emotional disturbances develop. The situation parallels those in human depression in which there is helplessness and threat outside the subject's control. Students with mild depression have been found to show some learning deficits analogous to those found in 'learned helplessness', in animals, but the equation is far from direct.

Lewinsohn and colleagues (1976) have conducted a series of studies based on a hypothesis relating depression to absence of positive reinforcement. They suggest that a low rate of response-contingent positive reinforcement may produce depression; that various environmental stresses such as loss may lower reinforcement, and that reinforcement from the social environment may be lacking because of poor social skills and because of the depressed person's actual behaviour.

A more clinical approach is that of Beck (1976). He has emphasized cognitive aspects of depression, and especially the content of thought, with low self-esteem, self-reproach and pessimism. He suggests that these depressed cognitions may be important in producing and maintaining depression, instead of being secondary consequences of the emotional disturbance, and has presented evidence that tangible demonstration of successful performance is beneficial. From this has evolved a therapeutic approach, cognitive therapy, combining behavioural techniques with discussion of the negative cognitions.

24
Genetics of the affective psychoses

THEODORE REICH,
C. ROBERT CLONINGER,
BRIAN SUAREZ,
JOHN RICE

Introduction

Emil Kraepelin, in his 1921 monograph, defined manic-depressive insanity very broadly. Included was an episodic course of illness, the presence of affective symptoms, and remission without serious personality defect. Involutional melancholia along with some cases of neurosis or psychopathy were part of the disorder. Kraepelin noted that the disorder was more common in women, that it was associated with a 'morbid temperament' which corresponded to the illness itself, and that a 'heredity taint' could be demonstrated in the vast majority of cases. Patients might have both manic and depressive episodes, or only depressive episodes.

Many epidemiological surveys have used a Kraepelinian definition or a variant of it. The illness has been found to be more common in women; the average male/female ratio is 0.69. The individual estimates of expectancy, however, are quite variable; 0.4 to 1.8 per cent in men and 0.4 to 2.5 per cent in women. This is due in part to the inclusion or exclusion of uncertain cases, probable cases, depressive neuroses, and psychogenic psychoses. For example, the morbidity risk for manic-depressive psychosis in a sample of the Icelandic population (certain + uncertain diagnoses) was 2.18 per cent for males and 3.28 per cent for females, and the morbidity risk for depressive neurosis for males was 2.25 per cent and for females, 4.14 per cent. If one assumes that all these subgroups are part of the same disorder, the risk is 5.39 per cent for males and 9.19 per cent for females (Helgason, 1964).

Slater (1971) modified and recalculated the expectancy of manic-depressive disorders in the first-degree relatives of manic-depressive index patients collected by Zerbin-Rudin (1967). These data were collected from 25 different studies by 11 investigators. If certain cases, probable cases and suicides were included, the expectancy was 11.7 per cent in parents, 12.3 per cent in sibs and 16.0 per cent in children. It seems that the affective psychoses are familial and that, unlike schizophrenia, the expectancy is similar in parents, siblings, and children. This similarity may indicate that the affective disorders are under less selection pressure. As a check on the validity of these studies, we note that the expectation of schizophrenia in the families of patients with affective disorder is not elevated above the population level.

Kringlen (1967) reviewed seven twin studies in order to determine whether manic-depressive illness is genetically determined. Unfortunately, the number of twins in each group is small, the methods of sampling variable, and the criteria for diagnosis uncertain. Over all, however, the concordance between monozygotic twins (33–96 per cent) is greater than for same-sexed dizygotic twins (0–39 per cent). If it can be assumed that the non-genetic causes of similarity between same-sexed twins are equal in monozygotic and dizygotic pairs, the evidence strongly suggests that manic-depressive illness is in some measure a genetic disorder.

Leonhard (1959), in Berlin, subdivided manic-depressive patients into bipolar (mania and depression) and unipolar (depression only) forms. In a family study reported by Leonhard, Korff, and Schulz (1962), it appeared that bipolar patients tended to have bipolar relatives and unipolar patients, unipolar relatives. They also found that cyclothymic personalities with high and low mood swings occurred in the bipolar families and depressive personalities more often in the unipolar families. Finally, the morbidity risk for endogenous affective psychosis was higher in the first-degree relatives of bipolar than unipolar probands (39.9 per cent versus 27.7 per cent). These findings suggest that manic-depressive illness can be divided into at least two subgroups, one in which mania and depression occurs, and a second in which only depression is manifest. Winokur and Clayton (1967) compared the family histories of consecutively admitted affective patients with two generations of affective disorder ($n = 112$) and affective patients without a family history of any psychiatric disorder ($n = 129$). They found that patients with mania were significantly over-represented in the two-generation group, supporting the Leonhardian subdivision.

Population and family data

A number of recent studies have estimated lifetime risks for unipolar and bipolar disorders in general populations (table 24.1). As with earlier estimates, marked variation is seen. In general, bipolar illness is less common than unipolar illness and females are over-represented in both categories. Figures from Italy (Smeraldi *et al.*, 1977) are taken from an official registry as are those from New Zealand (James & Chapman, 1975). The estimates from Israel (Gershon & Liebowitz, 1975) are derived from first admissions to a Jerusalem hospital. The English estimates were prepared by Shields (1978) using data from the Camberwell and Salford cases registers: first-ever contacts with patients diagnosed as schizophrenia or depression (Wing & Fryers, 1976). The depressives are divided into severe, moderate or not otherwise specified (n.o.s.) and these estimates have been cumulated to age 65.

The first set of estimates from the United States, collected by Weissman and colleagues (1978) during the third follow-up of the Yale–New Haven household survey, are based on approximately one-half of the original sample of 1095 adults interviewed in 1967. The instruments used by Weissman and colleagues (1978) were the Schedule of the Affective Disorders and Schizophrenia of Spitzer and Endicott (1979), and the Research Diagnostic Criteria of Spitzer, Endicott and Robins (1978). The second set of American estimates were collected by Cloninger and colleagues (1979) from first-degree relatives of psychiatric patients with illnesses that are not correlated with unipolar or bipolar depression.

Unfortunately, the diagnostic criteria in the table are variable; Gershon and Weissman labelled patients who had a major depression and hypomania as having a bipolar illness (bipolar II), whereas Cloninger used the criteria of Feighner and colleagues (1972), which required a major manic and depressive episode for a diagnosis of bipolar illness (bipolar I).

In addition to different ascertainment methods

* Supported in part by USPHS grants AA-03539, MH-31302, MH-25430, MH-00048 and MH-14677.

Table 24.1. *Lifetime risk for unipolar and bipolar disorders – as percentage*

Region	Author	Male Unipolar	Bipolar	Female Unipolar	Bipolar	Total Unipolar	Bipolar
Italy	Smeraldi					0.4	0.05
New Zealand	James & Chapman	1.0	0.2	2.0	0.27		
Israel	Gershon					1.32	1.08
England	Shields						
	severe	1.61	0.25	2.28	0.25		
	moderate	4.77		8.37			
	n.o.s.	1.71		2.84			
United States	Weissman	9.1	0.9	22.0	1.4		
United States	Cloninger					3.09	0.2

and variable criteria, the lifetime risks are further biased because 5 per cent to 16 per cent of unipolar patients develop manic symptoms. Perris (1966) has reported that even after more than four consecutive depressive episodes, 4 per cent of unipolar patients have a manic attack and are reclassified as bipolar. As recently shown by Akiskal and colleagues (1977) the conversion from unipolar to bipolar illness is not confined to severe or endogenous depression. In a four-year follow-up of 100 in- and out-patients with neurotic depression, 18 per cent become bipolar. The switch in polarity should most seriously bias estimates from the Camberwell and Salford case registers, since the diagnoses were those made at first contact.

In table 24.2 the morbid risk for the major affective disorders in the first-degree relatives of bipolar probands is displayed. Except in the data of Mendelwicz and colleagues (1974) and Perris, the morbid risk for unipolar illness is higher than that for bipolar illness. The anomalous results of Perris (1966) may be explained by his requirement of three separate unipolar episodes before a diagnosis of unipolar affective disorder was made. Since both Perris and Angst (1966) report that 16 per cent and 13 per cent of unipolar depressed patients become bipolar, the figures may change with time.

In table 24.3 the morbid risk for the major affective disorders in the first-degree relatives of unipolar probands is displayed. The risk for bipolar illness is approximately equal to the population prevalence, whereas the risk for unipolar illness is more variable and elevated above the population prevalence. These data therefore support the view that bipolar and unipolar affective disorder are independent familial disorders.

Gershon and colleagues (1976) have presented a table summarizing the morbid risk for a major affective illness in the first-degree relatives of bipolar probands, subdivided by the sex of the proband and relative. In some studies, such as that of Stenstedt (1952), there is a relative deficiency of opposite-sexed pairs of affected individuals implying that there is independence between the illnesses in males and females. In the study by Helzer and Winokur (1974) there appears to be a deficiency of male-to-male transmission not evident in the other data sets. However, it seems clear that different diagnostic criteria and ascertainment biases have led to heterogeneous data sets, and a unitary formulation of the mode of transmission is unlikely.

Gershon has presented a similar table for unipolar probands. An excess of affected females is present in about half the studies and in the remainder males and females are either equally at risk or the risk to males is higher. In several studies there are fewer opposite-sexed than same-sexed relatives. As with the other family data, the risks are very variable and do not lend themselves to unitary explanations. Unipolar affective disorder is familial but the effect is attenuated when recent population prevalence figures are used. By contrast the risk in the families of bipolar probands is higher, implying a stronger familial effect.

Table 24.2. *Bipolar probands: morbid risk for the major affective disorders in first-degree relatives (Expanded from Gershon et al., 1976)*

Study	Siblings At risk	Morbid risk (%) BP	UP	Parents–offspring At risk	Morbid risk (%) BP	UP	Total At risk	Morbid risk (%) BP	UP
Angst (1966)	84	4.7	15.5	77	3.9	10.4	161	4.3	13.0
Perris (1966)	315	13.6	0.3	312	6.7	0.7	627	10.2	0.5
Winokur & Clayton (1967)	82	11.0	18.3	85	9.4	22.4	167	10.2	20.4
Helzer & Winokur (1974)	91	5.5	8.8	60	3.3	13.3	151	4.6	10.6
Goetzl et al. (1974)	86	3.5	8.1	126	2.4	17.5	212	2.8	13.7
Gershon et al. (1975b)	164	4.3	7.3	177	3.4	6.2	341	3.8	6.8
James & Chapman (1975)	–	–	–	–	–	–	265	6.4	13.2
Mendelwicz et al. (1974)	268	21.2	–	377	11.9	–	605	17.7	–
	236	–	18.6	308	–	25.3	544	–	22.4
Smeraldi et al. (1977)	71	8.5	9.8	102	3.9	9.8	173	5.7	9.8

Table 24.3. *Unipolar probands: morbid risk for the major affective disorders in first-degree relatives (Expanded from Gershon et al., 1976)*

Study	Siblings At risk	Morbid risk (%) BP	UP	Parents-offspring At risk	Morbid risk (%) BP	UP	Total At risk	Morbid risk (%) BP	UP
Angst (1966)	470	0.64	5.1	341	0.0	5.0	811	0.3	5.1
Perris (1966)	348	0.3	8.9	336	0.3	3.9	684	0.3	6.4
Gershon et al. (1975b)	40	2.5	15.0	56	1.7	9.0	96	2.1	11.5
Smeraldi et al. (1977)	78	1.3	16.6	107	0.9	7.5	185	1.1	11.4

Assortative mating

If unipolar and bipolar types of affective illness were independent, the relatives of bipolar probands would not have an elevated risk for unipolar disorder. Since this risk is elevated, independence cannot be assumed. Some association between the two disorders may be the consequences of assortative mating. In table 24.4 the morbid risk for affective disorder in the spouses of affectively ill patients is displayed. Comparing the risk in spouses with the population prevalence, it is clear that a great deal of assortative mating occurs. Even if this degree of assortative mating has been going on for many generations, it is not known whether it is sufficient to explain the association of unipolar and bipolar disorder (Gershon et al., 1973).

Twin data

Bertelson and colleagues (1977) have conducted an excellent twin study using the Danish twin register, which includes all same-sexed twins born in Denmark in the years 1870 to 1920. By comparing the twin and psychiatric registers, it was possible to ascertain approximately 110 pairs of same-sexed twins where at least one member of each pair had an affective disorder. A catamnestic investigation was carried out by personal interview and zygosity established by blood tests.

The probandwise concordance for bipolar illness in monozygotic twins is 0.79 and in dizygotes 0.19. For unipolar illness the concordance is 0.54 in monozygotic twins and 0.24 in dizygotic twins. Since the concordance for monozygotic is higher than for

Table 24.4. *Morbid risk for affective disorder in spouses of affectively ill patients, systematic interview data (Gershon et al., 1973)*

	Number	Number at risk[a]	Affective disorder[b]
Wives of:			
Bipolar males	23	17	*41.2*
Unipolar males	8	6	*15.4*
Control Males	14	11	*0.0*
Husbands of:			
Bipolar females	24	17	*6.0*
Unipolar females	15	11	*27.6*
Control females	11	9	*0.0*

[a] Age-corrected
[b] All had unipolar illness.

dizygotic twins, a genetic factor is suggested for both forms of illness. In addition some overlap between unipolar and bipolar illness is found.

The concordant monozygotic co-twins of 27 bipolar probands were bipolar in 21 cases and unipolar in 6. By contrast the co-twins of 19 monozygotic unipolar probands were bipolar in 4 cases and unipolar in 15. Since the genotypes of monozygotic twins are identical, a bipolar genotype sometimes manifests as unipolar illness and a unipolar genotype as bipolar illness. A similar overlap is shown among the dizygotic twins. Other twin studies also support these conclusions (Price, 1968).

Adoption data

Mendelwicz *et al*. (1977) studied the families of adult bipolar probands who had been adopted early in life. All available parents were interviewed by researchers blind to the adoptive and clinical status of the offspring. A structured interview based on the criteria of Feighner and colleagues (1972) was used. As can be seen in table 24.5 the incidence of affective disorder in the biological parents was much higher than the adoptive parents.

Three control groups were used in this study. The first were bipolar non-adoptees, the second were normal adoptees, and the third were biological parents of patients with poliomyelitis. The rate of affective disorder in the biological parents who had not given their children up for adoption was similar to that in biological parents who had given them up. The rate of affective disorder in the biological parents and adoptive parents of normal adoptees was not elevated, nor was the rate in the biological parents of patients with poliomyelitis. This study strengthens the view that bipolar and unipolar affective disorder can to some extent be transmitted by a common genetic mechanism.

Cadoret (1978) conducted a small study of parents and offspring separated early in life by adoption. The results of this study also support the hypothesis of a genetic factor, primarily in unipolar depressive illness.

The intact family data, twin, and adoption studies support the view that unipolar and bipolar affective disorders are at least two independently transmissible genetic illnesses but that the psychopathological mechanism for producing a bipolar illness may sometimes produce a unipolar one. The

Table 24.5. *Manic-depressive illness in parents and offspring separated by adoption (Mendelwicz et al., 1977)*

	Bipolar adoptees (N = 29)		Bipolar non-adoptees (N = 31)	Normal adoptees (N = 22)		Poliomyelitis (N = 20)
	Adoptive parents	Biological parents	Biological parents	Adoptive parents	Biological parents	Biological parents
Bipolar	1	4	2	0	0	0
Unipolar	3	12	11	3	1	4
Total	4	16	13	3	1	4

p < 0.05.

Table 24.6. *Major linkage studies of the affective disorders*

Disorder in probands	Mode of Transmission	Method of linkage analysis
Primary affective	none assumed	sib pairs
Primary affective	none assumed	sib pairs
Pure depression	none assumed	sib pairs
Pure depression	autosomal dominant (NAC)	pedigrees/maximum likelihood
Depression spectrum	none assumed	sib pairs
Depression spectrum	autosomal dominant (AC)	pedigrees/maximum likelihood
Bipolar	X-linked dominant (NAC)	Recombinant v. non-recombinants
Bipolar	X-linked dominant (NAC)	Recombinant v. non-recombinants
Bipolar	X-linked dominant (NAC)	Edwards
Bipolar	X-linked dominant (NAC)	Edwards
Bipolar	X-linked dominant (NAC)	Edwards
Bipolar	X-linked dominant (NAC)	Edwards
Bipolar	X-linked dominant (NAC)	Edwards
Schizo-affective	X-linked dominant (NAC)	Edwards
Bipolar	X-linked dominant (AC)	Edwards
Bipolar	X-linked Dominant (?)	?
Bipolar	autosomal dominant (NAC)	pedigrees/maximum likelihood
Bipolar	incompletely penetrant X-linked dominant (AC)	pedigrees/maximum likelihood
Bipolar	X-linked dominant (AC)	pedigrees/maximum likelihood
Bipolar	X-linked dominant (AC)	pedigrees/maximum likelihood

AC = age-corrected, NAC = not age-corrected
[a]Collaborative study with two centres reporting evidence of linkage to colour-blindness loci and two centres failing to find linkage.

separation is also favored by the observations that patients with the bipolar illness are younger, have more episodes, respond differently to lithium carbonate, are relatively less often female, and have more frequent post-partum episodes (Winokur *et al.*, 1969; Zerbin-Rudin, 1979).

Linkage and association studies

Table 24.6 lists the major linkage studies of the affective disorders. The table does not include studies that use sex as a marker for X-linkage. The original papers should be consulted for a description of the criteria used to define the illness in the probands.

Without explanation, all linkage studies of bipolar affective disorder assume that unipolar relatives are affected with the same disorder as the proband. Many of the studies listed are not independent since, as new families were brought into a study, previously reported families were again reported. Under the heading 'Linked to' are included those loci claimed by the respective investigators to be linked to the disorder under study regardless of the strength of the evidence.

Within any diagnostic category the reports are often inconsistent and difficult to compare because different modes of transmission are assumed (modes

Linked to	Not linked to	Reference
–	ABO	Tanna & Winokur (1968)
HLA	–	Smeraldi *et al.* (1978)
Gc	ABO, Rh, Kell, MNS, Duffy, Kidd, Lutheran, AK, PGM₁, GPT, C₃, α-Hp	Tanna *et al.* (1976a)
Gc		Tanna *et al.* (1977a)
C₃, α-Hp	ABO, Rh, Kell, MNS, P, Duffy, Kidd, Gc, Lutheran, 6-PGD, ADA, PGM₁, GPT	Tanna *et al.* (1976b)
α-Hp	C₃	Tanna *et al.* (1979)
Xg	Duffy, MNS, ABO, Kidd	Winokur & Tanna (1969)
Protanopia, Deuteranopia	–	Reich *et al.* (1969)
Protanopia, Deuteranopia	–	Mendelwicz *et al.* (1972)
Xg	–	Fieve *et al.* (1973)
Protanopia, Deuteranopia	–	Mendelwicz *et al.* (1974)
Xg	–	Mendelwicz *et al.* (1974)
Protanopia, Deuteranopia	–	Fieve *et al.* (1975)
Xg	–	Mendelwicz *et al.* (1975)
Deuteranopia	–	Baron (1977)
–	Deuteranopia	Johnson & Leeman (1977)
G6PD	–	Mendelwicz & Linkowski (1978)
–	HLA	Targum *et al.* (1979)
–	Xg	Leckman *et al.* (1979)
–	Protanopia, Deuteranopia	Gershon *et al.* (1979)
Protanopia, Deuteranopia	–	Mendelwicz *et al.* (1979)

that are undoubtedly too simple especially in the light of the heterogeneity) and because assumptions inherent in the method are often ignored (for instance, the sib pairs studies count all possible pairs of sibs – a violation of the independence assumption – while some of the pedigree studies fail to take proper account of non-random ascertainment by selecting bipolar cases with an X-chromosome marker as probands). In still other cases the lod scores have been miscalculated. When multiple marker systems have been assayed, no account of the number of statistical tests performed was made so the reported level of significance is incorrect. Finally, many of the studies testing an X-linked hypothesis selected as probands patients with bipolar illness and an X-chromosome

marker which results in a sample of dubious 'generalizability'.

The search for a major single locus for any of the affective disorders is important but, as the evidence stands, none has conclusively been identified using the linkage strategy.

Table 24.7 lists the studies that have reported significant association between the affective disorders and the ABO blood groups or the HLA complex. The reported HLA associations are inconsistent across studies and the statistical significance of all but one of the reported associations (i.e., with BW16) disappears when corrected for the number of alleles tested. It is noteworthy that in some studies not a single BW16-positive affectively ill patient was identified,

Table 24.7. *Association studies of the affective disorders*

Disorder	Positive association	Negative associa-tion	Reference
Bipolar	0[a]	–	Masters (1967)
Bipolar	0[a]	A[a]	Mendelwicz *et al.* (1974)
Bipolar	–	B12	Stember & Fieve (1976)
Bipolar	BW16	–	Shapiro *et al.* (1976)
Bipolar	BW17	–	Bennahum *et al.* (1976)
Bipolar	0[a]	–	Shapiro *et al.* (1977)
Bipolar	–	B7	Beckman *et al.* (1978)
Bipolar	B14	B27	Targum *et al.* (1979)
Unipolar	A[a]	–	Shapiro *et al.* (1977)
Unipolar	A10	A1	Beckman *et al.* (1978)
Bipolar & unipolar	B[a,c]	–	Tanna & Winokur (1968)
Bipolar & unipolar	A3, B7, BW16	B8	Shapiro *et al.* (1976)
Bipolar & unipolar	B5, B13	–	Stember & Fieve (1976)
Bipolar & unipolar	B5	B15	Govaerts *et al.* (1977)
Bipolar & unipolar	A29, BW22	A10, A30	Smeraldi *et al.* (1978)
Bipolar, unipolar & cycloid	(A3, B18, B22)[b]	–	Perris *et al.* (1979)

[a] Refers to ABO blood groups.
[b] In patients relapsing on lithium therapy.
[c] In patients with one or more affected first-degree relatives only.

thereby casting doubt even on this association.

Among the ABO association studies the most consistent finding is an increase in blood group O among bipolar patients. Parker and colleagues (1961) and Irvine and Miyashita (1965) both report an increase of blood group O in bipolar patients but, in the former case, the increase failed to reach statistical significance while in the latter case, no properly chosen normal control group was available for comparison. In addition to these ABO and HLA association studies, Perris (1976) has reported that the frequency of SS homozygotes is significantly increased in bipolar patients compared to normal controls and that there are significant differences between unipolar and bipolar patients with respect to the Lewis blood group phenotype Le(a$^+$b$^-$). Since, however, over 30 marker systems were assayed, the possible significance of these two associations must await full publication of the data.

The association between bipolar affective disorder and blood group O appears to be the strongest reported to date. None the less, a study of this association should be replicated on a larger sample of bipolar patients diagnosed according to strict diagnostic criteria. Such a replication study could shed some light on the hypothesis that bipolar affective disorder is mediated, in part, by a membrane disorder.

Mode of transmission

Although the above results support the hypothesis that genetic factors play a role in the transmission of the affective disorders, no single mode of inheritance has been unambiguously established for any subtype of the disorder. This must be attributed both to unresolved clinical issues and, until recently, the lack of appropriate genetic models.

Current models postulate an underlying continuous liability scale together with a threshold value so that an individual manifests the disorder if his liability score is above the threshold value (Falconer, 1965). Multiple thresholds may be used to model sex differences (Kidd *et al.*, 1973) or subforms of intermediate severity (Reich *et al.*, 1972), or may be used as a vehicle to resolve phenotypic heterogeneity among subforms (Reich *et al.*, 1979). Gershon and his colleagues (1975a, b & c), using thresholds in their analysis of affective disorders in the Jewish population of Jerusalem to subtype diagnoses as moderate depression, unipolar illness, and bipolar illness, concluded that bipolar illness was a more severe form of unipolar illness.

The two models which have been used to describe the transmission of a threshold character are the single major locus model (SML) and the multifactorial model (MF). In the SML model (Reich *et al.*, 1972; Gershon *et al.*, 1976) a normally distributed liability is assumed for each genotype of the major locus, with the proportion of the genotype distribution above the threshold determining its penetrance (i.e. the probability that an individual with that genotype is affected). Using the method of Elston and Stewart (1971) and Elston (1973), the SML may be used to analyse large pedigrees for a trait with variable age of onset.

Winokur and colleagues (1969) analysed data on 62 bipolar probands and postulated that bipolar illness was transmitted as an X-linked dominant. Crowe and Smouse (1977) reanalysed their data incorporating age-dependent penetrance and found the X-linked hypothesis to hold after taking into account variable age of onset. However, father-to-son transmission has been reported by others (Gershon *et al.*, 1975c; Goetzl *et al.*, 1974; James & Chapman, 1975; Mendelwicz & Rainer, 1974; Stenstedt, 1952). Bucher and colleagues (1980a & b) have reanalysed the data of Winokur and colleagues and concluded that neither a single Mendelian autosomal or X-linked gene is adequate to describe the transmission of affective disorder in these families. An unsuccessful attempt was also made to fit a two-gene model. Mendelwicz and Rainer (1974), assuming that the bipolar and unipolar relatives of bipolar probands were genotypically identical, analysed families obtained from bipolar probands and reported X-linkage. Van Eerdewegh and colleagues (1980) have found that these data do not fit the X-chromosome SML model under this assumption, although they could not reject X-linked transmission using the data of Winokur and col-

leagues (1969) or using the data of Gershon and colleagues (1975a, b & c). However, these results do not rule out the X-linked hypothesis for bipolar illness since it is possible that only a portion of the unipolar relatives manifest the bipolar genotype and that this clinical heterogeneity accounts for the lack of fit.

The MF model assumes that many factors of small effect contribute additively to an individual's liability score. Resemblance between relatives is measured by the correlation between their liability distributions. Gershon and colleagues (1975a, b & c) found both the SML and MF models adequate to describe their data set obtained through both unipolar and bipolar probands. James and Chapman (1975) analysed the families of 46 bipolar probands and found that polygenic inheritance (the special case of the MF model when the transmissible factors comprise only additive genes) adequately described their data, but that an X-linked dominant hypothesis was inadequate. More recent formulations of the MF model use path analysis to allow systematically for polygenic inheritance, cultural inheritance, assortative mating, and a common environment of rearing (Rice *et al.*, 1978; Cloninger *et al.*, 1979a & b), but this newer formulation has yet to be applied to the affective disorders. The SML model precludes environmental sources of resemblance between relatives.

A strategy which complements the fitting of models of transmission is the search for biological or pharmacological markers to identify homogeneous subtypes of affective disorder prior to genetic analyses. Gershon (1978) provides a thorough review of such data, including MHPG, MAO, COMT, THR stimulation of TSH, and sleep studies. He found no marker that consistently distinguished between unipolar, bipolar, and normal subjects. Another strategy is to develop alternative diagnostic schema (such as the depressive spectrum concept proposed by Winokur and his colleagues) in concert with genetic analysis in order to clarify the mode of transmission.

Familial relationship to other psychiatric disorders

There is strong and consistent evidence from family studies that there are specific factors for the familial predisposition to affective disorders that are different from other types of psychiatric illness. Cloninger and his associates (1979c) recently reviewed the familial aggregation of primary affective disorders with other psychiatric disorders in 8 family interview studies carried out in St Louis. Both bipolar and unipolar disorder were increased in the relatives of acute schizophrenics but neither was in the relatives of chronic schizophrenics, hysterics, or sociopaths (antisocial personality). Slater and Roth (1969) and Gottesman and Shields (1972) have noted that schizophrenia and affective disorder have never been reported together in monozygous co-twins. Blind family interview data confirm the independence of affective disorder from most other psychiatric disorders (Tsuang, 1978; Gershon *et al.*, 1975b, c).

The relationship of typical affective disorder to schizo-affective psychoses in which features of affective disorder and schizophrenia are simultaneously combined is at present uncertain. Frequently, symptoms characteristic of chronic schizophrenia may occur acutely during some episodes of a disorder that is otherwise typical of bipolar or unipolar affective disorder in terms of both prognosis and family history (Goodwin & Guze, 1979). However, there is also a slight increase in schizophrenia in such cases which may reflect either the imperfect reliability of diagnosis in atypical cases, cases combining two disorders, variable expressivity of a disorder different from typical affective disorder, or some combination of these (Robins & Guze, 1970).

The relationship between alcoholism and affective disorder is complicated (Cloninger *et al.*, 1979; Morrison, 1975). Unipolar depression, but not mania, is increased in the relatives of primary alcoholics. Winokur has suggested that some cases of alcoholism and unipolar depression may be sex-typed variants of the same unitary genetic factor, but this hypothesis has been shown to be inadequate as a general explanation (Cloninger *et al.*, 1979c). Adopted-away daughters of alcoholics showed no increased risk of affective disorder (Goodwin *et al.*, 1977). First-degree relatives of unipolar depressives have the same morbid risk of alcoholism regardless of the presence or absence of parental affective disorder (Winokur & Clayton, 1967). Genetic factors which predispose specifically both to alcoholism and to affective disorder appear negligible, but living with an alcoholic seems to be an adverse experience which increases the risk of developing depression. This will be discussed further in the section on adverse childhood environments.

Since the predisposition to affective disorders is different from the predisposition to other psychiatric disorders, it is useful to distinguish cases in which there is no pre-existing psychiatric disorder (i.e., primary affective disorders) from cases in which another psychiatric illness preceded the onset of the affective disorder (i.e., secondary affective disorder) (Robins & Guze, 1972). The primary affective disorders are by definition more homogeneous aetiologically than secondary affective disorders, which include affective disorders coincident with other psychiatric disorders due to chance, due to symptomatic overlap, or due to adjustment reactions associated with reduced coping ability or increased situational stress as a complication of the primary disorder. The natural history of secondary affective disorders is often dominated by the primary psychiatric illness (Weissman *et al.*, 1977) and much evidence for neurobiological differences between primary and secondary affective disorder has accumulated (Akiskal *et al.*, 1979). Secondary depressions have been claimed to be situational reactions not associated with parental affective disorder (Akiskal *et al.*, 1979) but empirical data are sparse and contradictory (Guze *et al.*, 1971; Winokur, 1978).

Heterogeneity in predisposition to mania

Variation among manics in pre-morbid personality, age of onset, and frequency and type of episode may be related to familial factors. Perris (1966) compared the relatives of 138 bipolar manic-depressives with those of 17 unipolar manics who had never had a depressive episode. The morbid risk for bipolar illness was 16.3 ± 1.5 per cent and 7.6 ± 2.4 per cent respectively. The unipolar manic probands had no unipolar depressive relations. The risk of unipolar depression in relatives of the bipolar probands was 0.8 ± 0.4 per cent.

It is surprising that all the manic relatives of manic probands were bipolar (that is, they also had had depressions), whereas none of the bipolar probands had any unipolar manic relatives. Compared to the data in table 24.2, the low risk of unipolar depression in the relatives of bipolar and unipolar manic probands is compensated for by increased risk for unspecified depressions (7.9 per cent) and of suicide (7.6 per cent). These findings are supported in part by data obtained by Taylor and Abrams (1973). Dividing probands into those with onset before and after age 30, they found that late-onset probands had a unipolar manic course in half of 22 cases and in 11 per cent of 28 early-onset cases. Relatives of early- and late-onset probands had affective disorder in 31 per cent and 8 per cent of cases respectively ($p < 0.05$).

The authors suggested that late-onset mania may either be a milder form of the same illness or a heterogeneous group of different mania-like psychoses. They preferred the latter hypothesis because of the significant excess of unipolar mania in the late-onset group. Forty-six per cent of the bipolar probands described by Perris had onset at age 30 or later, but unfortunately he did not report the ages of his unipolar manics.

Others have also observed the correlation between positive family history and age of onset in mania and interpreted it as evidence for hereditary predisposition in early-onset cases and brain damage in late-onset cases. Dalén (1965) related electroencephalographic abnormalities to family history and observed that 56 per cent of those with a negative family history had paroxysmal theta activity compared to 11 per cent of those with a positive family history. He further observed that a history of perinatal trauma was correlated with late onset and EEG abnormality and concluded that late-onset mania may reflect perinatal brain damage. This has been supported by later work by Hays (1976) and Kadrmas and Winokur (1979) but not by Small and her associates (1975). The association between perinatal brain damage with late-onset mania rather than congenital behavioural disturbance seems dubious. Rare manic-like syndromes due to viral encephalitis (Steinberg *et al.*, 1972) or lesions in the vicinity of the hypothalamus (Slater & Roth, 1969; Fish, 1967) have been documented but the differences between early-onset and late-onset mania appear to be quantitative rather than qualitative in the vast majority of cases.

Severity of illness does not seem closely related to familial predisposition to mania. In the same families, the spectrum of severity in bipolar illness ranges from individuals with cyclothymic personality but no incapacity or need for treatment to individuals incapacitated both by the depressive and by the manic episodes (Leonhard *et al.*, 1962; Gershon & Liebowitz, 1975). Akiskal and associates (1977) have compared the families of psychiatric out-patients diagnosed as cyclothymic personality with those meeting explicit criteria for mania (Feighner *et al.*, 1972). The patients with cyclothymic personality had sought out-patient treatment for various personality maladjustments but had never had a psychiatric hospitalization, and failed to meet full criteria for hypomania or depression in terms of the duration and number of symptoms. The bipolar subjects met full criteria for mania and depression and had required hospitali-

zation for mania. When the families of the two groups were compared, the same high ratio of bipolar and unipolar affective disorder and suicide was observed in both groups of relatives. These rates were higher than in a control group who reported mood swings but had no behavioural signs of mania, such as hyperactivity, push of speech, flight of ideas, or decreased sleep. The correlation between personality type and polarity or psychosis is high (Leonhard *et al.*, 1962), but about one out of every four or five bipolar psychotic patients does not have a cyclothymic personality (Winokur, Clayton & Reich, 1969).

The findings on differences in pre-morbid personality in affective disorder provide important support for the bipolar–unipolar dichotomy. Furthermore, age of onset seems correlated with severity of familial predisposition to some extent in both bipolar and unipolar psychoses; and yet differences persist when late-onset manics and early-onset depressives, who should be most similar in terms of degree of familial predisposition, are compared.

Heterogeneity in unipolar depressives

The presence of parental affective disorder is weakly correlated ($r < 0.2$) with early onset and recurrent episodes of depression in their children in two studies (Winokur, 1979; Schlesser *et al.*, 1979). Thus, individuals with late onset and isolated episodes tend to have fewer affected relatives than those with early onset and/or multiple episodes (Kay, 1959; Hopkinson & Ley, 1969; Woodruff *et al.*, 1964; Pollitt, 1972). Sex, severity and type of symptoms (including so-called 'endogenous' depressive symptoms such as diurnal variation, early morning awakening, self-reproach, and psychomotor retardation) do not significantly differentiate depressives with and without familial affective disorder (Winokur & Clayton, 1967; Woodruff *et al.*, 1964; Winokur, 1979; Schlesser *et al.*, 1979; Andreason, 1979).

Dichotomizing depressives into endogenous/-reactive or neurotic/psychotic types does not yield groups that segregate in a homotypic fashion (i.e., they do not breed true) (Stenstedt, 1952, 1959 and 1966). Clinical subdivisions of neurotic, involutional, and endogenous depressives differ in the proportion of affected relatives in some studies (Stenstedt, 1952, 1959 and 1966) but not in others (Winokur & Pitts, 1964). However, the presence of certain types of precipitating factors do seem to influence the risk of manifestation in susceptible individuals; this will be discussed in the section on precipitating factors.

Favorable response to electroconvulsive therapy (Winokur, 1979; Mendels, 1965) or to tricyclic antidepressants (Winokur, 1979) is weakly correlated with family history of affective disorders. However, the sensitivity and specificity are so low (50 per cent and 70 per cent respectively) that this difference by itself is of limited clinical utility.

Adverse childhood environment

Many studies of childhood bereavement and other adverse experiences have compared subjects with affective disorder to other controls with contradictory results, as reviewed by Perris (1966). Interpretation is difficult owing to the fact that uncertainty about diagnosis is a confounding variable. Stenstedt (1952, 1966) found an increased risk of affective disorder in sibs reared under unfavorable conditions if the proband was manic-depressive but not if the proband was a neurotic depressive. Perris (1966) found that the only difference between bipolar and unipolar probands in terms of unfavorable childhood environments was due to parental psychiatric illness, not to parental death or separation. Parental affective disorder may well account for the results of Stenstedt and Perris.

However, recent adoption and family data suggest that the experience of living with an alcoholic parent may increase the risk of developing depression in offspring independent of genetic factors. Goodwin and associates (1977) observed that daughters of alcoholics had an increased risk of depression if they were reared in the parental home but not if they were adopted away. The effect of living with an alcoholic could be mediated through cultural inheritance such as learned helplessness (Akiskal & McKinney, 1975) or through increased susceptibility and exposure to precipitating factors. Cross-fostering studies, in which alcoholics reared the biological children of normals, would be needed to evaluate the interaction of inherited and acquired personality variables. Particularly significant is work suggesting that it is possible to distinguish patients with a familial diathesis for depression from those with a low genetic predisposition for depression who have had the adverse experience of living with an alcoholic or sociopath. Several investigators have found that hyperactivity of the hypothalamic-pituitary-adrenal (HPA) axis is characteristic of many but not all depressions (Ettigi & Brown, 1977). The best-documented and most specific measure of HPA-axis overactivity in depressives is the dexamethasone-suppression test, which shows early escape from suppression in about half of primary or endogenous depressives but not in most other psychiatric controls (Butler & Besser, 1968; Carroll et al., 1970 and 1976; Schlesser et al., 1979; Brown et al., 1979). In addition non-suppression is correlated with the familial loading for depression. When the remarkably similar results of Carroll and Davies (1970) and Schlesser and associates (1979) are combined, 80 per cent of 40 depressives with a family history of depression were non-suppressors as compared with 40 per cent of 73 depressives with no family history of depression and no adverse childhood environment. Furthermore, depressives with adverse childhood environments (such as having a family member with alcoholism or sociopathy) were non-suppressors in only 6 per cent of 32 cases. Brown and colleagues (1979) observed specificity for depression but failed to observe any relationship with family history of psychiatric illness in general. However, they did not specify the extent of information available to them about familial depression. Negative results with the dexamethasone-suppression test have been reported (Langer et al., 1979; see also Carroll et al., 1976) but did not control for family background of the subjects.

Factors precipitating depressive states

Pollitt (1972) and Akiskal and McKinney (1975) have described a diathesis-stress model of affective disorder in which certain specific types of somatic and psychological factors precipitate affective disturbance in susceptible individuals. Pollitt considers premorbid personality as an intervening variable which influences the individuals ability to cope with psychological stress. It is hypothesized that the risk of depression may be influenced by degrees of both genetic predisposition and stress, so that those episodes precipitated by severe stress are associated with lower morbid risk in relatives. Pollitt studied a series of depressives with a single episode (116 cases) or one prior episode more than four years earlier (26 cases) according to type of precipitant. Severe viral or bacterial infections, other physical stressors, and, to a lesser extent, severe psychological stress were associated with a lower morbidity risk than in those with no or doubtful psychological stress or puerperal psychoses. The lack of reduction in the puerperal psychoses confirms the earlier work of Protheroe (1969). Other work has indicated an increased incidence of herpes simplex virus antibodies in patients with psychotic depression (Rimon et al., 1971).

Reserpine can precipitate depression primarily in genetically predisposed individuals (Goodwin & Bunney, 1971; Jensen, 1959; Mendels & Frazer, 1974) but seldom in others (Bernstein & Kaufman, 1960). Each of these somatic precipitants, and also physical stress such as gross overwork, depletes brain monoamines (Akiskal & McKinney, 1975) and this may be the common pathway by which affective disorder is triggered off in susceptible subjects. Studies of psychological stress are considered in chapter 23.

Little information about precipitants in mania is available, though Perris (1966) observed that the incidence and type of precipitants in bipolar and unipolar subjects did not differ significantly. He presented no data on the relationship of precipitants in probands to morbid risk in relatives.

Given the ubiquity of the precipitants implicated there is need for blind prospective follow-up and family studies in order to clarify the specificity of both the putative precipitants and the host variables such as familial predisposition and personality factors. At this time such blind multivariate work is lacking, but the magnitude of the effects observed by Pollitt merits attempts at replication.

Summary and conclusions

(1) Affective disorders aggregate in families but the extent is uncertain because lifetime rates in the general population and in families vary markedly, owing to different diagnostic criteria and assessment procedures.

(2) Twin and adoption data indicate that some forms of affective disorder have substantial genetic determination but no specific mode of inheritance has been established for any subtype of the disorder. Neither mathematical models nor data on linkage and association have produced consistent conclusive results.

(3) Sibs, parents, and offspring all have about the same morbid risks for affective disorder, which suggests that affective disorder is not under much pressure from genetic selection despite a high suicide rate.

(4) The genetic diathesis for affective disorders is independent of that for other psychiatric disorders. Family and twin data indicate that bipolar manic-depressive illness is aetiologically distinct from most cases of unipolar depression, but the genotype underlying bipolar illness may sometimes produce either unipolar depressive illness or cyclothymic temperament.

(5) Morbid risks in relatives of manic probands vary with age of onset and EEG abnormalities but not with sex or severity of symptoms in the proband.

(6) Morbid risks in relatives of unipolar depressive probands vary with age of onset, responsiveness to treatment, and severity of precipitating factors, but not with severity or type of symptoms in the proband. Some data suggest a deficiency of cross-sex transmission (father–daughter, mother–son) but this varies between studies.

25

Biochemistry and pathology of the affective psychoses

GEORGE ASHCROFT

Suggestions that biochemical changes may be important in the aetiology of certain depressive and manic disorders were made before the time of Kraepelin, who reviewed the evidence than available (Kraepelin, 1921).

In recent years three major areas have received attention: the role of the biogenic amines, the importance of endocrinological changes, and changes in ion distribution and transport across cell membranes.

Several difficulties have been encountered in the interpretation of such studies in addition to the central problem presented by the relative inaccessibility of the brain to biochemical investigation, in particular, the following:

(1) The differentiation between changes that are directly linked to the aetiology of the disorders and changes secondary to the disorders or to the changes in activity level consequent on the changes in mood.

(2) Lack of information on the changes to be expected during normal mood responses.

(3) Difficulty in defining the clinical characteristics that need to be investigated biochemically. Should we be looking for correlations with accepted clinical disorders (e.g. bipolar depression, mania, or puerperal psychosis) or with specific features of disorders (such as retardation, agitation, depressed mood, or sleep disturbance) the occurrence of which cut across the established syndromes? Alternatively we

might seek to use biochemical markers as predictors of response to treatment.

(4) Many of the biochemical assays have undergone progressive improvement in accuracy, sensitivity, and specificity so that it is difficult to compare the results of early studies with those of more recent investigations.

As a background to the clinical studies, there has been an increase in understanding the functional significance of cerebral transmitter systems, including the regulation of transmitter release and metabolism and the influence of drugs on the systems. It is not surprising, therefore, that aetiological hypotheses are in a constant state of modification and development. All that is possible is to review the present state of the subject, giving most attention to studies which appear technically acceptable, which seem to be pointing the way to future developments, and which have led to replication.

Biogenic amines in the affective disorders

It was recognized in the 1950s that amines might be involved in the aetiology of the affective disorders when the antidepressant properties of the tricyclic and monoamine-oxidase inhibitor (MAOI) groups of drugs and the apparent precipitation of depression by the anti-hypertensive and tranquillizing drug reserpine were discovered.

It was discovered from animal experiments that reserpine reduced the cerebral concentrations of the amines noradrenaline, dopamine, and 5-hydroxytryptamine and that the antidepressant drugs were capable of raising the concentration of the amines (in the case of the MAOIs) or potentiating their effects at central synapses by blocking their re-uptake into the neurones. These findings provided the basis of the theory that depression could result from a reduction in the activity of amines at central synapses whilst mania could follow an increase in such activity (Coppen, 1974; Schildkraut, 1978). Studies over the past twenty years have led to a clarification of the role of the amines as synaptic transmitters and to progress in the understanding of the function of the neuronal systems in brain utilizing these transmitters.

These animal studies provide only indirect evidence of the involvement of changes in amine systems in the affective disorders and the possibility remains that the antidepressant drugs may be acting on systems which are not directly involved in their development. By analogy, the anticholinergic drugs which have a therapeutic action in relieving the symptoms of Parkinsonism are now recognized as not acting directly on the degenerating dopaminergic neurones primarily concerned in the development of the disease.

Direct evidence of the involvement of changes in cerebral amine systems in patients with affective illness has understandably been difficult to come by but the following types of study have been undertaken:

(1) Changes in amine metabolite concentrations in cerebrospinal fluid;

(2) Post-mortem changes in the cerebral concentrations of the amines and their metabolites;

(3) The effects of manipulation of amine synthesis by the administration of amine precursors;

(4) Measurement of blood hormone levels, e.g. prolactin, as an index of changes in amine-mediated hypothalamic hormonal control systems.

Peripheral indices, such as 3-methoxy-4-hydroxy phenylethyline glycol (MHPG) urinary excretion and platelet 5-hydroxytryptamine uptake mechanisms have been used to investigate or predict response to treatment.

Changes in amine metabolites: amine metabolites in cerebrospinal fluid

The amine metabolites 5-hydroxyindolacetic acid (5HIAA), homovanillic acid (HVA), and MHPG do not readily cross the blood-CSF barrier. Lumbar fluid CSF levels will, therefore, reflect changes in central nervous system metabolism and/or release of the amines. There are, however, many problems in interpreting the significance of lumbar fluid metabolite concentrations (Moir *et al.*, 1970).

First, it is difficult to distinguish the contribution of different parts of the nervous system. Second, there is a gradient in the concentrations of the acid metabolites, HVA and 5HIAA, which have high levels in the cerebral ventricles and lower concentrations at the cisterna magna and in the lumbar space as a result of an active transport of acid metabolites from CSF to blood in the choroid plexus of the IVth ventricle (Guldberg *et al.*, 1966). The transport mechanism is blocked by the uricosuric agent, probenecid. An ingenious attempt to obtain a more accurate reflection of cerebral amine metabolism has been made by the pre-treatment of patients with probenecid prior to lumbar CSF sampling (van Praag, 1973) but the interpretation of 5HIAA levels after probenecid is complicated by the fact that the drug can displace tryptophan from its binding to plasma protein and hence may influence the production of the amine 5-hydroxytryptamine (Korf *et al.*, 1972).

Summarizing the results of CSF amine metabolite studies is difficult as many of the studies have failed to differentiate between unipolar and bipolar disorders or between depressives of different severity.

Cerebrospinal fluid and post-mortem brain studies of 5-hydroxytryptamine and its metabolite 5-hydroxyindolacetic acid

Basal lumbar fluid levels of 5HIAA have been measured in a number of studies in depressed patients. Compared to controls, low levels are reported in some studies (Ashcroft *et al.*, 1966; Coppen, 1974; Denker *et al.*, 1966), whilst other investigators report normal levels (Bowers *et al.*, 1969; Sjöström & Roos, 1972). Asberg and colleagues (1976) report a bimodal distribution of levels in depression, one group with low levels having an increased risk of suicide compared to the other group with normal levels. Ashcroft and colleagues also reported different levels in different clinical syndromes; normal levels in bipolar patients and low levels in those with unipolar illness. Amongst those reporting low 5HIAA levels in depression, there seems to be a general agreement that levels do not rise to normal coincidentally with remission of depressive symptoms.

Probenecid has been used in a number of studies to block transport of 5HIAA from CSF and this is claimed to give a better reflection of levels in the nervous system. Most authors using this technique report decreased 5HIAA accumulation in depressed patients (Goodwin & Post, 1973; van Praag & Puite, 1970).

Studies of brain tissue obtained at post-mortem in patients who died by suicide compared to controls have also given variable results. Shaw and colleagues (1967) found low 5HT but normal 5HIAA concentrations in hind brain tissue of depressive suicides. Similar results were reported by Bourne and colleagues (1968) and Pare and colleagues (1969) with normal 5HT levels but low 5HIAA. More recently Lloyd and colleagues (1974) studying small areas of brain found low levels of 5HT in some brain areas, including the raphe nuclei in which is to be found one of the main concentrations of cell bodies of 5HT-containing neurones.

If we accept that low 5HIAA levels in the CSF are found in some depressed patients and that these may reflect low levels in the CNS, the low CSF levels

may result from a reduced rate of 5HT production or, alternatively, a reduction in the functional release of the amine. Reduction in synthesis might result from a reduced availability of the precursor amino-acid tryptophan or a change in the enzymatic mechanisms involved in synthesis.

Attempts have been made to investigate some of these possibilities. Brain and CSF levels of L-tryptophan are dependent on the plasma free levels of the amino-acid. Coppen and colleagues (1972b) have reported low levels of free tryptophan in plasma in depressed patients and also low CSF levels (Coppen *et al.*, 1972a) although normal levels of the amino-acid are reported by Ashcroft and colleagues (1973a).

A possibility remains that changes in plasma free tryptophan levels may be involved in some depressed patients, possibly in a group of premenopausal depressed women (Aylward, 1973; Coppen & Wood, 1978), but it does not appear to represent a general defect in depression.

The capacity of the CNS to synthesize 5HT when presented with a loading dose of the precursor L-tryptophan (Ashcroft *et al.*, 1973b) has been tested by measuring the rise in 5HIAA in lumbar CSF produced in depressed and in non-depressed controls by the loading technique. The rise in 5HIAA was comparable in the two groups suggesting that there is no general failure in the synthesis of the amine in depression.

In mania, CSF results are even less clear-cut than in depression. Normal and reduced levels have been reported (Ashcroft *et al.*, 1966; Bowers *et al.*, 1969; Denker *et al.*, 1966).

Dopamine and noradrenaline systems and depression: CSF and brain changes

The concentration of HVA reflects the metabolism of dopamine in the brain as there is no contribution from the spinal cord. Elevation of HVA levels following probenecid treatment is not complicated by any effects of the drug on dopamine turnover.

Basal lumbar fluid HVA levels have been shown to be decreased in most studies of depression (Bowers *et al.*, 1969; Denker *et al.*, 1966). Probenecid pretreatment studies indicate that this results from a decrease in dopamine turnover (Roos & Sjöström, 1969). Van Praag and Korf (1971) have suggested that the low HVA levels are more directly related to motor retardation than to depressed mood.

The main metabolite of noradrenaline in the nervous system is 3-methoxy-4-hydroxyphenylethylene glycol (MHPG). In man this exists in the CSF mainly in the free form with only 20 per cent present as the sulphate ester. Most studies of lumbar CSF levels have failed to show any direct correlation with mood, but high levels in mania and agitated depression suggest a relationship with behavioural arousal (Ashcroft *et al.*, 1974).

Measurements in urine and blood: urinary MHPG

Studies have suggested that the contribution of brain to urinary MHPG may be greater than 50 per cent. Schildkraut and colleagues (1973) have suggested that low levels of MHPG are to be found in depressive episodes in patients with bipolar affective illness and Maas and colleagues (1972) have suggested that patients with low MHPG excretion show a good response to treatment with imipramine and demethylimipramine.

5-HT transport in blood platelets

A study of transport of 5-HT in the platelets of depressed patients showed a reduction in the rate of transport although the affinity for the membrane carrier was unchanged (Tuomisto & Tukiainen, 1976). Coppen and colleagues (1980) reported similar results and showed that the abnormality is corrected by both short- and long-term lithium therapy.

Behavioural effects of precursor loading

Precursor loading studies have been carried out with levo-dopa, which increases dopamine levels in the basal ganglia in both human and animal subjects. In Parkinsonism the administration of levo-dopa results in improvement in the movement disorder and often an improvement in mood. Depression may, however, occur as a complication of levo-dopa treatment (Charington, 1970).

In patients with depressive illness levo-dopa shows no reliable antidepressant activity. However, Murphy and colleagues (1971) report the interesting finding that levo-dopa may precipitate manic episodes in patients with bipolar affective illness.

Two precursors of 5-hydroxytryptamine are available, L-tryptophan and 5-hydroxytryptophan (5HTP). No convincing evidence has been produced for an effect of 5HTP on mood. L-tryptophan has been used in a number of clinical trials in depression, either alone or in combination with mono-amine oxidase inhibitors or tricyclic antidepressants. There seems to be general agreement that the amino-acid increases

the efficacy of treatment with MAOIs (Coppen *et al.*, 1963) and the tricyclic compound clomipramine (Wålinder *et al.*, 1975). Whilst there is some disagreement, it seems that L-tryptophan may also have antidepressant properties when given alone (Coppen *et al.*, 1967), although, of course its action may depend on properties other than its ability to promote increased synthesis of brain 5HT. A claim that L-tryptophan has an antimanic effect has not been substantiated.

Amine hypotheses – a personal view

The evidence reviewed in the previous sections suggests that the changes in amine metabolism in unipolar depression may reflect an underactivity in the amine systems in the illness but does not suggest a primary disorder in the systems. Animal studies indicate the importance of the systems in mediating the behavioural components involved in exploratory activity. Such activity can be increased by drugs acting on the amine systems and it could be postulated that in man the increase might facilitate recovery from depression. This suggestion would imply that the antidepressants facilitate a behavioural pattern that predisposes to recovery from depression rather than reversing any hypothetical pathophysiological abnormality.

In bipolar illness, the evidence suggests the possibility of a primary disorder in amine systems with the probability that this involves a change in stability of the mechanisms which control the sensitivity of post-synaptic receptors.

Hormonal changes in the affective disorders

Abnormalities in endocrine secretion have been reported in depression since the 1960s with most of the early studies concentrating on the adrenal cortico-steroids. Cortisol excretion and cortisol secretion rates are increased in some depressed patients (Gibbons, 1964). It is difficult to separate out clearly the cortisol hypersecretors on clinical grounds, but in general they are severely depressed, anxious, suicidal, and suffering from unipolar depression (Bunney *et al.*, 1965; Bunney *et al.*, 1969). In these patients there is a disturbance of the circadian rhythm of cortisol secretion (Sachar *et al.*, 1973b).

In an attempt to distinguish between a non-specific response to emotional distress and a change in central controlling mechanisms, Carroll and colleagues (1976a,b) have studied the suppression of cortisol secretion following the administration of the synthetic steroid dexamethasone. In normal subjects following administration of dexamethasone, endogenous cortisol secretion is inhibited for 24 hours. In many depressed patients there is a failure of such suppression. Carroll and colleagues (1976a,b) have suggested that the effect is specific to endogenous depression and that the response to dexamethasone returns to normal following remission of depressive symptoms. Using the classification of depression into unipolar and depression spectrum disease proposed by Winokur and colleagues (1975), Schlesser and colleagues (1979) showed that 82 per cent of patients with familial pure depressive disease were resistant to suppression with dexamethasone as compared with only 4 per cent of patients with depressive spectrum disease.

In animal studies it has been suggested that noradrenaline systems in the central nervous system act as an inhibitor of the hypothalamic pituitary adrenal axis in a manner similar to the effect of dopamine systems in inhibiting prolactin release. Response to methylamphetamine (Checkley, 1979), which acts in the brain by release of both noradrenaline and dopamine, is reported to be reduced in patients with endogenous but not reactive depression. A possible involvement of central cholinergic systems in the abnormal response to dexamethasone is suggested by the studies of Carroll and colleagues (1978). In normal subjects pre-medication with the cholinesterone inhibitor physostigmine prevented cortisol suppression by dexamethasone, the physostigmine effect in turn being blocked by atropine but not by scopolamine.

These results suggest that there may be an underactivity in central noradrenergic systems and/or an increase in the activity in the central cholinergic systems concerned in the control of cortisol secretion in the group of patients suffering from endogenous depression.

Release of growth hormone in depression
Hypoglycaemia provoked by insulin results in increased release of growth hormone into peripheral blood. Impaired release in response to insulin stimulation has been demonstrated in a series of studies in depressed patients (Gruer et al., 1975; Sachar et al., 1971) whilst stimulation of release by the dopamine agonist apomorphine (Caspar et al., 1977) is normal.

Growth hormone response to clonidine, believed to act as a central noradrenergic agonist is reported to be reduced in depression (Malussek, 1978).

Summarizing these findings, the evidence indicates that as far as the control of growth hormone release is concerned, there is evidence of normal sensitivity of dopaminergic receptors but reduced sensitivity of noradrenergic receptors.

Other hormones in depression
Prolactin. Inhibition of prolactin secretion by administration of bromocriptine and levo-dopa has been shown to occur normally in depressed subjects indicating normal sensitivity of hypothalamic dopamine receptors (Coppen & Ghose, 1978; Sachar et al., 1973a).

Thyroid hormones. Indices of thyroid function have revealed no abnormalities in depression. Less directly, however, tri-iodothyronine (Prange et al., 1969) has been claimed to potentiate the antidepressant effects of imipramine and amitriptyline although this effect may be brought about by changes in plasma binding of imipramine induced by tri-iodothyronine. A transient antidepressant effect has been reported on administration of thyroid-releasing hormone.

Electrolytes and affective disorders
Gibbons (1960) reported a reversible retention of water and sodium in depressed patients. Coppen and Shaw (1963), using an isotope dilution technique, showed no over-all change in sodium balance but produced evidence of an increase in residual sodium, considered to be composed of intracellular sodium and exchangeable bone sodium, in both depressed and manic patients, with the latter showing the greater abnormality. The same workers failed to confirm the results in a subsequent study (Shaw & Coppen, 1966). Using ^{22}Na and total body counting, Coppen and colleagues (1962) measured exchangeable body sodium after equilibration for 6–7 days. There was a small but non-significant decrease in total exchangeable sodium on recovery from depression.

The rate of uptake of isotopic sodium into cerebrospinal fluid was shown in depression in a study by Coppen (1960) and there was an increase with clinical improvement following treatment with electroconvulsive therapy. This finding was not confirmed in two subsequent studies (Carroll et al., 1969; Fotherby et al., 1963). However, it seems possible that apparent low rates of uptake into lumbar fluid in patients with psychomotor retardation may be explained by poor mixing of cerebrospinal fluid of the cerebrospinal axis.

Studies of post-mortem brain material (Shaw *et al.*, 1969) showed lower sodium concentrations in patients dying from suicide as compared with controls. In another study (Ueno *et al.*, 1963) a small but significant decrease in CSF sodium concentration was reported in depressed patients.

The results of these studies are not consistent. There are many methodological difficulties in measuring the size of different fluid compartments which may account for the different results reported. There is, however, some general indication of a change in sodium distribution with a retention of 'intracellular' sodium during the depressed phase with return to normal in remission.

Naylor and his colleagues have utilized a different approach to the study of changes in electrolyte distribution – studying the concentration and transport of electrolytes. They reported (Naylor *et al.*, 1970) low red cell concentrations of sodium and potassium in patients with neurotic depression as compared to patients with endogenous depression and controls. There was a significant fall in sodium levels with recovery but no change in the patients with neurotic depression (Naylor *et al.*, 1971). They have extended these studies by attempting to assess the mechanisms by which sodium and potassium are transported across the red cell membrane. They report (Naylor *et al.*, 1973) that in patients with depressive psychosis ouabain-sensitive potassium influx and sodium-potassium-activated adenosine trysphosphatase activity (thought to represent activity of the sodium pump) increase significantly with improvement of mood.

Glen and colleagues (1968) studied the concentration of sodium in saliva and found it to be raised in depressive psychosis, concluding that this indicates a failure in membrane transport of sodium.

Calcium and magnesium in depression
Plasma concentrations of calcium are reported to be normal in depression (Gour & Chaudrey, 1957)

whilst magnesium levels have been reported to be raised in one study (Cade, 1964) and low in another (Frizel *et al.*, 1969). Using balance techniques and radioactive calcium (Faragalla & Flach, 1970), a decreased bone resorption rate and an increased retention of calcium was reported following recovery from depression.

Electrolytes in mania
There have been relatively few studies in mania. Serum and CSF sodium, potassium, and calcium levels have been reported normal (Ueno *et al.*, 1963; Coppen *et al.*, 1966). Intracellular or residual sodium levels are higher even than those in depression (Coppen *et al.*, 1966), but this finding was not confirmed by Baer and colleagues (1970).

Pathological changes in the affective disorders
No definite pathological changes have been reported in the main groups of patients with affective disorders.

There have been reports of manic syndromes in association with organic brain pathology, e.g. in a patient with a parasagittal meningioma (Oppler, 1950) and with a glioma of the diencephalon (Stern & Dancey, 1942).

Less clear-cut associations have been reported between brain damage and depression.

Post (1962) reported in elderly depressed patients that focal cerebral pathology occurred more frequently than was to be expected. Corsellis (1962) reported that the incidence of depression was lower in patients with senile dementia (6 per cent) than in those with vascular disease (20 per cent). Roth (1955) commented on the frequency with which depressive symptoms occurred in patients with organic cerebral disease.

Perhaps one of the most interesting observations was made by Flor-Henry (1969) who reported that patients with non-dominant temporal lobe lesions tend to present with manic-depressive symptoms whilst those with dominant lobe lesions present with symptoms of schizophrenic type.

Section 6

CHAPTERS 26–28

Treatment

26
Medication and physical treatment of affective disorders

E. S. PAYKEL

Good treatment of affective disorders involves detailed assessment and balanced eclectic employment of all types of treatment, including physical, psychotherapeutic, and social. This chapter is concerned particularly with physical treatments. The decision as to whether to use physical treatments can be difficult in mild depression but for severe depression and mania they are almost invariably required. The extensive literature on pharmacology and controlled evaluation is reviewed in Paykel and Coppen (1979). This chapter will focus on the clinical aspects of treatment.

Treatment of acute depression

The main treatments available for acute depression are tricyclic antidepressants, monoamine oxidase (MAO) inhibitors, and electroconvulsive therapy (ECT). There are numerous studies of factors predicting a good outcome with different kinds of treatment (Paykel, 1979). ECT is most effective in severe endogenous or psychotic depression, where it is more effective than any other treatment. Tricyclic antidepressants are generally regarded as more effective in endogenous than neurotic depression. However, there is evidence that the most severe depressions with delusions do not respond well and, on the other hand, there are many controlled trials indicating that tricyclics are superior to placebo for neurotic depressions. MAO inhibitors appear of particular value in outpatients with mixed anxiety-depressions

Table 26.1. *Tricyclic and related antidepressives*

Generic name	Trade name (UK)	Usual daily dose range (mg)
Iminodibenzyls		
Imipramine	Tofranil, etc.	75–300
Desipramine	Pertofran	75–300
Trimipramine	Surmontil	50–100
Clomipramine	Anafranil	75–200
Dibenzocycloheptenes		
Amitriptyline	Tryptizol, Lentizol	75–300
Nortriptyline	Allegron, Aventyl	50–150
Protriptyline	Concordin	15– 60
Butriptyline	Evadyne	150–300
Other tricyclics		
Doxepin	Sinequan	50–300
Opipramol	Insidon	150–300
Dibenzepin	Noveril	160–560
Dothiepin	Prothiaden	75–225
Tetracyclics		
Maprotiline	Ludiomil	75–300
Mianserin	Bolvidon, Norval	30–120
Other drugs with similar presumed action		
Nomifensine	Merital	50–200
Iprindole	Prondol	45–180
Viloxazine	Vivalan	150–300

and phobic states; controlled trials in in-patients have mainly been negative. Previous history of response is a useful guide. Biochemical predictors are emerging but are not yet suitable for general use.

In practice, severity is the best guide to initial treatment. For the most severe depressions with marked retardation or agitation and depressive delusions, and where there is refusal of food and fluids, ECT is the first choice unless there has been very clear previous tricyclic response. For moderate or milder depression tricyclic antidepressants are the first choice in most cases. In milder depressions with marked phobic symptoms some would use MAO inhibitors first, others tricyclics in view of their greater safety. When initial treatment fails, second choice can be guided by similar considerations but the results of prediction studies do not always prove reliable in clinical practice.

Tricyclic and related antidepressants
Since their introduction in the late 1950s, tricyclic antidepressants have become firmly established. Those available in the UK at the time of writing are listed in table 26.1.

Pharmacology is reviewed by Klerman and Cole (1965). In normal human beings the tricyclics produce mild sedative effects. In animals many of the actions are phenothiazine-like. Antidepressant effects are believed related to potentiation of CNS amines. These drugs potentiate the peripheral effects of noradrenaline and serotonin and reverse the reserpine syndrome by inhibiting re-uptake of released amines from the synaptic cleft. However, other pharmacological effects may be important.

The majority of the many controlled trials against placebo have shown significant differences (Morris & Beck, 1974). However, despite exceptions in some patients, overall these drugs are not strikingly effective, perhaps producing 30 per cent more recoveries than might occur spontaneously.

There are some differences between the drugs in pharmacological effects. Secondary amines such as nortriptyline and desipramine predominantly affect noradrenaline re-uptake, while tertiary amines and clomipramine predominantly affect serotonin. Clinically the differences are small. Amitriptyline, doxepin, and trimipramine are more sedative and useful where insomnia is a problem. Protriptyline, nortriptyline, and desipramine are less sedative and better tolerated with marked daytime anergia. Mianserin has fewer anticholinergic side effects. All take between one and four weeks to produce antidepressant effects, although anticholinergic and sedative effects develop early.

There are some differences in dose for dose potency, but what really matters is the ratio of efficacy to side effects, or the effectiveness at maximum tolerated doses, and here the differences are small. Principles of clinical use are the same for all these drugs. It is best to start with a moderately low dose and to warn the patient to persist in spite of early dry mouth, drowsiness, and delayed therapeutic effects. Lower starting doses are required in the elderly, who readily develop side-effects.

The tricyclics are broken down relatively slowly. Anticholinergic and sedative effects diminish to some extent 12 hours after the last dose, but antidepressant effects fall off much more slowly. Therefore at least half the daily dose should be given at night to diminish side-effects and avoid the necessity for night sedation. Reasonable blood levels can be achieved by a single daily dose, but one further dose in the morning is probably better, and some patients prefer multiple doses.

A major fault of non-psychiatrists is to prescribe too low a dosage. Doses below the equivalent of 100 mg of imipramine daily are usually inadequate, except in the elderly. However, there is remarkable pharmacokinetic variability, with up to 40-fold variation in blood-levels produced by the same dose on different individuals (Peet & Coppen, 1979). Some of this is genetic; some may be the results

of enzyme induction by other drugs such as barbiturates, which should be avoided. Benzodiazepines lack this effect and are much safer in overdose. Phenothiazines increase blood-levels. A better clinical response occurs with higher blood-levels. For nortriptyline, and possibly for other secondary amines, the effect is curvilinear, with poor response at very high blood-levels. Measurement of blood-levels may prove useful in the future.

Side-effects, particularly anticholinergic ones, tend weakly to parallel blood-levels. Clinically, doses should be increased to a point where side-effects are moderate but still tolerable. Sometimes this level may be well above the usually recommended dosage. In length, four weeks represents a minimum adequate trial, but unless severe illness mandates other treatment, six weeks is better. In controlled trials effects appear at about three weeks. If there is no response, the drug should be stopped. If response is partial, it may be worth continuing.

The most common side-effects are drowsiness and atropinic effects. Caution is required where urinary obstruction or glaucoma are present. Driving should be avoided until the extent of the drowsiness is clear. Alcohol and sympathomimetic agents are potentiated. Tremor is not uncommon and convulsions occasionally occur. Confusion and delirium may occur in the elderly. Arrhythmias may be precipitated and caution is required in the presence of cardiac disease. Increased appetite may develop after several weeks.

Tricyclic overdose is increasing as a method of suicide, death resulting from cardiac effects. When tricyclics are used properly for a well-developed persistent depressive syndrome, the benefits outweigh the risks, but appropriate precautions should be taken.

Monoamine-oxidase inhibitors

Although the MAO inhibitors were introduced into therapeutics before the tricyclic antidepressants, their place remains less secure, and they are used mainly by psychiatrists. Those available in the UK are shown in table 26.2. All inhibit MAO irreversibly, so that effects persist up to two weeks after cessation, until new enzyme is formed.

Clinical aspects are reviewed by Tyrer (1976). Evidence for efficacy is less impressive than for tricyclics, but best for phenelzine, which is the drug of choice in milder cases. Probably the most effective,

Table 26.2. *Monoamine oxidase inhibitors*

Generic name	Trade name (UK)	Usual daily dose range (mg)
Hydrazines		
Phenelzine	Nardil	45–75
Isocarboxazid	Marplan	20–30
Iproniazid	Marsilid	50–100
Non-hydrazines		
Tranylcypromine	Parnate	20–30

and the MAO inhibitor of choice for severe or resistant depression, is tranylcypromine, although also more prone to toxic interactions. Isocarboxazid appears comparable to phenelzine. Iproniazid is effective, but carries a high risk of liver damage.

Starting doses are in the lower range indicated in the table, and they should be increased over two or three weeks. Response is delayed, and the time is inversely related to dose. For phenelzine, 45 mg daily for three weeks is below the borderline, and it is best to allow at least six weeks, with a dose increasing to 60–75 mg daily. Hydrazines are acetylated, and fast acetylators (about 40 per cent of the population) require doses in the higher ranges.

Tranylcypromine produces amphetamine-like stimulation and should not be taken after mid-afternoon. The situation for other MAO inhibitors is not clear, and they are often used in divided doses through the day.

Minor side-effects are mainly autonomic, particularly postural hypotension. The major clinical problem is the risk of interactions with other substances. The best known is the hypertensive crisis resulting from pressor amines (particularly indirectly acting) either therapeutically (including amphetamine, levo-dopa), or through diet. Foods containing tyramine or other pressor amines include cheese, Marmite and other yeast extracts, some alcoholic drinks (particularly red wine), broad beans and, less commonly, pickled herrings, chocolate, yoghurt, cream, and game. The patient experiences sudden onset of palpitations and a severe throbbing headache spreading from the occipital region, with nau-

sea, vomiting, neck stiffness, and photophobia. Intracranial haemorrhage and death have been reported. Phentolamine is the treatment of choice. MAO inhibitors are contra-indicated in the presence of phaeochromocytoma or intracranial aneurysm.

Tricyclic-MAO inhibitor combinations can cause coma with hyperpyrexia and in routine practice should be avoided, with 10 days off drug when changing from tricyclic to MAO inhibitor, and two weeks in the opposite direction. Opiates, particularly pethidine, can be potentiated, as can insulin. The patient should be provided with a card indicating the drug being received, and the substances to be avoided.

Electroconvulsive therapy

Convulsive therapy was introduced in the 1930s, originally by chemical means. The standard procedure is cerebral electroshock induction of a major fit modified by short-acting muscle relaxant under barbiturate anaesthesia.

The mode of action is still uncertain. The convulsive cerebral discharge appears to be an essential component (Cronholm & Ottoson, 1960). Recent animal experiments suggest the possibility of post-synaptic enhancement of action of amine neurotransmitters.

Comparisons with antidepressant drugs among in-patients show ECT either superior or equal to the antidepressant drugs, without any studies showing antidepressant superior (Turek & Hanlon, 1977). Unilateral application of current to the non-dominant hemisphere produces less disturbance of verbal memory than bilateral ECT, but appears a little less effective. Double-blind comparisons of ECT with placebo treatments have recently been undertaken.

Recommended standards of administration include informed consent, presence of an anaesthetist, a special room or suite, adequate surveillance during recovery, treatment preferably twice weekly with an initial course of about six treatments, but with more often necessary (Royal College of Psychiatrists, 1977). Frequent courses, and more than 12–14 treatments in one course, should be avoided.

There is a low risk of anaesthetic mortality, between three and nine per 100 000 treatments, appreciably less than that of suicide in such patients. Memory loss is well documented, but most studies have failed to show any objective evidence of long-term loss (Squire & Chace, 1975).

Other drugs

The place of tryptophan as an antidepressant is still uncertain. There is good evidence that it enhances MAO inhibitors and serotoninergic tricyclic antidepressants, but only equivocal evidence that it is effective by itself.

Phenothiazines have a place in combination with tricyclics in the treatment of agitated depression and schizo-affective states. There is some evidence that in-patient anxious depressives may respond to phenothiazines alone and clinically an occasional patient does well on them.

Intermediate in structure between phenothiazines and tricyclics is the thioxanthene, flupenthixol. Evidence of antidepressant effect is not yet definitive and its place is yet to be established. Depot injections may be useful where there is marked mood lability and suicidal risk.

Benzodiazepines are of considerable value in acute crises for daytime tranquillization and night sedation. They may also provide adjunctive sedation with stimulant MAO inhibitors. They are not a definitive treatment, and they are over-used.

Resistant depression

Only a small proportion of patients with severe depression fail to show some improvement after treatment with ECT, tricyclics, MAO inhibitors, singly or consecutively. Persistent milder symptoms are not uncommon, but only a few patients show severe resistant depressions.

Shaw (1977) has suggested guide-lines for their treatment. Full clinical reassessment should include physical examination and laboratory testing for endocrine and neoplastic disease. Some patients improve if all drugs are withdrawn, except night sedation. A full course of bilateral ECT, tricyclic antidepressant or tranylcypromine should then be given if not used recently. If there is no response, tryptophan can be combined with tranylcypromine or with a serotoninergic tricyclic drug.

Next, or earlier, a tricyclic-MAO inhibitor combination should be tried, starting with low doses and working up. Amitriptyline and trimipramine are safer tricyclics, and clomipramine should be avoided. Many prefer to avoid tranylcypromine.

At some point phenothiazines can be tried, and lithium, either alone or in combination with other classes of antidepressant. It may be worth while to combine tricyclics with tri-iodothyronine or methyl-

phenidate. If these fail, a wait for natural remission may be useful, or a second trial of a treatment previously used. Some patients finally respond to ECT after a year or more. A very small group show a persistent severe depression, for which ultimately leucotomy is indicated (Bridges & Bartlett, 1977).

Special problems

On general principles antidepressants should be avoided in the first trimester of pregnancy. Lithium should be avoided throughout in view of evidence of teratogenicity. If antidepressants are required, tricyclics are generally safer. At delivery the dose should be decreased in view of possible transplacental transfer with neonatal sedation and withdrawal effects. Breast feeding is better avoided.

Tricyclics should be used cautiously where there is pre-existing cardiac disease. Amitriptyline should be avoided; doxepin, mianserin and nomifensine are safer. The commonest cardiovascular effects are postural hypotension and tachycardia. ECG changes can occur, particularly T-wave changes, conduction defects and arrhythmias.

The combined treatment of hypertension and depression presents difficulties. Reserpine and methyldopa can induce depression. Clonidine, guanethidine and propranolol, although suspect, probably do not (Paykel *et al.*, 1982). Intraneuronal blocking agents such as guanethidine are antagonized by tricyclics which block neuronal uptake. Control can still sometimes be achieved, but care must be taken when stopping the tricyclic to reduce also the dose of antihypertensive to avoid hypotension. Clonidine also interacts. Beta adrenoceptor-blocking drugs are useful, neither causing depression nor interacting with antidepressants.

Treatment of acute mania

Pharmacotherapeutic choice in mania is limited to the neuroleptic drugs and lithium. ECT is used by some but has not been adequately evaluated. Controlled studies suggest that neuroleptic drugs are superior to lithium in severe mania, but lithium is superior in mild mania (Johnson, 1975). Often a combination is required and lithium cannot be administered until excited and uncooperative behaviour has been controlled by injectable neuroleptics and dehydration corrected. The neuroleptic used in most controlled comparisons has been chlorpromazine, which is valuable for its sedative properties. If large doses are required haloperidol is less likely to produce hypotension. Neuroleptics are also superior to lithium where there is a schizo-affective element.

Lithium

Lithium was first used for mania by Cade in 1949, but took 20 years for general adoption. It shares properties with sodium and potassium but is more evenly distributed extracellularly and intracellularly. It is readily absorbed from the gastro-intestinal tract, with a peak in one-half to two hours unless in slow-release preparations, and a half-life of 18–24 hours. Excretion is renal and lithium is dealt with like sodium, but without distal tubule reabsorption. Lithium retention tends to occur with sodium retention in circumstances such as dehydration and use of diuretics.

Pharmacology, mode of action and clinical use are reviewed in Johnson (1975). Among possible modes of action are effects on amine neurotransmitters, and on membrane excitability. Efficacy has been demonstrated in acute mania, prevention of mania, bipolar and severe unipolar depression. There is suggestive evidence of an acute antidepressant action during bipolar depression, and although this is not conclusive, lithium is probably indicated in these circumstances. It may be worth a trial in other resistant depressives.

A usual starting dose for a healthy patient is 800–1600 mg daily. Sustained released preparations are preferable to avoid peaks in the toxic range, although with some of these the absorption is not much delayed so that twice daily administration is preferable. Renal function should be normal and checked if there is any doubt. The drug is contra-indicated in heart failure, and disorders such as Addison's disease which disturb sodium balance.

Administration must be controlled by blood-levels, initially every three to four days during rapid stabilization in manic illness, or every week in initial out-patient treatment. During maintenance after stabilization, a check on blood-levels every two to three months will suffice. Blood should be taken at least 12 hours after the last dose. The therapeutic range lies between 0.5 and 1.5 millimoles per litre, and preferably between 0.8 and 1.2.

Mild tremor, anorexia, nausea are common dose-related side-effects. With toxic levels these reach vomiting, diarrhoea, ataxia, coma, convulsions, cardiac arrhythmias, death. In long-term use there may be lethargy and impaired concentration, polyuria due to renal diabetes insipidus, weight gain and hypothyroidism. Thyroid function should be assessed periodically. Possible evidence of irreversible renal changes has recently been reported. Diuretics should be avoided.

Maintenance treatment

Two different situations must be distinguished in treatment after acute illness: routine continuation therapy as part of active treatment, and longer-term maintenance. In the last few years three double-blind studies found that high relapse rates (30–50 per cent) after early withdrawal of tricyclics were halved by continuation treatment for six months or one year longer (Coppen & Peet, 1979). Improvement during acute treatment is not necessarily due to the drug, particularly if the response is very rapid, occurs on low doses, or is concurrent with major environmental changes. However, where a patient shows response which is pharmacologically more typical, particularly with incomplete remission or previous relapses, treatment should routinely be continued for a further six months. The dose may be reduced a little and compliance improved by a single daily dose. After six months the drug can be withdrawn in two or three steps at intervals of two weeks. Abrupt withdrawal from high doses of tricyclic antidepressants can produce a withdrawal syndrome, with influenza-like and gastro-intestinal symptoms.

There is not such clear evidence regarding MAO inhibitors, but similar principles probably apply. There is also an appreciable risk of early relapse after ECT, which is reduced by treatment with a tricyclic, MAO inhibitor, or possibly lithium, for about six months (Paykel & Coppen, 1979).

The course of affective illness is variable and there may be long periods between, or complete freedom from, further episodes, so that decision to use longer-term maintenance therapy depends on frequent recent episodes, perhaps two in two years or three in five years. Bipolar illness tends to have a worse spontaneous course and to respond better to lithium, so that indications for maintenance will be stronger. The destructive social consequences of mania strongly indicate lithium maintenance after a single episode. Length of maintenance depends on circumstances. Where illness is prevented during maintenance treatment but recurs repeatedly on its withdrawal, maintenance may become indefinite.

There is clear evidence that lithium is superior to placebo and to tricyclic antidepressants in the maintenance treatment of bipolar patients (Johnson, 1975). It should be administered for several months even if apparently ineffective, but some cases are refractory and here tricyclics may be useful, some-times in combination with phenothiazines. For uni-polar depressives both lithium and tricyclic are superior to placebo, and either is a reasonable first choice (Johnson, 1975). Most studies have been carried out in patients with severe illnesses and for recurrent neurotic depressions tricyclics or MAO inhibitors are probably indicated.

27
Management and rehabilitation of affective psychoses

D. H. BENNETT

In discussing the management of severe affective disorders, it is difficult to improve on Lewis' statement that 'to hinder suicide, prevent irritation and to provide nutrition, sleep or rest, and in due course occupational interest have long been the objects of judicious treatment, conscious that of the factors potent to heal, time is more important than any kind of interference so far attempted' (Lewis, 1934). Since 1934, when Lewis made this statement, the scope of management has been enlarged by the availability of effective pharmacotherapy and new knowledge about the social factors that maintain or ameliorate affective disorders.

Management
Before one can plan management in a sensible fashion it is necessary not only to assess the patient's mood, thought, and physiological functions but also the level at which he functions socially, including the performance of social roles. Impairment is found most commonly in work performance and in the intimate relationships of marriage and parenthood. In making assessments of social adjustment clinicians cannot rely simply upon a patient's own report. If depressed he may report greater impairment, and if hypomanic, less than is observed by others. Weissman and Paykel (1974) believe that, in depression, social disturbances and impairments are, in part, an indirect reflection of the severity of symptoms although there is, of course, a direct relationship as well. When

assessment is complete the first decision to be made is whether the sick individual can be managed in or out of hospital. This will be decided not only on the basis of symptoms, but on the extent of social impairments and their effect on the family or significant others. Much, too, will depend on the individual's psychological resources, coping responses, and the supports available. If the patient is suffering from the extremities of depression or hypomania, a point will be reached where feelings of hopelessness and worthlessness, or alternatively superiority and omnipotence, make co-operation with family, friends and doctor, impossible. In the presence of such gross disturbance, management becomes a matter of control rather than of support and advice. In the past such social control was often exercised by compulsory hospital admission. Today, in an era distrustful of psychiatry and jealous of the individual's rights, there is an increase in the threshold at which compulsory measures can be taken. This may have led to some increase in the difficulties of management. However, some hypomanic patients have always harmed themselves and distressed other people because of their overspending or promiscuous sexual relationships without quite reaching a severity of disturbance that justified admission on order. To these problems are added the danger of the motor car for the depressed or hypomanic patient. The psychiatrist, or family member or a friend should, if possible, persuade the patient with severe disorder to hand over car keys, credit cards, and cheque book at the first sign of illness. Even so it may be too late to prevent damage. It is often advisable therefore, in the case of individuals with means, who suffer repeated hypomanic episodes, to persuade them, when well, to put their affairs in the hands of a solicitor, a friend, or the Court of Protection. In some circumstances one should attempt to secure an agreement that family members should have the censorship of mail or, if the patient is in hospital, that he will allow a doctor or staff member to undertake this function.

Certain patients deny that there is anything wrong with them when they are becoming severely ill. They cease to take medication, become more elated or more depressed and have to be admitted time after time on compulsory orders. Under such circumstances, an attempt should be made by the responsible psychiatrist to obtain the co-operation of the spouse or family, who can be excellent informants, in reporting the early symptoms of relapse. In this way social damage may be limited until the patient's disorder can be brought under control. However, success on one occasion is no predictor of success on another. Even long-standing relationships with patients are no guarantee against irresponsibility or attempts at suicide during periods of relapse. Weissman and Paykel (1974) suggest that the closer the relationship the more likely it is to be characterized by hostility during an episode of illness.

Thus great judgement is required in the handling of patients with severe depression or hypomania. Too great a restriction may exacerbate the over-activity of the hypomanic patient or alternatively increase the depressed patient's despair and hopelessness. Many clinicians, following the suicide of one of their patients, may regret that they were not more restrictive. Yet there is no clear evidence that more permissive forms of management have increased the suicide rate in depression. The evidence from different countries and different hospitals is conflicting. A study of suicides at Dingleton Hospital in the ten years before, and the ten years after, the introduction of the open door system showed that there was no increase in in-patients or in patients recently discharged (Ratcliff, 1962). The need for long-term restriction and control is less frequent, now that treatment is not only more effective, but also more accessible and acceptable in out-patient departments or day hospitals. There are, however, other reasons for hospital admission. While only a minority of patients need social regulation by control, a much larger number, especially those who do not have families, need hospital admission if they are unable to care for themselves or take their medication reliably.

Social support

Personal relations within or outside the family or marital life can be a source of stress or support. Recent research has demonstrated the importance of social support in preventing and reducing symptoms and effecting more rapid recovery in a wide variety of medical and psychological conditions (Cobb, 1976). Lowenthal and Haven (1968) demonstrated how a single intimate relationship buffers the aged against the stress of social disengagement and the associated depression. Brown and Harris (1978) have suggested that a close and confiding relationship with a male confidant protected from mild depression women experiencing severe life events. Similarly Pearlin and

Johnson (1977) investigating a greater disposition of unmarried people to psychological disturbance – depression in particular – thought that this resulted from the greater exposure of single people to hardship or strain. They expected that single and married individuals contending with life strains would be similarly inclined to depression. In fact they found that the effects of stress were more penetrating among the unmarried. They concluded that marriage can 'function as a protective barrier against the distressful consequences of external threats'.

Since it is impossible to avoid life's strains, and since maintenance treatment with amitriptyline does not protect against the effects of them (Paykel & Tanner, 1976), the provision of support is vital in the management of manic-depressive disorder. For those who are unmarried, lonely, or lack family it may be necessary to provide an 'artificial' confidant using volunteer befrienders. Many doctors and social workers play this role whether or not they intend to do so. Depressed people have formed self-help groups although these have not yet achieved the same influence as other such groups of distressed and disabled people.

Family and marriage

Marriage and parenthood are inevitably affected by mania and depression and it may be difficult to make up one's mind whether the family situation is the result, or the cause, of the defined patient's affective disorder (Briscoe & Smith, 1973). Depressed or hypomanic patients, unlike patients with schizophrenia, are not socially isolated, so that their impairments have an immediate effect on the many persons with whom they have intimate contact. There are stresses for the family whether the patient is in hospital or at home (Grad & Sainsbury, 1968). In both situations the illness forces role adjustment for family members. Not all relatives are able to cope with such role reversals and children are likely to be particularly affected (Fabian & Donohue, 1956). Rutter (1966) suggests that if the family recognize that the abnormal behaviour is due to illness, family adaptation may be easier. Adjustment is difficult when irritability, moodiness and hostility are seen as the normal feelings of a relative who has inexplicably turned against the family. Deykin, Weissman and Klerman (1971) suggest that a family conference is useful if the patient and family members are given the opportunity to express their perception of the illness, their expectations of treatment, and their hopes for the future. Some families try to avoid such open discussion, since they fear it may lead to the exposure of intolerable and unacceptable subjects such as suicide. Yet a forthright discussion of the situation between the family, the patient, and the clinician serves many useful purposes. It is not only important that the psychiatrist knows what the patient is thinking; it is equally important that the family knows that the patient realizes that his distress is being taken seriously. An exploration of taboo subjects opens the way for discussion of other forbidden subjects; especially those which have to do with unacceptable hostility and aggression. This approach is less likely to succeed with the hypomanic patient.

Casework with the patient's family can be useful in increasing the understanding of the effects of medication and motivating the family to persuade the patient to continue taking whatever is necessary and helpful (Weissman, 1972). When the patient remains at home, social casework, when undertaken, is primarily supportive in the early stages using advice, encouragement, reassurance, the reduction of guilt, ventilation, and direct help to modify the environment. While the reduction of symptoms is achieved through the use of medication, casework is more important in the restoration of the patient's social functioning. It also has an important part to play in exploring the patient's maladaptive patterns of behaviour. The social workers who were involved in the Boston/Yale collaborative studies of depression found that when it comes to the stage of recovery, some patients are interested in intensive casework, some are mildly interested, while a few show mixed attitudes (Deykin *et al.*, 1971).

Employment

While depression and hypomania in the acute stages may make it impossible for the individual to work, this phase may not last long. The clinician must use his discretion, but he should not be too eager to recommend that the depressed patient stops work if he or she has not already done so. Weissman and Paykel (1974) noted that women at work out of the home are likely to show less impairment following depression than housewives. They suggested that outside employment could have a protective effect. Brown and Harris (1978) report a similar finding that paid employment reduced the vulnerability of the women in their study to mild depression.

Rehabilitation

There is no doubt that in a number of cases of affective disorder the condition results in or is associated with, persisting disability.

These disabilities have often been overlooked, perhaps because, by and large, they are not so massive nor so fixed as those found in schizophrenia. It has often been believed that such disabilities are reversible, although the evidence is inconclusive. Paykel, Weissman, Prusoff and Tonks (1971) suggest that in recovery from depression the improvement in social functioning may stop considerably short of complete restoration of normal adjustment, with a residuum of diminished work performance and friendships, disturbed interpersonal relations, or marital breakdown. Mann and Cree (1976) found that 15.8 per cent of 400 'new' long-stay patients under the age of sixty-five in ten mental hospitals in England and Wales were suffering from affective disorder. This is only a third of the 44.4 per cent suffering from schizophrenic disabilities. These patients, nevertheless, form the second largest disabled group in the long-stay mental hospital population.

Patients with manic-depressive disorder are equally likely to be handicapped by the frequent recurrence of episodes of depression and hypo-mania. Repeated illnesses have a devastating effect on career prospects, employment, and family life. In time confidence and motivation too are undermined. Since stressful life-events occur with some regularity, any defects in an individual's psychological resources or coping capacity (Pearlin & Schooler, 1978) and any lack of family or marital support, will reduce a person's capacity to master these strains and in fact precipitate further depression or hypomania (Brown & Harris, 1978; Ambelas, 1979). They may also determine the quality of social adjustment after discharge from hospital (Burke, Deykin, Jacobson & Haley, 1967). Even in those cases where endogenous mood rhythms or other psychological or physiological changes seem to determine the course of disorder, the social outcome depends on coping capacity, personality and social support.

While the outline of a rehabilitation strategy for manic-depressive psychosis is beginning to develop it is by no means as well developed as that for schizophrenia (see chapter 14). While the latter provides a useful model (Bennett, 1978) further research and clinical innovation is necessary in order to establish the specific principles of long-term management of the severe affective disorders in the era of partially effective pharmacotherapy.

28
Medico-legal issues
ANTHONY W. CLARE

Introduction

Academic lawyers and criminologists, as well as psychiatrists, have shown considerable interest in notions of psychosis and insanity. The existence of mental disorder in a defendant calls into question two fundamental principles of the criminal law. That law is still founded on the premise that the best way of achieving acceptable standards of behaviour from the majority of society's members is by prohibiting certain actions and punishing those who disobey such prohibitions. Disobedience, however, is presumed to involve two distinct mental processes. The first is the knowledge of what is prohibited and the consequences of taking prohibited action. The second is the deliberate decision to go ahead regardless of prohibition and consequences. Only then does punishment appear to be both rational and morally acceptable. Nearly two hundred years ago it was decided that an individual defendant could not claim ignorance of the law as a defence, since this would make it too easy for someone to choose which laws he would obey and which he could conveniently fail to learn. The second proposition, however, became central to the criminal law. Built into the definition of most prohibited acts is the concept of *mens rea* or guilty mind. The actual state of mind differs from offence to offence but the minimum generally required is foresight of the effects of one's actions, and either an intention to produce these effects or recklessness as to whether they occur. Theoretically, the prosecution has to prove *mens rea,* although it is often possible to infer it simply from proof of the offending deed. But any defendant may put forward lack of *mens rea* as a defence to any offence of which it forms part – the so-called insanity defence.

The existence of mental disorder, however, has medico-legal implications over and above the consideration of criminal responsibility. The concept of *informed consent,* the chief covenant or canon of loyalty between patient and doctor (Ramsey, 1970), rests on the supposition that the patient has a full and proper understanding of the nature, procedure, and risks of a proposed treatment and consents to undergo it. Informed consent in turn depends on so-called 'voluntariness', which is usually defined as the absence of internal and external restraints (Faden & Faden, 1977). The degree to which a mental disorder, particularly a severe one such as schizophrenia or manic-depressive psychosis, may act as an internal restraint affecting not merely the individual's ability to decide on issues such as treatment but his freedom to do so without constraint is a judgment circumscribed by legal as well as psychiatric considerations. A related medico-legal issue is the question of who should be entrusted with safeguarding the legal rights of a patient whose 'voluntariness' is in doubt on account of his mental state. These issues reflect the fact that many mental disorders can affect an individual's judgment and reason, and thereby his responsibility, to such an extent as to require, in certain circumstances, external intervention and the imposition of hospitalization and treatment against the individual's expressed desires and intentions.

The insanity defence

The history of insanity as a defence in serious criminal cases illustrates the considerable difficulty that lawyers have had in comprehending the effects of mental disease and in relating these effects to the basic principles of the criminal law (Ormrod, 1977). A landmark was the case of Daniel McNaughton, a Scottish wood-turner, who, acting under the influence of delusions of persecution, and apparently under the impression that he was attacking the Prime Minister, Sir Robert Peel, shot and killed Sir Edward Drummond, Peel's private secretary. In view of the medical evidence presented, the judge interrupted the trial and directed the jury to find McNaughton not guilty on the ground of insanity. So much controversy was provoked by this verdict that the House of Lords asked the judges to give opinions on the sev-

eral points of law involved. These opinions, known as the McNaughton Rules, were destined to influence the law on insanity in English-speaking countries for more than a century. The relevant Rules are as follows:

(1) *Criminal responsibility of persons labouring under partial delusions*

A person labouring under partial delusions only, and not otherwise insane, who did the act charged with a view, under the influence of redressing or revenging some supposed grievance or wrong, or of producing some public benefit, is punishable, if he knew at the time that he was acting contrary to the law of the land.

If a party labouring under an insane delusion as to existing facts, and not otherwise insane, commits an offence, he must be considered in the same situation as if the facts in respect to which the delusion exists were real.

(2) *Direction to the jury in such cases*

To establish a defence on the ground of insanity it must be clearly proved that, at the time of committing the act, the party accused was labouring under such a defect of reason from disease of the mind, as not to know the nature and quality of the act he was doing, or if he did know it, that he did not know that what he was doing was wrong.

If the accused was conscious that the act was one which he ought not to do, and if that act was at the same time contrary to the law of the land, he is punishable.

Since the 1957 Homicide Act and the abolition of capital punishment in Britain the use of the insanity defence in cases of murder (formerly its main application) is rare. Not guilty by reason of insanity may still be invoked as a defence against other charges and where such a verdict is recorded the court must order that the accused be admitted to a hospital to be specified by the Home Secretary, which is almost always a special hospital. In the United States, the McNaughton Rules occupy only a portion of the law on insanity and, as Goldstein (1967) has pointed out, several tests now compete. Nevertheless, the rules remain the sole definition in 21 States; in another 11 States they are part of a formula which adds some form of 'irresistible impulse' or 'control' rule.

The interpretation of the McNaughton Rules has been fraught with controversy, not least on account of disagreements over the precise meaning of crucial words contained in them. There has, for example, been virtually no judicial definition of mental disease and what little law does exist on the subject is found in cases which reject the effort to assert insanity by persons whose mental states appear marginal, such as cases involving alcohol intoxication, narcotics withdrawal, or borderline mental defects. Another problem is the tendency to equate psychosis and insanity, an equation believed to reflect the widespread assumption among lawyers that insanity describes medical entities and among psychiatrists that psychosis is the only entity which satisfies the law's requirements (Goldstein & Marcus, 1977). The word 'know' has also provoked argument with critics of the Rules reading it as referring to formal cognition or intellectual awareness alone, thereby distinguishing it from what they understand to be a fuller and more 'psychiatric' meaning, involving emotional as well as intellectual awareness. A number of other legal rulings refer to knowledge fused with affect and some, particularly in North America, include some notion of 'irrestible impulse'. In Britain, the concept of 'diminished responsibility' (Homicide Act, 1957) includes the situation wherein the overwhelming difficulty the accused found in controlling his impulse to commit a physical act was substantially greater than an ordinary man, not suffering from mental abnormality, would experience in similar circumstances. The jury decides on the basis of the medical evidence whether the accused was suffering from

> such abnormality of mind (whether arising from a condition of arrested or retarded development of mind or any inherent causes or induced by disease or injury) as substantially impaired his mental responsibility for his acts and omissions or being a party to the killing.

Substantial, in this instance, need not mean total but means more than trivial and the usual sentence is hospitalization under Sections 60 and 65 of the Mental Health Act 1959, although the judge may specify any of a range of sentences from probation to life. A related notion of impaired responsibility is contained in the Infanticide Act 1938 which rules that a woman who kills her child within a year of its birth may have a charge of murder reduced to that of infanticide and dealt with as if guilty of manslaughter thus avoiding automatic life sentence, if it can be shown that the 'balance of her mind was disturbed . . . by . . . the effects of giving birth or by . . . lactation consequent upon the birth.'

In Britain, the report of the committee on the mentally abnormal offender (the Butler committee) took note of the criticisms that have repeatedly been made of the McNaughton Rules and of the various attempts that have been made to reform the rules, particularly in the United States, such as the New Hampshire Rule, the American Model Penal Code, and the Durham Formula. In general, these modifications sought to excuse an offender if his act were the consequence of substantial impairment of judgement or control by reason of mental disorder. The committee noted that such revisions had not succeeded in improving the situation since the psychiatrist was still expected to give opinion on the question of responsibility. After lengthy consideration, the committee recommended a new special verdict of 'not guilty on evidence of mental disorder'. This would mean that the psychiatrist would have to produce detailed evidence of severe mental disorder and leave to the jury the question of what weight such evidence should carry. The evidence of severe mental disorder which the committee would recognize includes the following:

> A mental illness is severe when it has one or more of the following characteristics:
> (a) lasting impairment of intellectual functions shown by failure of memory, orientation, comprehension and learning capacity;
> (b) lasting alteration of mood of such degree as to give rise to delusional appraisal of the patient's situation, his past or his future or that of others or the lack of any appraisal;
> (c) delusional beliefs – persecutory, grandiose or jealous;
> (d) abnormal perceptions associated with delusional interpretations of events;
> (e) thinking so disordered as to prevent reasonable appraisal of the patient's situation or reasonable communication with others.

Such an approach leaves the discussion of responsibility to the jury. The psychiatrist simply testifies to the state of mind of the accused at the time of examination and is not invited to speculate on the accused's state of mind when he committed the act or made the omission of which he is accused. The suggested criteria relate only to serious mental disorders and do not include psychopathic disorder or subnormality. The problem of crimes committed by intoxicated offenders deserves separate consideration. An individual could be so intoxicated as not to have the *mens rea* to commit the crime yet, if his intoxication were voluntary, he could be judged responsible for getting into a state in which he was not able to appreciate the effects of his actions. The Butler committee's recommendation is that where the accused is faced with a charge which, under circumstances, would be one of a dangerous offence, and then excuses himself on the grounds that he was so intoxicated by drink or drugs as not to know what he was doing, he should be acquitted of the original charge but should be convicted of an alternative charge of 'dangerous intoxication', carrying serious penalties.

Fitness to plead

The criteria for fitness to plead include the following:

(1) the ability to understand the charge and its consequences;
(2) the ability to understand the court proceedings;
(3) the ability to instruct counsel for the defence;
(4) the ability to challenge the jurors.

The Butler committee was doubtful whether the last criterion is essential. It also recognized that it is often difficult to determine, by examination in prison, whether or not a person is under disability and, furthermore, that some who are under disability would become fit to stand trial after a period of treatment. For these reasons, the committee recommended that an 'interim hospital order' be introduced, imposed by the courts, in those cases where there is a need:

(a) for a proper and lengthy assessment of the accused's mental condition, either for report or to determine whether a hospital order is appropriate;
(b) for a period of treatment so that someone under disability might become fit to plead;
(c) for medical care during a custodial remand.

Compulsory hospitalization and treatment

A review of involuntary hospitalization undertaken for the World Health Organization (Curran & Harding, 1978) reported that in the great majority of jurisdictions the relevant legislation requires a finding that the patient, owing to mental illness, constitutes a danger to himself or to others around him or to the community at large. In a number of jurisdictions, this type of 'dangerousness' criterion was the exclusive ground for compulsory hospitalization. In the remainder, it was an additional ground, usually accompanied by another criterion such as the person's need for treatment, his refusal to accept it, or his inability to understand his need for it.

In the United Kingdom, compulsory hospitalization rests on two main grounds. First, the patient must be found to be suffering from a 'mental disorder' being (a) 'mental illness' or 'severe subnormality' in a patient of any age, or (b) 'psychopathic disorder' or 'subnormality' in any patient under 21 years; such disorder warranting detention for medical treatment.

Second, compulsory detention is 'necessary' in the interests of the patient's health or safety or for the protection of other persons.

These criteria, unlike those governing compulsory hospitalization in, for example, the State of Massachusetts, avoid a particular definition of dangerousness. Whether or not an individual is likely to be dangerous by reason of mental disorder is an extremely difficult judgement to make. Apart from clinical judgement there are few specific guidelines. In such discussions, harm is often implicitly intended to mean physical harm, an assumption which poses particular problems in those cases of psychotic illness, such as mania, in which the question of physical dangerousness may not arise but in which harm of a less physical nature, such as financial harm or serious damage to one's professional reputation, is by no means an uncommon hazard. Basing the indications for compulsory hospitalization on a criterion of possible dangerousness in the future and/or violent behaviour in the past, as is advocated by some critics of current British mental health legislation (Gostin, 1975), would exclude these patients from consideration of compulsory hospitalization and treatment.

Competency and consent

The 1959 Mental Health Act, which is currently the subject of Governmental review, does not make a clear distinction between compulsory hospitalization and compulsory treatment, the assumption being that any person adjudged to require the one requires the other. It is the treating physician who determines the competency of the patient to accept or refuse treatment although a number of critics have argued that judicial rather than medical decision-making should be involved in the removal of a patient's rights concerning treatment (Gostin, 1979; Steadman, 1979). However, the Royal College of Psychiatrists, in its review of the British White Paper on the Mental Health Act, makes its position clear:

. . . . the responsibility for invoking compulsory powers (in relation to admission and treatment) is a clinical matter and the College considers that the professional background and higher professional training of psychiatrists prepare them to make fundamental decisions in the field of clinical psychiatric practice, and to take the primary responsibility for these decisions.

The question of consent also arises in relation to particular treatments used in contemporary psychiatry, such as ECT, long-acting drugs, and psychosurgery. Valid consent implies the ability, given an explanation in simple terms, to understand the nature, purpose and effect of the proposed treatment. Before giving treatment, it is accepted good professional practice to seek consent wherever the patient is capable of giving a valid consent. The Government's view is that if a detained patient who is capable of giving valid consent refuses to give it the doctor should not be able to impose any treatment (except in an emergency) without a concurring second opinion. Certain treatments, described as 'irreversible', 'hazardous', or 'not fully established', raise particular concerns. The White Paper appears to favour review by multi-disciplinary panels before such treatments are administered to detained patients. However, psychosurgery apart, it is not clear what treatments would be so regarded at the present time. Public anxiety concerning ECT conflicts with professional confidence that the treatment is safe and effective in those conditions for which it is indicated. The Royal College of Psychiatrists has issued a memorandum which, in addition to reviewing evidence concerning the efficacy of ECT, its associated morbidity and mortality, and the various methods of administration, also considers the question of consent. It advises psychiatrists that consent is a matter between the patient and doctor and that it is a 'medical responsibility' to ensure that the patient has been given an explanation of the procedure, benefits, and dangers of the treatment. The memorandum makes no mention of independent advisers or tribunals with powers to oversee the administration and prescription of ECT.

The situation with regard to psychosurgery appears somewhat different. Most jurisdictions support the idea of an independent medical 'referee' or panel whose assessment of the indications for intervention and agreement to it has to be registered before treatment can proceed. The most extensive recent review of psychosurgery, based on evidence accumulated over the decade 1965–75 and from a number of studies performed under contract to a National Commission (Report on Psychosurgery prepared by the US National Commission for the Protection of Human Subjects of Biomedical and Behavioral Research, 1977), recommended that such procedures should only be performed at approved institutions on properly assessed, informed and consenting patients. A New South Wales Report, which like the American one, was provoked by massive adverse publicity, made a similar recommendation and added that, where there is a doubt about the quality of the patient's consent, the case should be referred for a ruling to a justice of the Supreme Court. In Britain, the practice is for patients being considered for psychosurgery to be assessed by an independent professional panel but such a procedure is entirely voluntary and not laid down by legal statute.

Summary

As indicated by Curran and Harding (1978), the trend of the law in most countries is towards preserving the rights of the mentally ill. This is part of the civil rights movement, according to which any deprivation of rights must be fully and individually justified. The presumption, even in the case of seriously psychotic patients, must be that the individual is legally competent and entitled to the rights and privileges and obligations of other citizens. Any restriction placed on mentally disturbed persons must be proved on its merits, and limits in scope and time must be placed on the restrictions. Ethical as well as medico-legal issues are involved, lending support to appeals to professionals (Thompson, 1976) to involve themselves not merely in the construction of codes of conduct but in the demanding task of clarifying the nature of the fundamental ethical principles which form the moral base of clinical action. The participation of the World Health Organization in exercises designed to harmonize international approaches to classification and mental health legislation is but one professional response. The appearance of a Declaration of Ethics from the World Psychiatric Association is another, the issue precipitating it, namely the abuse of psychiatric power in the detention of political dissidents, being an issue of psychiatric practice as much as an ethical and legal issue.

PART III
Psychoses of early childhood
Edited by L. Wing & J. K. Wing

Section 7

CHAPTERS 29–33

Clinical

29
Development of concepts, classification, and relationship to mental retardation

LORNA WING

Historical background

Although accounts of children with strange behaviour, such as the story of the wild boy of Aveyron (Itard, 1801, 1807; Lane, 1977) and the boy described by Haslam (1809), were published early in the nineteenth century, the idea that 'insanity' could occur in children was first introduced by Maudsley (1867). Early classifications of childhood psychosis utilized concepts derived from adult psychiatry. It was not until the second half of the present century that the relevance of work on language and cognitive development became apparent, at least so far as the early childhood psychoses were concerned.

The search for specific syndromes

A number of writers described subgroups of children who, they believed, had in common an identifiable pattern of abnormal behaviour. These hypothetical syndromes were thought by their authors to be distinct varieties of childhood psychosis.

De Sanctis (1906) adopted Kraepelinian nomenclature and coined the term 'dementia praecocissima' for a rather wide range of conditions beginning before puberty and leading to behavioural deterioration. He also used the name 'dementia praecocissima catatonica' (de Sanctis, 1908) to refer to a condition that seems to have had much in common with the 'dementia infantilis' of Heller (see the translation of Heller's paper in Hulse, 1954). The children concerned regressed markedly in behaviour after a period of normal development. Within a few months they lost language and self-care skills, became socially withdrawn, and developed odd postures and stereotyped movements, though retaining mobility and an intelligent facial expression.

Earl (1934) described a condition he observed in mentally retarded people, which he called 'primitive catatonic psychosis of idiocy'. The 34 adults he studied all functioned as profoundly retarded, with no speech or self-care, but with some motor skills above this level. Echolalia and echopraxia were present in some. They were all solitary, uninterested in other people or their surroundings. Stereotyped, repetitive movements involving twisting and turning of the hands and flicking of the fingers, or of pieces of string, or other materials, were characteristic. Periods of excitement and laughter, or of weeping and apathy, or vague anxiety occurred for no obvious reason. Reduced response to pain was noted in many of the group.

Mahler (1952) gave an account of a behaviour pattern she referred to as 'symbiotic psychosis'. Her descriptions contain more inferences from than details of actual behaviour. The important points appear to be an abnormality of social relationships characterized by 'affectionless clinging', echolalia, repetitive speech on bizarre, sometimes frightening, themes, and attacks of 'abysmal affective panic'.

Kanner's work in this field has been of major importance, due, at least in part, to the clarity of his descriptions of the cluster of behavioural abnormalities he named 'early infantile autism' (Kanner, 1943, 1946, 1949, 1951, 1968, 1973). From among the various items making up this cluster he selected five as particularly characteristic (Kanner, 1949). These were a profound lack of affective contact; an anxiously obsessive desire for the maintenance of sameness as shown by repetitive activities as well as by dislike of change in specific aspects of the environment; a fascination with objects, which were handled with dexterity; mutism, or language that did not seem to serve interpersonal communication; and retention of good cognitive potential, shown by feats of rote memory, or non-verbal skills such as rapid completion of the Séguin form board. Later, Kanner and Eisenberg (1956) suggested that the first two points in the above list should be regarded as primary and, of the two, the lack of affective contact was considered the more fundamental. It was this aspect of the syndrome that influenced Kanner to use the word 'autism', previ-

ously chosen by Bleuler as a name for the social withdrawal seen in adult schizophrenia. The borrowing, once again, of a term from adult psychiatry led to a confusion of the two conditions based on semantics rather than clinical observation (see chapters 1 and 30).

At first Kanner believed autism was always present from birth, but Kanner and Eisenberg (1956) reported the typical behaviour pattern in children who had had up to 20 months of apparently normal development. Later authors have extended the possible age of onset up to 3 (Rutter, 1968; Kolvin, 1971) or 4 to 5 (Lotter, 1966, 1967) or even to 6 years (Brask, 1967; 1972). For this reason the term early *childhood* rather than *infantile* autism seems more appropriate and will be used hereafter.

The year following Kanner's original paper on autism, Asperger (1944) published his first account of a group of children he called 'autistic psychopaths'. The essential characteristics of this group were: a lack of inuitive understanding of the rules of social interaction, leading to naive, tactless behaviour; a pedantic, literal understanding and use of language, and a tendency to talk at rather than with other people; difficulty in co-ordinating complex movements, producing an odd gait and poor performance in games needing motor skills; unusual circumscribed interest patterns, involving, for example, maps, astronomy, or the routes of trains, which absorbed most of the attention of the child or adult concerned. There are close similarities between this picture and that seen in the mildly handicapped autistic person, but Asperger considered his to be distinct, viewing it as a fixed personality trait, and autism as a psychotic process with a definite course. Since the terms 'personality trait' and 'psychotic process' have not been defined empirically, it is difficult to make the distinction (Wing, 1981b). Van Krevelen (1971) suggested that childhood autism could be the result of some cerebral pathology, perhaps from birth trauma, in a child who, if it were not for such an accident, would have had Asperger's syndrome.

The unitary hypothesis

While some authors were attempting to identify specific syndromes, others took the view that all childhood psychoses could be grouped together as one single condition; the clinical variation, due to such factors as age or type of onset or environmental pressures, masked an underlying unity (Bender, 1947, 1961; Rank, 1949; Szurek, 1956; Goldfarb, 1970;

O'Gorman, 1970). Such authors tended to emphasize the links they saw between childhood psychosis and adult schizophrenia. The working party chaired by Creak (1961), which produced a list of nine points for the diagnosis of 'childhood schizophrenia', was influenced by this unitary hypothesis.

Kanner (1959) discussed and firmly rejected the idea that no useful distinctions could be made between different types of childhood psychosis. But Anthony (1958a) pointed out how much overlap there was between the so-called syndromes named by different workers. The lack of agreement on definitions was shown by the way in which the terms childhood psychosis, schizophrenia and autism were used interchangeably. The last came to be used much more widely than Kanner intended. The description of autistic children given by Ornitz and Ritvo (1976), for example, overlaps with that of Kanner, but emphasizes different aspects from those Kanner considered to be of special importance.

Recent approaches to classification
Grouping by age of onset

A major advance in classification came when the clinical pictures associated with different ages of onset were examined (Anthony, 1958a, b; Rutter, 1972a). Kolvin and his colleagues (Kolvin, 1971; Kolvin, Garside & Kidd, 1971; Kolvin, Humphrey & McNay, 1971; Kolvin, Ounsted, Humphrey & McNay, 1971; Kolvin, Ounsted & Roth, 1971; Kolvin, Ounsted, Richardson & Garside, 1971) compared three groups of children; those in whom abnormalities began, respectively, from birth or within the first 3 years of life, from 3 to 5 years, and over 5 years of age. The first group, referred to as infantile psychosis, was the commonest of the three. The children included had a behaviour pattern identical to or sharing many features in common with early childhood autism. The second group, which was extremely rare, appeared to consist of a mixture of conditions, many with an identifiable organic aetiology. The term 'disintegrative psychosis' has been suggested for the clinical picture in which deterioration of cognitive skills and behaviour occurs after three to four years of apparently normal development (Rutter, Shaffer & Sturge, 1975) but it is doubtful how far a separate category can be justified (see page 189). The last group, less rare than the second, but still much less common than infantile psychosis, contained children showing the symptoms and signs of adult schizophrenia, including hallucinations and delusions. 'Psychotic' behav-

iour associated with neuro-degenerative disorders beginning after age 5 (Corbett, Harris, Taylor & Trimble, 1977), and affective illnesses (see volume 4, chapter 5) have also been reported in children, but were not included in Kolvin's study.

The authors found too few children with onset from 3 to 5 years for detailed consideration, but those with early and late onset were compared, and a number of significant differences were found. A higher proportion of the parents of the late-onset group had schizophrenia. The early-onset group were more likely to have detectable evidence of cerebral dysfunction, and many more had an intelligence quotient in the mildly or severely retarded range.

The early childhood psychoses

The rest of this chapter will be concerned only with the conditions referred to as the early childhood psychoses. Childhood schizophrenia and affective psychoses are discussed in chapters 7 and 18 respectively (see also volume 4, chapter 5).

The differentiation of the early childhood psychoses from the adult psychoses occurring in childhood did not solve the problem of the subclassification of the former. Anthony's (1958a) comment concerning the overlapping of the features of the various named syndromes was an accurate summary of the situation. In some children, the clinical picture changed with increasing age from that of one syndrome to that of another. Descriptions of all the various forms of early childhood psychosis had the following aspects in common; absence, or marked impairment of the ability to take part in reciprocal social interactions; mutism, or characteristic abnormalities of both verbal and non-verbal language; absence or marked impairment of the development of imaginative pursuits such as pretend play, and the substitution of repetitive, stereotyped activities. The precise way in which these problems were manifested varied, but all could be identified in the clinical accounts.

Associated organic conditions and mental retardation. A history of identifiable conditions likely to affect the central nervous system is found in many children with early childhood psychoses, including autism (see chapter 38).

Aspects of the behaviour of early childhood psychosis have been reported in a substantial minority of mentally retarded people, especially those in the severely retarded range (IQ below 50) (Earl, 1934;

Forrest & Ogunremi, 1974; Haracopos & Kelstrup, 1978). Conversely, detailed psychological testing of children with early childhood psychosis, including autism, has shown that the majority score as mildly or severely mentally retarded (Lotter, 1966; Rutter & Lockyer, 1967; Kolvin, Humphrey & McNay, 1971; DeMyer *et al.*, 1974; Carr, 1976; Wing & Gould, 1979). The argument that the low scores are due to refusal rather than inability to perform, and that the results of testing are too unreliable to be meaningful (Kanner & Lesser, 1958) is refuted by the finding that the children willingly complete items within their range of capability, and fail in areas that can be predicted from a knowledge of their specific impairments (DeMyer *et al.*, 1974; Clark and Rutter, 1977). Furthermore, IQ has been shown to be highly correlated with prognosis (Rutter, 1970; Lotter, 1974; DeMyer, 1976).

Kanner, writing in the early 1940s, believed that the children with his syndrome were essentially physically normal and of good cognitive potential. Since that time there have been advances in techniques of neurological examination, methods of psychological testing, and understanding of cognitive and language development. Follow-up studies have shown that evidence for neurological disorder, such as epileptic fits, may first appear in adolescence or early adult life (Rutter, 1970; Lotter, 1974). It is now clear that behaviour exactly like that described by Kanner, as well as other forms of early childhood psychosis, can be associated with low intelligence and cerebral pathology.

Classification based on an epidemiological study

Having regard to this historical background, Wing and Gould (1979) carried out an epidemiological study designed to examine the relationship of early childhood psychosis to mental retardation and organic conditions affecting the central nervous system, and to consider systems of subclassification. These authors examined a complete population of children from one area of London who were selected because they functioned as severely mentally retarded, or because they had at least one of the three features listed earlier in this chapter as occurring in all forms of early childhood psychosis. Many children were included on both these criteria. It was found that, regardless of IQ, associated organic conditions, or additional handicaps such as deafness or blindness, the group could be divided into those whose two-way social

interactions were appropriate in the light of their mental ages, and those with impairments of reciprocal social interaction. The latter also had the other features of early childhood psychosis, namely, abnormalities of non-verbal and verbal language developed in the normal child. If, later, his mental age place of pursuits needing symbolic language and imagination. This cluster of abnormalities will be referred to as the triad of language and social impairments.

Many of the sociable, severely retarded children had problems with spoken language, but were able to use non-verbal communication to compensate. Some had simple repetitive activities such as rocking, arm-flapping, or flicking objects, but these occurred mostly in the children with mental ages below 20 months, that is before pretend play has developed in the normal child. If, later, his mental age matured beyond his level, the sociable retarded child developed imaginative play, and his repetitive activities tended to diminish or disappear. The study also corroborated the previous reports in the literature of an association between early childhood psychosis and the particular organic conditions mentioned in chapter 38.

Identification of named syndromes. The authors considered that the 74 children in the study with the triad of language and social impairments represented the range of conditions covered by the term early childhood psychosis. An attempt was made to identify, among this group, the syndromes named by past workers. Although aspects of the behaviour listed by all these writers could be found in different children within the population studied, the only subgroup that could be reliably identified was Kanner's early childhood autism, using the criteria of social aloofness and indifference, and maintenance of sameness shown by elaborate repetitive routines (Kanner & Eisenberg, 1956), both being present from early childhood up to at least 7 years of age. However, as Kanner reported (1973), some of the children became more inclined to accept and initiate social approaches in later childhood and adult life.

Seventeen children in the study had a history of the behaviour pattern described by Kanner, although some of these had also had identifiable conditions likely to impair brain function, and a few had additional physical handicaps. When those with a history of typical autism were compared with the rest showing the triad of language and social impairments, certain differences were found. Two-thirds of the former had age-related quotients above 50 on standardized tests of visuo-spatial skills, compared with only one-third of the latter. This was not surprising since, by definition, the autistic children had elaborate repetitive routines, often involving the organization of objects into complex patterns or constructions. Those in the autistic group who had sufficient speech had a history of reversal of pronouns and the use of words or phrases in idiosyncratic, stereotyped ways. The capacity for intense concentration on a narrow range of repetitive activities (though not on other pursuits) was also characteristic of the autistic children. Otherwise, the two groups did not differ in the clinical picture, nor on types or frequency of associated organic conditions.

Classification by degree of social impairment. Independently of the presence or absence of a history of typical autism, the socially impaired children were subdivided on the quality of their social interaction. Three subgroups were identified, namely those who were aloof and indifferent to others, and avoided contact except for obtaining needs or simple physical pleasure, such as tickling; those who made no spontaneous social contacts, but passively accepted approaches and allowed themselves to be pulled into other people's activities; and those who did initiate contact in an odd, one-sided way, which was unaffected by the response of the person approached. Children with a *history* of typical autism were found in all three social impairment groups, as the latter classification was based on behaviour current at the time of assessment.

There were highly significant differences between the three groups in the severity and type of behavioural abnormalities shown, level of language and non-verbal abilities, and associated organic conditions. There appeared to be a gradation of severity of handicap, the aloof group being most severely impaired, tending to be lowest in intelligence and the most likely to have an identifiable gross organic aetiology, the passive group being intermediate, and the odd group having a less global impairment, but still markedly abnormal in behaviour. It was felt that this method of subdivision had more value in relation to studies of aetiology, and to education and management, than the division into early childhood autism and other early childhood psychosis.

In the children studied, no differences in behaviour and course could be observed between those with an onset before 3 years and those with an onset between 3 and 5 years of age. However, there were too few of the latter for reliable comparisons to be made.

Impairments underlying early childhood psychosis

Recent formulations of the nature of early childhood psychosis relate it to cognitive and language impairments (Ricks & Wing, 1975; DeMyer, 1976; Hermelin, 1976; Churchill, 1978; Rutter, 1978a,b,c) and are very different from the early theories that linked it to adult psychosis. The most striking of the observable clinical phenomena is the triad of problems affecting reciprocal social interaction, verbal and non-verbal language, and imaginative activities. What are the impairments underlying these abnormalities? It can be hypothesized that an essential aspect of normal brain function is the attribution of significance to experiences, whether these are of external, or internal, bodily origin. Understanding of the past, planning for the future, and creative imaginative activities all depend upon an intuitive grasp of meaning which the normal child, from the beginning of life, attaches to people, objects and events. For the child with early childhood psychosis, experiences seem to be wholly or partially devoid of meaning. Simple, often superficial, connections between events may be established through conditioning, but a true comprehension of more complex associations, and especially the subtleties of the rules of symbolic language and social interaction would be impossible to achieve, as would any truly imaginative activity.

This idea was first put forward by Rimland (1965), and more recently Damasio and Maurer (1978) have suggested a possible neurological basis for such an impairment.

This central problem could occur as the sole impairment, resulting in a classically autistic child with good skills in areas not dependent on creative language and imagination – that is, visuo-spatial tasks and rote memory. Much more commonly, it could occur in association with more widespread brain damage, due, for instance, to encephalitis, producing a child with early childhood psychosis and retardation of all aspects of cognitive development. The central problem itself could vary in degree of severity, which would also affect the clinical picture. Conversely, other cognitive impairments could occur without the central problem, giving a sociable but retarded child.

This formulation must be regarded as a tentative hypothesis, but the importance of language and cognitive development in early childhood psychoses is no longer in doubt. It is to be hoped that the vague and ill-defined terms 'autism' and 'psychosis' will soon be abandoned, and more suitable names found which will be related to the special impairments underlying these conditions.

30

Clinical description, diagnosis, and differential diagnosis

LORNA WING

Diagnosis: the clinical picture

In the absence of any knowledge of the specific underlying pathology, even where the gross aetiology can be identified, early childhood psychosis must be defined and diagnosed solely on the past and present behaviour. Some authors include age of onset before 3 years as a diagnostic criterion (Rutter, 1978c). In the great majority of cases, these conditions do begin before 3 years of age, but there are a few children for whom the reported age of onset is between 3 and 5 years and in whom the clinical picture is closely similar to that found with an earlier onset (Wing & Gould, 1979). Very rarely, the abnormalities of behaviour appear to begin after 5 years (Brask, 1967; 1972). In any case, the possibility of error in reporting, especially when making a diagnosis in an older child or adult, argues against the use of age of onset as an essential aspect of diagnosis.

A multi-axial diagnostic formulation is the most appropriate (Rutter *et al.*, 1969, 1975; Wing, L., 1970; Rutter, Shaffer & Sturge, 1975). The psychiatric condition (that is, the overt behaviour pattern), any associated organic conditions of possible aetiological significance, any additional handicaps, and intelligence level are recorded separately, since they can vary independently of one another. A number of detailed descriptions of the behaviour in early childhood psychoses can be found in the literature (Kanner, 1943, 1973; Rutter, 1966, 1967; Wing, L., 1976, 1980; DeMyer, 1979). The most vivid have been written by parents (Junker, 1964; Park, 1967; Hundley, 1971).

As explained in chapter 29, the behaviour patterns in all forms of early childhood psychosis overlap to a considerable extent, so that it is possible to give a general description of the main features, while indicating the variations which have led some authors to try to identify specific subgroups.

The first year of life

Accounts of behaviour at this stage have all been obtained retrospectively from parents, since the diagnosis of early childhood psychosis is rarely made before 2 years of age (Wing, L., 1971). If the abnormality is present from birth, the mother may feel that something is wrong without being able to specify the reason. Such anxieties should be treated seriously and the baby's development watched carefully, even if no problems can be detected on first examination.

The baby may show little or no interest in social interaction, apart from the simple pleasure derived from physical contact such as tickling or bouncing up and down. He may fail to engage in pre-verbal 'conversational' exchanges with his mother, clearly seen in the normal baby from around 2 months of age (Schaffer, 1974; Trevarthen, 1974). Failure to get ready to be picked up, by, for example, lifting the arms has been reported as characteristic of autistic babies (Kanner, 1943).

Around 10 months of age, normal babies begin to point things out to their parents in order to share the interest. The toddler will bring objects to give or show to his parents and others, as part of the process of social interaction. In early childhood psychosis this behaviour is often reported to be absent. Imitation and subsequent spontaneous initiation of actions such as waving good-bye, clapping, pulling funny faces, and making sounds are characteristic of the normal baby around one year of age, but may fail to appear if early childhood psychosis is present from infancy. Later, perhaps by 4 or 5 years, a small minority of the affected children develop automatic copying without understanding (echopraxia).

Babbling may be absent or limited in quality and quantity. Speech is characteristically delayed, or never develops at all and the child does not use gesture to compensate. Sometimes a child is reported to have begun to speak at the usual age and then to have lost this skill. In some cases the child did have a period of normal development before the impairments appeared. In others, careful questioning shows that the speech was immediate or delayed echolalia, without real meaning.

Repetitive behaviours are part of normal baby development, but sometimes these are reported as abnormal in intensity and persistence in a child who is later shown to have early childhood psychosis, especially autism. For example, such a child may be fascinated by a pattern on the wallpaper (Hundley, 1971) or by an electric light and become very distressed if placed where these objects cannot be seen.

One to five years

Unless the child has some years of normal development, the behaviour problems tend to be most marked from the time he or she is able to walk, up to age 5 or 6 years.

The clinical features include the triad of social impairment, language abnormalities, and repetitive activities in place of imaginative pursuits, described in chapter 29, but there are other abnormalities in addition to these, as described below. It is not yet possible to explain how all the items are related, but that they tend to occur together is a matter of clinical observation (Wing & Gould, 1979).

The extent of handicap varies widely among different children. The characteristic features may occur in more or less severe form and some aspects may be more prominent than others. The number and severity of associated abnormalities will markedly affect the clinical picture. Interaction between the child's primary disabilities and his environment plays an important part, though the limits within which such factors can operate are much narrower than for children with the potential for symbolic thought and language. The external manifestations of the basic handicaps change with age, there being a tendency for some improvement to occur, though with adolescence there may be a temporary regression to more difficult behaviour.

Impairment of social interaction. This varies from aloofness, through social passivity, to odd one-sided social approaches as described in chapter 29. It is important to emphasize that a child may pass from one group to another during the course of maturation. When and if the stage of aloofness and indifference is passed, there may be a positive desire to interact with others, but the lack of awareness of the rules of social conduct makes this difficult or impossible. Diagnosis depends not upon lack of affect, but upon lack of ability to initiate and carry on a reciprocal interaction. These problems are especially marked with age peers, and true friendships are rarely if ever formed. Sometimes a normal, or a sociable retarded child 'adopts' a child with early childhood psychosis and they might refer to each other as friends, but the initiative is entirely with the non-psychotic child. More able, older, socially impaired children may wish to have friends, and will describe all their acquaintances, or even strangers, as 'friends' because they lack any understanding of the nature of friendship.

Abnormalities of language and communication. These affect understanding and use of non-verbal as well as verbal methods of communication (Ricks & Wing, 1975). Speech problems include mutism in about half of the affected children. In those who do speak, one or more of the following problems can be seen: immediate echolalia; delayed echolalia (repeating words and phrases first overheard or learned days, weeks, even years previously, sometimes with the exact accent and tone of voice of the original speaker); repetitive, stereotyped, inflexible use of words or phrases; and, in the most able children, a grammatical but inappropriately pedantic style of speech. Problems similar to those in the specific developmental speech disorders, such as missing out, or inappropriate use of, prepositions and conjunctions and other small linking words, and confusion of word order, may occur.

Reversal of pronouns (you instead of I, and so on) and a peculiar, idiosyncratic use of words and phrases are particularly characteristic of Kanner's syndrome (Kanner, 1946; Rutter, 1966; Wing & Gould, 1979).

Understanding and use of gesture are limited and may be confined to pulling others by the hand, or simple pointing. There is poor comprehension and use of information conveyed by facial expression, bodily movements, posture, and vocal intonation.

The making and breaking of eye contact is another aspect of nonverbal communication that is abnormal in early childhood psychosis. This may take the form of lack of eye contact or even gaze avoidance. This is common, though not invariably present, in the young child with Kanner's syndrome. It may also be manifested by inappropriate rather than too little eye contact. In this case the child may look too long and too hard at times, but fail to meet someone's gaze when contact would have been expected,

such as in greeting, or when wishing to make a remark in conversation.

Impairment of imaginative activities. Most children with early childhood psychosis have no pretend play or other imaginative activities. A minority develop the ability to copy other people's activities, though without understanding of their significance, and a small number do have some apparently symbolic, imaginative interests (Wing, Gould, Yeates & Brierley, 1977). However, these are limited in scope and markedly repetitive, the child playing the same game over and over again, perhaps acting like a television character, or like teacher at school, regardless of suggestions from other children.

Rarely, children with early childhood psychosis seem to have a partial, distorted, fragmented, uncontrolled development of their imaginative abilities. They may talk on bizarre, frightening themes, which can give the superficial impression of a rich fantasy life. In a few such cases, much trouble can be caused because a child's stories of theft, murder or sexual assault are taken seriously by an adult who does not know him well. Longer contact with such children discloses the repetitive, stereotyped nature of the ideas expressed, and the lack of any ability to use symbolic thought to understand the present and plan for the future. This small subgroup should not be confused with schizophrenia occurring in childhood (see chapters 7 and 29).

Repetitive activities. When not supervised, children with early childhood psychosis tend to indulge in repetitive activities. At the simplest level these are entirely self-directed, for example rocking, teeth-grinding, grunting, eye-poking, flicking hands and fingers near the eyes, or self-injury. The repetitive pursuits can involve objects, such as flicking pieces of string, tapping or shaking, turning the wheels of toy cars, or dextrous spinning of such unlikely things as wooden blocks or wine glasses. More elaborate routines, such as making repetitive patterns from leaves, stones, even kitchen utensils, or insisting that everyone in the room sits with the right leg crossed over the left or that the route for the daily walk is never varied, are characteristic of Kanner's syndrome. Some children in this subgroup may collect objects to twiddle, arrange in patterns, or just to hold. These can include empty detergent packets, tin lids, pieces of photographic negatives, shoes, umbrella handles – nothing is too peculiar or useless to be of fascination to some autistic child. On the other hand, such a child may develop an intense fear, occasionally mingled with fascination, of some objects or experiences, such as having a bath, barking dogs, rooms with yellow curtains, red buses (but not buses of any other colour), which may cause great problems for the family.

Kanner classified all these repetitive activities and preoccupations as manifestations of a desire to maintain sameness in the environment. There may be intense dislike of change in such things as the furniture, the arrangement of ornaments, or the daily routine, shown by temper tantrums or great distress and fear. Quite often, a child will accept a totally new experience, such as moving house, without any fuss, but react strongly to a trivial change in his own room, his clothing, or his collection of objects.

In the most able children, the repetitive activities may take the form of apparently academic pursuits, such as learning and repeating large numbers of facts about the planets, wild flowers, the railways, meteorology. The essential point is that the facts are learnt by rote, and understanding of their significance falls a long way behind the accuracy of the recall.

Repetitive pseudo-imaginative play has already been described. Repetitive speech, especially repetitive questioning regardless of the replies received, is also quite common in children with large vocabularies and good executive speech.

Responses to sensory stimuli. There are often abnormal responses to sensory stimuli. The child may ignore many sounds, be distressed by some, yet delighted by others. He may be intensely fascinated with bright lights and shiny objects, or things that spin round. The same child may be indifferent to pain, heat, and cold in his early years, but later on become upset by trivial injuries. Some of the children like to touch surfaces such as smooth wood, plastic, or fur, and may touch the clothes of strangers in the street. They may also smell and lick objects or people.

When young, autistic children may seem to pay more attention to stimuli on the periphery rather than in the centre of the visual fields.

Imitation. Difficulty in imitation of other people's actions continues after infancy. The children can most easily copy a stationary model, but they have difficulty in remembering a movement they have seen and translating it into an equivalent action of their own bodies (DeMyer, 1976). This handicap contrasts oddly with the accurate but meaningless imitation observed in those with echolalia or echopraxia.

Motor control. Flapping and writhing movements of the arms and legs, facial grimaces, jumping, or a tense quivering of the flexed arms are often seen, especially when the child is pleasurably excited. Some of these movements are reminiscent of those seen in normal infants. Tip-toe walking, an odd 'disjointed' walk without arm-swinging, a tendency to stand in odd postures, and peculiar hand movements and postures with marked separation and extension of the fingers may be observed. Intermittent interruption of ongoing motor activities can occur. Damasio and Maurer (1978) point out that many of these phenomena are like those found in post-encephalitic states.

Spontaneous large movements, or fine skilled movements, or both, may be clumsy in some children, though others appear to be graceful and nimble.

Autonomic and vestibular functions. The children may have peculiar patterns of sleeping or feeding, and some consume unusually large quantities of fluid. They often show an unusual degree of interest in being spun round, as on a roundabout, or spinning themselves (Ornitz & Ritvo, 1968a,b) and may show no signs of vertigo.

Abnormalities of attention. It may be impossible to capture the attention of the most severely retarded children with early childhood psychosis. Some, including those with rather higher levels of skill, are distractible and may be over-active as well. The Kanner's syndrome child is characteristically non-distractible when he is engaged in his elaborate routines, but it is difficult to channel this capacity for intense concentration into tasks chosen by the teacher. The children may attend to one trivial aspect of a person or object, rather than to the whole (Koegel & Wilhelm, 1973).

Special skills. Children with early childhood psychosis typically have uneven profiles of skills and impairments, contrasting with the more or less equal backwardness in all areas of the sociable retarded child. In the majority, performance on all tasks is in the retarded range, though some areas are better than others. Children with higher than normal performance in one or a few skills do exist (Selfe, 1977), but form a tiny minority of those with early childhood psychosis.

The better areas of performance tend to be in non-symbolic fitting and assembly tasks, or those needing rote memory, such as recognition of music, arithmetical calculations, reproduction of maps, poems, or words of songs.

A small group of children can be found who score better on language than on performance tests (Rutter, 1966) but their speech is repetitive rather than spontaneous, and they have the usual problems with abstract meanings. This subgroup may present diagnostic problems until the odd social interaction and the impairment of symbolic language and imagination are recognized.

Socially inappropriate behaviour. This can include screaming, temper tantrums, grabbing things from counters in shops, laughing, or crying inappropriately, making naive, embarrassing remarks in a loud voice, and generally behaving in strange and unpredictable ways in public as well as at home.

As has been emphasized in chapter 29 the impairments of social interaction, communication, and imagination are the essential features of early childhood psychosis. The other aspects described above may be very marked, especially in the more severely handicapped children, or may be moderate, mild, or observed rarely or not at all. They may occur in the first few years and then fade away. This variability and tendency to change with age makes the obtaining of a detailed history of the child's behaviour essential for diagnosis.

Other aspects of multi-axial diagnosis

Once the diagnosis of early childhood psychosis has been made on the overt behaviour pattern, it may be of relevance to decide into which subgroup a particular child best fits. Different methods of subgrouping are discussed in chapter 29.

A detailed medical history and appropriate examinations and investigations are needed to establish the possible aetiology (see chapter 38) and to identify any additional handicaps such as impairments of hearing or vision.

The child's intelligence level is relevant for planning education and management, and as a guide to prognosis. A profile of visuo-spatial, verbal and practical skills is of more value than a single intelligence quotient. Methods of assessment are discussed in chapter 32.

Differential diagnosis
Adult psychoses occurring in children

The differences between schizophrenia and early childhood psychosis have been mentioned in chapter 29 (see also chapter 6). Affective psychoses have also been reported in childhood and can be diagnosed on the clinical picture (see chapter 18). Progressive cognitive deterioration due to conditions such as lipoidosis or of unknown aetiology, is rare, but does occur in childhood and the changes in behaviour may resemble those of early childhood psychosis. The diagnosis is made on the neurological signs (which may be late in developing) and the course (Corbett, Harris, Taylor & Trimble, 1977).

Obsessional illnesses and phobias can be distinguished from the repetitive activities and special fears of early childhood psychosis by examining the child's whole behaviour pattern and his cognitive, language, and imaginative development.

Adult psychiatric illness of all kinds can occur as an additional problem complicating early childhood psychosis, especially in adolescence and adult life. The commonest problem is depression, in the more mildly handicapped young adult, as a consequence of partial recognition of his own handicaps, or following unhappy experiences such as bereavement.

Mental retardation

The relationship between early childhood psychosis and mental retardation has been discussed in chapter 29.

Brain damage

This is an unsatisfactory, vague, general category. The diagnosis of early childhood psychosis depends on the behaviour pattern. The presence or absence of diagnosable brain damage is an independent axis of the diagnostic formulation, as explained above.

Hyperkinetic syndrome

Hyperkinesis and early childhood psychosis are different behavioural clusters that occasionally coexist. The diagnosis of the latter depends upon the presence of the characteristic impairments, whether or not the child is also over-active. If both are present, each should be mentioned in the diagnostic formulation. The aimless restlessness often seen in early childhood psychosis when the child is unsupervised and unoccupied should not be confused with the excessive unceasing activity of true hyperkinesis. The concept of the hyperkinetic syndrome has been critically reviewed by Shaffer and Greenhill (1979). See also volume 4, chapter 4.

Impairments of hearing

A young congenitally deaf child may appear socially withdrawn and show some repetitive activities, but once he develops gestural communication he becomes able to engage in two-way social interaction. Pretend play develops normally.

It is possible for deafness and early childhood psychosis to coexist, in which case the behaviour pattern of the latter will be present. In some mute autistic children, the equivocal responses to sound may make it difficult to decide even with formal testing whether or not they are also deaf.

Developmental receptive and expressive speech disorders

As with the young deaf child, social withdrawal and repetitive activities may be seen in these conditions, in the early years, especially if receptive problems are marked (Ingram, 1959; Wing, L., 1971). But, if the problems are specific to speech, gestural and other non-verbal communication develops, as does pretend play and other imaginative activities. Social interaction improves with increasing ability to communicate, although rather 'silly', immature behaviour is common.

These disorders and the early childhood psychoses shade into one another and aspects of the speech problems of the former are found in the latter. Some children are on the borderline between the groups (Bartak, Rutter & Cox, 1975; Cox, Rutter, Newman & Bartak, 1975; Wing, L., 1979a).

Impairments of vision, or vision and hearing

A few autistic children are so unresponsive to visual stimuli that they are thought to be blind. Careful observation may show that the child can make some fine visual discriminations in areas related to his repetitive activities. Blindness and early childhood psychosis can coexist (Wing & Gould, 1979).

Congenitally blind or partially sighted children may twist and turn their hands near their eyes, and show other stereotyped movements such as rocking (Freedman, 1971). This may occur as the only behavioural abnormality, or it may be part of the complete picture of early childhood psychosis.

A combination of visual and hearing impair-

ments, present from birth and due, for example, to maternal rubella (Chess, 1971), is particularly likely to be associated with this type of behaviour (Wing, L., 1969, 1971). In some cases, the problems diminish or disappear with maturation and the development of alternative methods of communication (Chess, 1977) but, in others, the psychotic behaviour proves to be permanent. Presumably, the prognosis depends upon the degree of brain damage produced by the condition that also caused the impairments of vision and hearing.

Visuo-spatial problems

Children with specific impairments of visuospatial skills may show fascination with visual stimuli, very similar to that seen in early childhood psychosis. Such children may also be socially withdrawn when in large groups of their peers. However, they interact appropriately with children they know well, and show imaginative play, (Wing, L., 1981a).

Visuo-spatial problems can be found in some children with early childhood psychosis, although many, especially those with Kanner's syndrome, are dextrous in fitting and assembly tasks.

Elective mutism

In this condition, the child speaks in some situations but not others. He may have speech problems and be difficult in behaviour in other ways, but he will use non-verbal communication and does not show the behaviour pattern of early childhood psychosis (Reed, 1963).

Psychosocial deprivation

This has been fully discussed by Rutter (1972b) and Clarke and Clarke (1976a).

Potentially normal children deprived of social interaction, interesting activities and opportunities for learning may be socially withdrawn, retarded in speech development, and show repetitive stereotyped movements. In cases of gross deprivation they may function as severely mentally retarded. When placed in an appropriate environment, they make rapid strides in social, language, cognitive, and imaginative development (Koluchova, 1972, 1976; Clarke & Clarke, 1976b).

The differences from children with early childhood psychosis become evident within a few days or weeks.

The major diagnostic problem arises if a child with early childhood psychosis happens to have been brought up in an understimulating environment. The behaviour pattern and the lack of progress with improvement in circumstances will establish the diagnosis.

Schizoid personality

Kretschmer (1925), who coined the term schizoid personality, defined it so widely that it could include the more able autistic adult. He presented a number of case histories, one or two of which were strongly reminiscent of the picture seen in autistic people who have made enough progress to become independent as adults, especially those with the features described by Asperger (1944).

Wolff and Barlow (1979) argued that Asperger's syndrome (see chapter 29) should be regarded as a form of schizoid personality. Although a case can be made for this classification, there are two disadvantages in doing so (Wing, L., 1981b). First, it suggests a relationship with adult schizophrenia, which is, as yet, an untested assumption. Second, it has no practical implications for education and management. Inclusion within the group of those with the triad of language and social impairment, on the other hand, emphasizes the need for an organized, structured, individual programme at home, school and work.

The differential diagnosis can be made only on the details of the childhood history and present state.

31

Epilepsy and the electroencephalogram in early childhood psychoses

JOHN A. CORBETT

Epidemiological studies suggest that, by the age of eleven years, four in every 1000 children have been diagnosed as suffering from nonfebrile epilepsy (Ross, Peckham, West & Butler, 1980).

Seizures in infancy are more common than in school-age children. Febrile convulsions affect 2.3 per cent of well babies and 6 per cent of those with cerebral palsy (Lennox-Buchthal, 1973). Perinatal complications may lead to fits in the neonatal period, and infantile spasms typically appear between the third and eighth month of life (Corbett, Harris & Robinson, 1975).

Epilepsy may make its appearance for the first time in later childhood or adolescence, particularly around the time of puberty.

The frequency of seizures of both early and late onset is much increased in children who suffer from severe intellectual retardation (Corbett, Harris & Robinson, 1975).

The prevalence of autism and other forms of early childhood psychosis is discussed in chapter 34. Estimates of the frequency of a history of seizures at any age in children with autism and related conditions range between 14 per cent (DeMyer *et al.*, 1973) and 42 per cent (Schain & Yannet, 1960). Factors likely to produce variations in the estimates include differences in the ages and severity of impairments of the children examined. Rutter (1970, 1979) studied a group of autistic children who had all attended the Maudsley Hospital. He found that one-third had had at least one seizure by the time they were adults. Virtually all of those with a history of epileptic fits had an intelligence quotient below 70. Rutter found that, in many cases, the onset of fits was in adolescence. This has also been reported by Deykin and Mac-Mahon (1979).

The calculation of exact prevalence rates is also complicated by the fact that the diagnosis of early childhood psychosis depends entirely, and that of epilepsy largely, upon the observation of specific patterns of abnormal behaviour. Overt signs of neurological disorder may be found in either, but these are less relevant as far as identification of the two conditions under discussion is concerned.

An epidemiological study of children with early childhood psychosis or severe mental retardation was carried out in the former London borough of Camberwell (Wing & Gould, 1979). Neurological investigation of this group was carried out by Corbett, Harris and Robinson (1975). It was found at a follow-up when the subjects were aged 9 to 23 years, that approximately one-third of all those with any form of early childhood psychosis had a history of one or more seizures since birth (unpublished data). Low levels of intelligence (especially IQ below 20), historical or current evidence of brain damage, and particularly marked social aloofness and indifference to others tended to cluster together, and were highly associated with the occurrence of epileptic fits. None of the children in the study with an IQ of 70 or above had had seizures at the time of assessment.

Neurological disorders and epilepsy

It seems likely, from the available evidence, that damage or maldevelopment of various kinds affecting different parts of the brain underlies both childhood psychosis and epilepsy. Many different disease entities and signs of brain damage have been described in autism and related conditions. One of the main problems in investigating the link between the neurological disorders and early childhood psychosis is that most of the published papers give isolated case reports, and the criteria for diagnosis vary considerably. However, some conditions tend to be reported fairly frequently in early childhood psychosis, whereas others, notably Down's syndrome, occur much more frequently in sociable though retarded children (Wing & Gould, 1979). Organic and possible genetic aetiologies are discussed in chapters 36, 37 and 38. Here, certain aspects of neurological disorder of particular relevance to epilepsy and early childhood psychosis will be discussed in more detail.

Infantile spasms

This form of epilepsy, with typical salaam spasms, may occur with a wide variety of identifiable pathologies affecting the brain, but, in approximately 50 per cent of cases, no cause can be found. These are referred to as 'idiopathic', but it seems likely that the proportion of cases so described will diminish with advances in knowledge of neuropathology.

The EEG characteristically shows hypsarrhythmia with high voltage spike and slow wave activity.

The prognosis for subsequent intellectual development is poor, although there is evidence that treatment with steroids may improve the outcome (Corbett, Harris & Robinson, 1975). The particular pattern of impairments that often follows infantile spasms was discussed by Illingworth (1955). He suggested that retardation in the personal–social abilities tended to be greater than that in motor skills. He pointed out that the failure of social responsiveness was so marked that the infant may appear to be blind.

Later authors, including Knobloch and Pasamanick (1966, 1975) and Kolvin, Ounsted and Roth (1971), who were interested in the psychiatric manifestations of cognitive dysfunction, recognized that the abnormal behaviour consequent upon infantile spasms could be classified under the general heading of early childhood psychosis and, in some cases, was that of typical autism.

The most detailed account is given by Taft and Cohen (1971). These authors described five children, diagnosed as autistic, whose EEGs showed hypsarrhythmia and who had suffered from infantile spasms. Four were mentally retarded, though two of these had 'islets of intelligence' in marked contrast to the retardation in social and language skills. Two had tuberose sclerosis. Taft and Cohen concluded that the encephalopathy associated with infantile spasms causes permanent brain damage of a specific kind, which underlies both the fits and the pattern of impairments and abnormal behavior.

In the Camberwell epidemiological study mentioned above, of the 165 children who were included, 9 had had infantile spasms; 4 following identifiable aetiologies, and 5 of unknown cause. Of these, 1 had the nuclear and 1 the non-nuclear autistic behaviour patterns and 5 had other forms of early childhood psychosis. The remainder (2) were totally nonmobile, with severe impairment of all functions including social interaction. None of the sociable severely retarded children had had a history of infantile spasms.

Childhood encephalopathies

Acute encephalopathies occurring after birth and caused by infective, toxic, traumatic, and other agents may lead to arrest in development and behavioural regression and, in some instances, may give rise to severe, persistent behavioural abnormalities. If seizures occur during the acute phase of the illness, the subsequent brain damage is more likely to be severe. The prevention of status epilepticus is of considerable importance for the child's prognosis. Whether or not the subsequent behaviour disorder and pattern of cognitive functioning are characteristic of early childhood psychosis appears to depend on the stage of development at which the cerebral insult occurred, its severity, and which parts of the brain are involved. There is strong evidence that early childhood psychosis is more likely to result if the original illness occurred under three years of age (see chapter 29).

Although not commonly associated with epilepsy, one particularly important and preventable cause of pre-natal brain damage is maternal rubella, in which the virus can affect the central nervous system of the developing foetus (Desmond *et al.*, 1970; Chess, 1971; Chess, Korn & Fernandez, 1971). Other viral encephalopathies which may cause the onset of early childhood psychosis after birth are those due to measles, herpes, chicken pox, and other acute infectious diseases that are common in the early years of life. There is now doubt as to whether pertussis immunization is a major specific cause of encephalopathy, but, unquestionably, anything that can provoke prolonged pyrexial convulsions may lead to brain damage.

It has recently been reported by Hauser, DeLong and Rosman (1975) and DeLong (1978b) that pneumoencephalograms in children with a history of retarded language development and autistic behaviour show dilatation of the temporal horns of the lateral ventricles, particularly on the left side. This suggests that temporal lobe dysfunction may be a factor in the pathogenesis of such conditions. The authors, however, did not clarify whether the children studied had any identifiable cerebral pathology which might have produced both the autism and the temporal horn dilatation. It is now well established that temporal lobe epilepsy, with mesial temporal scle-

rosis, affecting one or both temporal lobes, may follow prolonged infantile convulsions (Falconer, 1971). This may be associated with severe behaviour disturbances, although such problems usually take the form of hyperkinetic conduct disorder, rather than early childhood psychosis.

Rarely, features of early childhood psychosis are seen during the course of progressive neurodegenerative disorders which can also cause seizures, such as metachromatic leucodystrophy, Schilder's disease, or subacute sclerosing panencephalitis (Corbett, Harris, Taylor & Trimble, 1977). In the early stages, differential diagnosis is likely to be difficult, but the appearance of neurological signs and the long-term course of the illness clarify the nature of the problem. Some of the children described by Heller (see Hulse, 1954) probably had progressive conditions of this kind. This condition is referred to as disintegrative psychosis of childhood in the ninth revision of the *International Classification of Diseases*.

Minor status epilepticus

In both early childhood and adolescence, very frequent minor seizures or subclinical seizure discharge may lead to an organic confusional state with a fluctuating level of consciousness. In this condition the behaviour may resemble that of early childhood psychosis. Diagnosis depends upon a detailed clinical history and the EEG.

This type of epilepsy can be very difficult to treat with conventional anticonvulsant drugs. Occasionally a trial of ACTH or a ketogenic diet using medium chain triglyceride oil may be indicated.

Epilepsy with late onset

As with all forms of epilepsy, seizures which first appear in adolescence or adult life are considerably more likely to occur in those who are mentally retarded. There are few long-term follow-up studies and little information concerning management and prognosis.

An exacerbation of already existing epilepsy is often seen around puberty, so it seems likely that hormonal factors have an effect on the occurrence of seizures. Also, some of the psychotropic drugs, such as chlorpromazine, which may be given for the first time in adolescence to alleviate behaviour disturbance, are epileptogenic and it may be preferable to use a less epileptogenic drug such as haloperidol. The seizures may occur on only two or three occasions. Unless the EEG shows gross and persistent abnormality, it is often advisable to withhold anticonvulsant medication following the first or even the second attack.

If the seizures persist, carbamazepine, 20 mg/kg daily, may be given in two divided doses, the dose being adjusted to give a plasma level of 6 to 8 mg/l. If the seizures are of a minor type, sodium valproate, in a dose of 20 mg/kg daily in three divided doses may be used, adjusted to give a blood-level of 40 to 100 mg/l.

Psychomotor seizures originating from the temporal lobe may be particularly difficult to identify in adolescents with early childhood psychosis and mental retardation, as a precise clinical diagnosis depends to a large extent on a subjective account of experiences during the seizures. A description, by an observer, of acute changes in behaviour, with distress suggestive of an epigastric aura, or subjective terror which cannot be explained by any obvious external cause, is helpful. The diagnosis may be confirmed by the finding of focal spike, and spike and wave activity, recorded from surface electrodes over the temporal region. Such abnormalities are more likely to be seen if the recording is taken during sleep. It may be possible to distinguish clinically between the seizure itself, which may be quite brief, and more prolonged post-ictal confusion. This is important in managing the behaviour disturbance associated with such attacks.

Occasionally, the onset of seizures in adolescents with early childhood psychosis is associated with marked regression in behaviour and, rarely, there is progressive deterioration involving cognitive as well as social skills. While it is not usually possible to find a specific neurological cause for this, great care must be taken to exclude intoxication with anticonvulsant drugs. Phenytoin and barbiturates both sometimes cause deterioration. Anticonvulsant drugs can interact with each other and mimic the signs of progressive neurological disorder. For this reason, combinations of drugs should, if possible, be avoided.

Neurophysiological studies
Routine EEG recordings
It is often difficult to obtain reliable EEG recordings from children with early childhood psychosis, because they do not understand what is required of them and may not co-operate. Few EEG studies have been published and even fewer with adequate controls. Abnormalities in routine record-

ings have been reported, the frequency in different series varying from 10 to 83 per cent, with an average of 51 per cent (White, DeMyer & DeMyer, 1964; Fish & Shapiro, 1965; Hutt, Hutt, Lee & Ounsted, 1965; Small, 1968; Creak & Pampiglione, 1969; Ritvo, Ornitz, Walter & Hanley, 1970; Gubbay, Lobascher & Kingerlee, 1970). In each of the studies in which controls were used, there were more abnormalities in the psychotic children.

The findings with regard to the EEG patterns were inconsistent. For example, White, DeMyer, and DeMyer (1964) and Small (1975) reported prominent spike and wave abnormalities, while Stevens and Milstein (1970) described unusually persistent alpha rhythm, except during ritualistic or manneristic behaviour. Hutt, Hutt, Lee, and Ounsted (1965) reported an excess of fast frequencies, particularly during stereotyped behaviour.

There is also some disagreement between authors concerning the significance they attribute to the EEG abnormalities. Creak and Pampiglione (1969) found considerable variation in the EEGs of their series of children, but felt that the different patterns could not be used to predict clinical outcome. Ritvo, Ornitz, Walter, and Hanley (1970), Gubbay, Lobascher, and Kingerlee (1970), and Small (1975) on the other hand, reported that EEG abnormalities were associated with evidence of brain damage and more severe degrees of intellectual impairment, and thus with a poorer prognosis.

Specialized neurophysiological techniques
Ornitz and his co-workers have carried out all-night sleep recordings of the EEG in children with early childhood psychosis (Ornitz, Ritvo & Walter, 1965a, b; Ornitz et al., 1968). No special features were found in length of sleep, REM and non-REM periods. In one study (Ornitz et al., 1969) inactive wave forms were identified in some of the younger children.

This group of workers have described abnormalities in the inhibition of sensory evoked responses during REM sleep, which have added support to their hypothesis of an imbalance in central mechanisms of vestibular regulation of sensori-motor integration (Ornitz et al., 1968; Ornitz, 1970). Young children diagnosed as autistic on the criteria used by this group (Ornitz & Ritvo, 1976) (which would tend to select those with early childhood psychosis, not just typical autism, and those towards the lower rather than the upper end of the scale of severity of impairments) showed increased auditory evoked response amplitude during REM sleep, while normal controls showed a reduction in amplitude. Ornitz and Forsythe (1973) also showed that continuous vestibular stimulation produced significant increases in the duration and organization of REM bursts in autistic children. In another study, Ornitz et al. (1972) found few differences between autistic and normal children in other aspects of auditory evoked response functions.

Small, DeMyer, and Kendell (1969) and Small (1971), studying visual evoked responses in waking autistic and normal children, reported lower ampli-tudes, shorter latencies and more variability in the former, although they failed to show significant differences in auditory evoked responses.

In summary, data from evoked potentials recorded during waking and sleep periods indicate that autistic children show abnormalities in neurophysiological responsiveness both to internal regulatory mechanisms and to external stimuli. Quantitative EEG analyses suggest that spontaneous waking EEG activity in children with autism and related conditions is neither as variable nor as differentiated as in normal controls (Small, 1971).

32
Psychological assessment of early childhood psychoses

JUDITH GOULD

Psychological testing: uses and problems

There are two separate but equally important aspects to the assessment of cognitive skills in children with early childhood psychosis. The first is the measurement of level of over-all intelligence, which allows comparison with the norms for children of the same chronological age. The second is the detailed analysis of each child's specific impairments and skills.

Intelligence quotients (IQs) in handicapped children have to be assessed using the same standardized tests as those available for normal children (see below). The value of an IQ for a child with early childhood psychosis is limited, but it is a guide to educational placement. If he obtains a low total score on a test of intellectual function, he will need some form of special education. IQ is also an important indication of eventual outcome – the lower the IQ, the worse the prognosis.

Rutter (1970), in a follow-up of autistic children into adolescence and adult life, found that the fluctuations in IQ over time were about the same size in autistic children as they are in normal children. DeMyer and colleagues (1974) also came to the conclusion that the stability of IQ in autistic children was very similar to that found in the normal population. Studies relating to the predictive value of IQ tests in autistic children have been summarized and discussed by Carr (1976).

Standardized tests have the advantage that they

avoid the possible subjective biases in judgements of a child's ability based on informal observations (Warren, 1977). However, there are problems in using them with intellectually impaired children (Freeman, 1978). The tests are constructed on the assumption that abilities are normally distributed. The intelligence quotient is calculated from the degree of deviation from the average score for the relevant chronological age. None of the available tests has included mentally retarded children in the normative samples, so if a child's score falls well outside the expected range, his IQ has to be calculated by extrapolation.

An even more serious disadvantage arises from the use of a single numerical index to give an indication of a child's general intellectual functioning. This is an over-simplification even when applied to normal children (Sigel, 1963; Anastasi, 1968; Butcher, 1968; Sattler, 1974) but is a gross distortion of the true picture in a child with early childhood psychosis (Gould, 1976). Characteristically, in such children, there are very marked discrepancies between levels of development of different types of skills, the scores on visuo-spatial tasks tending to be considerably higher than those on tests requiring language comprehension and abstract thought. An intelligence quotient based on an average of all subtests obscures both the peaks and the troughs of performances.

Detailed analysis of the pattern of skills and handicaps is essential for planning a programme of education and management of behaviour problems. Psychological tests, combined with information from people who know the child well, and observation of his behaviour in his own familiar environment, are used for this type of assessment. Here the aim is not to derive a single quotient, but to examine function on different tests and subtests. Haywood (1977) discussed the alternatives to normative assessments, and the value of comparison between different aspects of a child's abilities, and measurement of progress by comparing results obtained at different times.

Administration of tests

Kanner and Lesser (1958) felt that, because of the children's lack of co-operation, the results of intellectual testing of autistic children were too unreliable to be of any use. As mentioned above, other workers (Rutter, 1970; DeMyer *et al.*, 1974; Lotter, 1974) have found that estimates of intelligence are reasonably stable over time in autism and other early childhood psychoses. Experimental work has shown

that such children are not deliberately uncooperative or negative if given appropriate types of tests (Alpern, 1967; Freeman, 1976; Clark & Rutter, 1977). Anecdotal accounts of large changes in intelligence over time in individual children may well be due to the use of unsuitable methods of assessment, or the comparison of the estimates of IQ derived from tests of different aspects of function. This emphasizes the importance of specifying the exact tests used in assessment, whether for an individual child or in reports of research work (Gould, 1977).

Reliable results can be obtained if tests are chosen and administered with care by a worker experienced in this field. The tester should obtain some information from the parent or teacher concerning the child's level of function in everyday activities, so that the assessment can begin with tests that are well within the child's capacity. These are likely to be simple fitting or assembly tasks. Children with early childhood psychoses often react badly to failure (Churchill, 1971), so it is important to make sure they achieve success at the outset of the assessment. Prior knowledge, also obtained from an informant, of the child's likes and dislikes is useful, in case rewards are needed to encourage him to perform.

Successful testing also depends upon detailed understanding of the impairments underlying the early childhood psychoses. Within the limits imposed by the necessity to present the tests in a standardized way, great care is needed to make sure that the child understands the instructions to the best of his ability.

The most suitable environment for testing is a quiet room, with comfortable and appropriately sized table and chairs, without too many visual distractions, where the child and the tester can be alone and undisturbed. However, if the child is too anxious to co-operate when separated from his mother or some other familiar person, it is necessary to compromise and ask her to be present, but as unobtrusively as possible.

It is preferable for the tester to sit beside and not opposite the child. Problems of imitating other people's movements or copying constructions are common, and are made worse if directions have to be reversed, as would be the case if the tester faces the child.

Perhaps the greatest advantage conferred by experience is the ability to know when to insist that the child tries to perform and when to cease to apply pressure and move on to another task.

Methods of assessment

In the rest of this chapter, methods of measuring IQ and of analysing patterns of impairments and skills will be considered for three different age-groups – the pre-school years (under 5), school age (5 to 14), and the school leaving period (15 to 19). When choosing tests for children with early childhood psychoses, the approximate mental age rather than the chronological age is the best guide. It is not, strictly speaking, good psychological practice to assess a twelve-year-old child using a test battery designed for normal children up to age six. But, if the twelve-year-old's skills are around the level of a normal two- to three-year-old, it is necessary to use methods suitable for the younger age group, and to make this clear in the report. In this situation, the calculation of a mental age is more appropriate than an intelligence quotient, but all such indices must be regarded as, at best, very rough approximations.

The aspects of function to be examined include gross motor skills, self-care, practical and domestic skills, visuo-spatial abilities, comprehension and use of verbal and non-verbal language, the development of symbolic, imaginative activities, the level of understanding of the rules governing social behaviour, and the quality of social interaction (see chapter 29). Formal tests are available for only some of these skills, and some tests cover only a limited age range.

Below five years old

General level of intelligence. Cognitive assessment of young children with various forms of language delay was discussed by Berger and Yule (1972). The batteries used for the early stages of child development emphasise motor and visuo-spatial rather than language skills. Children with autism and early childhood psychoses may score rather better on these scales than on the more language-dependent tests used at later ages. This should be taken into account in evaluating the results.

For very young or very retarded children, the Bayley Infant Scales of Mental and Motor Development (Francis-Williams & Yule, 1967; Bayley, 1969), which give separate mental and motor quotients, can be used. These were standardized on infants aged 1 month to 2 years 6 months.

The most widely used test designed for the young child is the Merrill-Palmer Scale of Mental Tests (Stutsman, 1931). It was developed for the age range 2 years to 5 years 3 months, but it can be used for handicapped children with mental ages between 1

year 6 months and 5 years 11 months. As the majority of items involve fitting and assembly tasks, the scale is especially useful for children with severe language problems. The attractive, brightly coloured materials and the emphasis on simple visuo-spatial skills greatly increase the probability that such children will enjoy the tests and co-operate with the tester. However, the danger of overestimating a child's abilities is particularly marked with this scale.

The brighter pre-school children can be assessed using the Wechsler Pre-School and Primary Scale of Intelligence (WPPSI) (1967) which covers the age-range 4 years to 6 years 6 months. The WPPSI has now been standardized on a British sample of children and various modifications made (Yule *et al.*, 1969). The structure of the test is like that of the WISC, to be discussed in the section on tests for school-age.

The Vineland Social Maturity Scale (Doll, 1953) allows a social age and a social quotient to be calculated. The latter should not be regarded as identical to an intelligence quotient, but does give a useful indication of the child's level of competence in everyday life.

The Vineland Scale is not a psychological test performed by the child, but an assessment based on information obtained by interview with someone who knows the child well. It was developed and standardized for use with mentally handicapped people, and covers the age-range 3 months to 30 years. It can be completed for any child, however retarded, or however uncooperative. It can be most useful in assessing children with early childhood psychosis, though it does have a number of limitations (Shakespeare, 1970; Gould, 1977).

Analysis of impairments and skills. Gross motor skills up to the 2 years 6 months level can be assessed by using the Motor Development Scale of the Bayley test.

The Vineland Scale, described above, can be used to examine development of self-care, practical, domestic and occupational skills, and level of independence from supervision by others. The Gunzburg Progress Assessment Chart of Social and Personal Development (Gunzburg, 1974) is also a measure of practical competence. A chart is filled in by an informant who knows the child, and gives a pictorial indication of levels reached in self-care, communication, socialization, and occupation. No normative data are available, so the chart can be used only to show the progress of an individual child by comparison with his past levels.

Ability with visuo-spatial skills can be estimated from the child's performance on the relevant subtests of the Bayley, Merrill-Palmer or WPPSI scales.

Assessment of language development and language abnormalities is a most important aspect of the analysis of impairments in early childhood psychosis, and should cover comprehension and use of non-verbal communication as well as speech.

Some tests are available for comprehension and use of speech, though they are far from satisfactory when used in early childhood psychosis. The Peabody Picture Vocabulary test (Dunn, 1959), which was standardized on subjects aged 2½ to 18 years, and the English Picture Vocabulary test (Brimer & Dunn, 1966), which consists of 2 tests, one for age-range 5 years to 8 years 11 months and one for 7 years to 11 years 11 months, can be used. There is also a pre-school supplement to the latter for age-range 3 years to 4 years 11 months. These tests give an indication of the number of words understood by a child, though not the size of his spoken vocabulary or his ability to use grammar. Autistic children and those with other early childhood psychoses may have quite large receptive or expressive vocabularies but little or no ability to use these words to form appropriate phrases or sentences, so these tests are of limited value.

The Reynell Developmental Language Scales (Reynell, 1977) aim to measure receptive language, that is, the process of interpreting what is heard, and expressive language, the ability to express ideas in words. The scales were standardized with English children and cover the ages 1 year 6 months to 7 years. They are considerably more useful, in early childhood psychosis, than the vocabulary tests, but do not provide a measure of the limited scope, repetitiveness, and pedantic quality that characterize the speech of such children, even if they have the ability to form grammatical sentences (Gould, 1976).

There are, to date, no standardized tests of non-verbal communication. The child's ability to understand and use vocal intonation, facial expression, bodily movement, gesture and mime has to be estimated by questioning an informant who knows the child well, and by direct observation, especially in a group with both children and adults. The structured interview schedule for rating the handicaps, behaviour, and skills of retarded or psychotic children (the HBS schedule), described by Wing and Gould (1978) can be used in order to obtain and record this information systematically. In the absence of detailed description of developmental norms, comparison with other children of similar mental age is necessary.

Absence or marked limitation of the development of imaginative activities is typical of autism and other early childhood psychoses (Ricks & Wing, 1975; Wing, Gould, Yeates & Brierley, 1977). Pretend play in normal children is considered to be the outward manifestation of imagination and the ability to manipulate abstract ideas (Sheridan, 1969; Piaget, 1972; Lowe, 1975). Much can be learned by observation of a child's spontaneous play, especially concerning the degree to which he co-operates with other children and joins with others in games involving imagination and pretence. Lowe and Costello (1976) have developed a test of young children's ability to play creatively with a set of minature objects including table and chair, cups and saucers, dolls, tractors, and so on. The test has been standardized on normal children and a symbolic play age can be obtained. The age-range covered is 12 to 36 months. Many children with early childhood psychosis fail to score at all on the test because they do not recognize what the miniatures represent. Those who do grasp the concepts necessary for recognizing the nature of the toys will demonstrate their practical uses, such as laying the table with crockery and cutlery, or sitting the man on the tractor seat, but, unlike normal children, will not devise little games with, and stories about, the dolls and the objects. In some of the brighter autistic and similar children, the score on the Reynell comprehension and expression scales is considerably higher than on the symbolic play test.

The quality of social interaction, that is, the child's desire to communicate and ability to take part in a two-way social interchange, in speech, gesture, or play, can be assessed only by observation and questioning an informant. As with non-verbal communication, the HBS schedule can be used to provide a framework for eliciting and recording information.

The last three aspects of development mentioned above, namely non-verbal communication, imaginative play, and quality of social interaction, are of crucial importance in the diagnosis of early childhood autism, and other early childhood psychoses, and differentiating them from other disorders affecting language (Wing, L., 1969; 1979a; Rutter, Bartak & Newman, 1971; Ricks & Wing, 1975).

Five to fourteen years
General level of intelligence. Many children with early childhood psychosis who are chronologically of school age function at a much lower level, at least in

some areas. The test batteries mentioned in the previous section have to be used in these circumstances.

For children who are sufficiently advanced in intellectual development, the Wechsler Intelligence Scale for Children (WISC) (Wechsler, 1949, 1974) is appropriate. This was standardized on an American sample of normal children and covers the age-range 6 years 6 months to 16 years 6 months. A 'verbal' and a 'performance', as well as a 'full scale' IQ can be calculated (see below).

The Stanford-Binet Intelligence Scale exists in various modifications. It covers the age-range 2 years to superior adult level, and has, in the past, been widely used for educational assessment. It is not to be recommended for children with early childhood psychosis because so many of the items require a high level of skill with language (Berger, 1970; Berger & Yule, 1972).

Analysis of impairments and skills. Gross motor skills can be assessed with the Lincoln–Oseretsky Motor Development Scale (Sloan, 1955). The age-range covered is 6 to 14 years.

The Vineland Scale can be used to record self-care and other practical everyday skills, as with the pre-school age group.

For children whose visuo-spatial skills have developed beyond the ceiling of the Merrill-Palmer scale, the WISC can be used to assess performance. The ten subtests in this battery are divided into five needing verbal comprehension and expression (the verbal scale) and five requiring visuo-spatial and motor skills, but no verbal expression (the performance scale). The problem is that three of the latter items involve the ability to understand abstract concepts, even though the child does not have to speak (Gould, 1976). They are not therefore truly language-independent, as are many of the Merrill-Palmer subtests. Characteristically, classically autistic children do well on the two tasks which can be completed using visuo-spatial skills only, that is 'block design' and 'object assembly', but do poorly on the other performance items such as 'picture arrangement' or 'coding' that require symbolic reasoning (Rutter 1968; Lockyer & Rutter, 1969; Tymchuk, Simmons & Neafsey, 1977).

The Columbia Mental Maturity Scale (3 years to 10 years) (Burgemeister, Hollander, Blum & Lorge, 1972) and the Leiter International Performance Scale (2 years to 18 years) (Leiter, 1952) were both designed to assess children with sensory or motor deficits, or who have difficulty in speaking and reading. They

both give an overall IQ, but their main use with children with early childhood psychosis is to show which types of concepts the child is able to understand and manipulate, and which are beyond his grasp. The tests examine, for example, concepts of shape, colour, number, and age as shown in human beings.

Various aspects of language development can be examined with the Illinois Test of Psycholinguistic Abilities (Kirk, McCarthy & Kirk, 1968; Paraskevopoulos & Kirk, 1969). This covers the age-range 2 years to 10 years. There are many problems in using the test in early childhood psychosis (Gould, 1976), but it can be helpful for those children who have sufficient use and understanding of speech to be able to co-operate.

Tubbs (1966) used the test to compare children with early childhood psychosis, normal children, and children who were severely retarded without psychotic behaviour. She found that the psychotic children were particularly poor in the tests requiring the expression of ideas in speech and, even more markedly, in gesture.

They were also impaired in transferring information across modalities, for example from a visual input to a spoken output. Other workers who have investigated and analysed different aspects of language development in autism and related conditions include Cunningham (1968), Churchill (1972, 1978), Ricks and Wing (1975), Boucher (1976), Cantwell, Howlin and Rutter (1977), and Pierce and Bartolucci (1977).

There are no formal tests of symbolic play for this age-range. This aspect of development, together with non-verbal communication and quality of social interaction, has to be assessed by interviews with informants and by observation.

Fifteen years and over

At this stage the aim of assessment changes. The major concerns are now vocational guidance, training in social and occupational skills, and the planning of suitable living arrangements, work and leisure activities in adult life. Over-all IQ becomes less relevant and specific skills comparatively more important.

Formal methods of testing are of little value for adolescents and adults who are handicapped by early childhood psychosis. The Wechsler Adult Intelligence Scale (WAIS) (Wechsler, 1955) is beyond the capacity of the great majority of such people. The only standardized method that remains generally applicable is the Vineland Social Maturity Scale.

A full assessment has to be made from the past history, results of past testing, and details of present performance in self-care and practical and social skills.

Following up the children into early adult life, the author has observed that, after a relatively stable period in later childhood, behaviour may become more difficult in adolescence, especially in the more severely handicapped group. The young person may become uncooperative and disinclined to use the skills he does possess. Attempts at testing during this stage can give a misleadingly low score, and pressure to perform can make behaviour problems worse. In this situation, knowledge of the child's past history of handicaps and skills is particularly important. From the evidence available so far it appears that improvement is likely after a varying period of time, and skills can then be used effectively.

Future developments

Early childhood psychosis, including classic autism, can occur in association with any level of intelligence as measured on formal tests. A low overall IQ because of severe language impairment does mean that the child will be unable to achieve independence as an adult, however good his non-language dependent skills. But it is important to identify and measure any potential the child might have so that he can develop as many useful skills as possible. Behaviour problems and the language impairments may combine to make identification of any abilities very difficult.

All the tests mentioned in this chapter have a place in assessing children with early childhood psychosis, but none was designed with the particular needs of this group in mind. Some authors have devised special methods of investigation specific to autism and related conditions. The work of Frith, Hermelin, and O'Connor is discussed in chapter 35. Churchill (1972, 1978) and Taylor (1976) have designed special non-verbal languages for studying and assessing language development in autistic and other language impaired children.

As mentioned above, the problem of reciprocal social interaction, leading to social naivety, is a handicap found in even the most able child with autism or a related condition. It is even more obvious in adult life, and causes much unhappiness for those who achieve a degree of insight into their problems. A method of analysing the nature and measuring the severity of this aspect of the problem might help in devising ways of alleviating the impairment.

33
Outcome and prognosis of early childhood psychoses

I. KOLVIN

Most work on prognosis has been carried out on children with typical or fairly typical early childhood autism. However, such evidence as is available suggests that the findings apply to the wider group of all children with psychosis of early onset.

Outcome

The clinical picture of childhood autism tends to vary with the age of the child and his stage of development. For instance, in early infancy, a characteristic feature is a failure to cuddle, whereas, in the toddler, profound social aloofness and avoidance of gaze are particularly marked. This is the peak period for the more florid symptoms of the disorder, which then slowly but irregularly decline over the next five years, although most older children retain their difficulties in interpersonal relationships, particularly outside the home. Thus, while the family often report that the child is now affectionate, this may not be substantiated in other environments. This is probably because the adults not in regular contact with the child are unaccustomed to interpreting his communications, or making allowance for his behaviour. Also important in this context is the inability of the older autistic children to appreciate the nuances in social relationships, or to understand other people's feelings. Often there is a desire for close friendships, but the lack of social skills and appropriate empathy make these impossible.

While other symptoms may diminish or even

disappear with increasing age, it is not uncommon for stereotyped behaviour and more complex repetitive routines not only to persist, but to expand.

When the child attends school, the educational difficulties become most evident. Lack of interest in learning and lack of initiative are then very marked. Some of the children are inactive and inert, while others show an aimless restlessness.

In spite of modern methods of treatment, the outcome in adolescence and adulthood is mostly poor in terms of intellectual development, over-all adjustment and work potential. Irrespective of whether the sample is drawn from a clinic or is epidemiologically based, the picture of the outcome is roughly the same (Rutter, Greenfeld & Lockyer, 1967; DeMyer et al., 1973; Kanner, 1971; Lotter, 1974). While two out of three autistic children remain severely handicapped, one out of four does moderately well, with some continuing social and relational problems. Only about one child in ten (Kanner, 1971) develops sufficiently in intellect and social adjustment to be able to survive in an unsheltered work situation (Rutter, 1970; DeMyer et al., 1973). Even those few who become independent in adult life usually show continuing difficulties of relationships and oddities of personality.

Factors related to prognosis

Because improvement is not uniform, it is important to identify indicators of likely outcome, in order to help clinicians when counselling parents and planning management. A summary of prognostic factors found in a follow-up study of 59 children was given by Rees and Taylor (1975).

Level of intelligence

The most important prognostic factor is the testable level of intelligence (Rutter, Greenfeld & Lockyer, 1967; Lockyer & Rutter, 1969). For purposes of prognosis the position can be over-simplified, with outcome being envisaged as closely tied to the degree of associated subnormality. For instance, DeMyer and colleagues (1973) have demonstrated that children remain in the same academic or work category to which they were initially assigned, rather than improving with time. However, while the mean IQ remains stable, these workers found that autistic children who were rated as having the best potential at initial assessment showed considerable gains in verbal IQ with the passage of time. As a rough guide, those within the lowest intelligence band (IQ below 50), constituting about 40 per cent of the autistic

population, will make a major contribution to those who remain severely handicapped; the next band (with an IQ ranging from 50 to 70), constituting about 30 per cent of the autistic population, contains a high proportion of those who make moderate progress, and the highest band (with an IQ above 70), constituting again about 30 per cent of the autistic population, comprises the majority of those who improve most. In the course of time some movement does occur between bands, but upward change is unusual and tends to be confined to adjacent bands. Such studies offer little support for the idea that all autistic children have latent intelligence, a belief which has prevented even experienced psychologists committing themselves about a psychotic child's intellectual potential (Kolvin, Humphrey & McNay, 1971). Careful psychometric assessment by an experienced child psychologist, therefore, is of major importance when considering prognosis (see chapter 32).

Organic factors

Inter-related with these cognitive factors are organic abnormalities – about one in two autistic children has demonstrable brain damage and the level of IQ is likely to be related to the severity or cumulative evidence of damage (Kolvin, Humphrey & McNay, 1971). For instance, it has been found that one in four autistic children develops fits in adolescence and these are highly related to the level of intelligence (Rutter, 1970) (see chapter 31).

Language and communication

Language and communication are important in assessing prognosis. It is well known that a better outcome is associated with the development of useful speech by the age of five years, but about one in two does not achieve this. The more communicative the child, or the better developed the speech or language at initial assessment, and the more constructive or symbolic the play (which reflects inner language), the better the development of conversational speech later (DeMyer et al., 1973). Mutism indicates a particularly poor prognosis. However, even where speech improves considerably, there are often residual difficulties with speech rhythm, repetitiveness, and abstract concepts (Rutter, Greenfeld & Lockyer, 1967; DeMyer et al., 1973).

Severity

Prognosis is also associated with the severity of the clinical picture (DeMyer et al., 1973) and a slow rate of losing the more florid autistic symptoms (Kolvin, 1972). If substantial improvement is to occur it will usually show itself by the age of seven years (Rutter, 1967).

Effects of treatment

The effects of treatment in relation to IQ have been studied by DeMyer and colleagues (1974). While treated children with initial IQs above 50 showed a greater increase in intelligence than untreated autistic children in the same IQ range, those with IQs below 40 showed no differential effect. Furthermore, after treatment, the gains in verbal IQ achieved during treatment tended to be maintained in the autistic children with high initial levels, but stagnated in the middle groups or were even lost in those in the lower IQ groups. Unfortunately, these researchers do not precisely specify the nature of the treatment and hence the value of these important findings cannot be adequately assessed.

Bartak and Rutter (1973) and Rutter and Bartak (1973) investigated the effects on autistic children of different educational approaches. They found improvements over the course of three years in speech and schoolwork skills. The greatest gains were made by children with IQ above 50, although those with IQ below that level did rather better in a school with a structured and organized routine. No information is yet available on the outcome in adult life for the children in this study. Schopler, Brehm, Kinsbourne, and Reichler (1971) also emphasized the importance of structured education.

Lovaas, Koegel, Simmons, and Long (1973) reported that behaviour modification produced improvement in behaviour and skills in autistic children, but regression to initial levels occurred if the programmes were not continued. The authors did not differentiate between children of different IQ levels, nor did the follow-up cover a period longer than four years.

Conclusions

The child with a comparatively good prognosis has an IQ in the normal range, little identifiable evidence of cerebral dysfunction, shows development of useful speech and language in the pre-school years, has mild symptomatology which shows rapid improvement, and is given appropriate schooling.

The major determinants of prognosis are the levels of cognitive and social skills. Environmental factors, such as an appropriate level of stimulation at home and at school, a harmonious atmosphere at home (Lotter, 1974), and a structured educational setting, also play a part, but their effects appear to be limited, and become progressively smaller with increasing severity of handicap.

Section 8

CHAPTERS 34–38

Aetiology and pathology

34

Epidemiology of early childhood psychoses

LORNA WING

In most studies of groups of children with early childhood psychoses (Creak, 1963; Mittler, Gillies & Jukes, 1966; Rutter, Greenfield & Lockyer, 1967; Rutter & Lockyer, 1967; Lockyer & Rutter, 1969; Kolvin, 1971; Kanner, 1973; Knobloch & Pasamanick, 1974; DeMyer, 1976), the samples consisted of children referred to certain services. Three large-scale epidemiological studies of early childhood autism have been published (Lotter, 1966, 1967; Brask, 1967, 1972; Wing, Yeates, Brierley & Gould, 1976). These were based on defined geographical areas (Middlesex County, England; Aarhus County, Denmark; and the Camberwell area of London, England, respectively). The authors examined specified groups of children and made their own diagnoses. Brask and Wing attempted to use the definitions previously adopted by Lotter. The main criteria were social aloofness, especially to peers (at least in the early years), repetitive, ritualistic behaviour (excluding those who showed only simple self-directed activities such as hand-flicking, rocking and self-injury), and abnormalities of speech (Lotter, 1966). Children were included as autistic if they showed these problems, whatever the reported age of onset and level of intelligence on psychological tests, and regardless of the presence or absence of identifiable organic aetiology or associated handicaps. Thus the groups covered a wider range than would be included by Kanner (in theory, if not in practice).

Two epidemiological investigations of the

prevalence of all forms of early childhood psychosis, one carried out in Camberwell, London (Wing & Gould, 1979), and one in Aarhus, Denmark (Brask, 1967; 1972) have been reported.

Treffert (1970) surveyed children in contact with specified services in Wisconsin, but he selected only those already diagnosed by the agencies. The overall rate for early childhood autism found by this author was half that reported in the three epidemiological studies mentioned above. Wing and colleagues (1976) studied the reasons why a prevalence rate based on diagnosed cases listed in local authority records in an area of London was only half that found in their epidemiological study of the same area. The discrepancy was due to a combination of the uncertainty of the processes of referral, the lack of any consistent rules for classifying and filing diagnostic groups in the records and simple clerical errors. For this reason, the results to be quoted in this chapter will be based mainly on the three epidemiological surveys of early childhood autism, for which the findings were closely similar.

Age-specific prevalence

The age-specific prevalence for early childhood autism (as defined above) in children aged under 15 years is between 4 and 5 in every 10 000. Approximately 2 of these 4 to 5 children have typical or 'nuclear' autism, closest to Kanner's syndrome. Both Lotter and Wing identified such a group. The criteria they used differed somewhat but they both described the nuclear children as showing relatively more elaborate, complex, repetitive, routines. The remainder were said to have 'non-nuclear' autism.

The Camberwell study of early childhood psychoses (Wing & Gould, 1979) gave a prevalence, for children aged 0–14, of 4.9 per 10 000 for childhood autism, and 16.3 for other early childhood psychoses (defined as discussed in chapter 29); a total of 21.2 per 10 000.

Dividing the children on their quality of social contact, as described in chapter 29, 10.6 per 10 000 were aloof, 5.7 were passive, and 4.9 odd, in social interaction.

Unpublished work by the same authors suggested that, whereas the prevalence of nuclear and non-nuclear autism may be similar in different areas, rates for other forms of early childhood psychosis may be significantly higher in Camberwell than in areas that do not have the same demographic characteristics. The rate for the latter reported for Aarhus (Brask,

1967, 1972) was only 1.7 per 10 000. This dramatic difference was due partly to lack of commonly agreed criteria for diagnosis, but marked social contrasts between the two areas may also have contributed.

At the time of writing, no prevalence studies have been published concerning people with early childhood psychosis who have reached adult life. Differential mortality of the most handicapped groups, especially those with gross organic aetiology, might make the rates lower than in childhood, but nothing is known for certain.

Age of onset

Early childhood psychosis is present from birth or is manifested within the first few years of life. In both the Middlesex and Camberwell studies, 94 per cent of the autistic children were reported to be abnormal before age 3 and in the rest onset between 3 and 5 years of age had been reported. The proportions for other forms of early childhood psychosis were almost the same. Wing and Gould (1979) noted that 47 per cent of the autistic children were said to be abnormal from birth as compared with 77 per cent of those with other early childhood psychoses.

Sex

Kanner (1954) found a ratio of 4 boys to 1 girl in his series of 100 autistic children, and an excess of boys has been consistently reported since then, although the ratios vary, many being lower than Kanner's. Brask for example, found a boy–girl ratio of 1.4 to 1.

Lotter and Brask noted that the excess of boys was more marked among the autistic children with higher IQs. Wing and Gould (see Wing, 1981c) found the same bias in all forms of early childhood psychosis. The cause of these sex differences is not known.

Social class

Kanner emphasized that the great majority of the parents of the children whom he diagnosed as typically autistic had occupations that placed them in Social Class I or II (Kanner, 1954). Other authors have reported a similar significant social class bias, though less marked than in Kanner's series (Creak, 1963; Rimland, 1965; Rutter, 1966; Kolvin, Ounsted, Richardson & Garside, 1971). All these were studies of children referred to services. Ritvo and colleagues (1971) using somewhat different and wider criteria for the diagnosis of autism, did not find any social class bias in the parents of 274 hospitalized children.

Of the epidemiological investigations, Brask was sceptical concerning the social class differences usually reported, but gave no details from her own study. Lotter found 60 per cent of the parents of his nuclear group in the Registrar General's classes I and II compared with 31 per cent of the non-nuclear autistic children.

Wing (1980) on the other hand, found no tendency for parents of either autistic or other children with early childhood psychoses to be of higher social class than those of sociable severely retarded children, or the general population.

Schopler, Andrews, and Strupp (1979) and Wing (1980) found that parents asking for referrals to centres with a special interest in autistic children were more likely to be of higher social class than those whose children were referred to local services. This may explain some of the discrepancies between different studies, but does not account for Lotter's findings. Whatever the position with regard to Kanner's syndrome, there appears to be no particular social class bias for other forms of early childhood psychosis.

Ethnic group

From clinical experience, it is clear that early childhood psychosis can occur in children from a wide variety of ethnic groups.

The three epidemiological studies were carried out in European countries. Lotter (1978) also studied childhood autism in six African countries, and identified nine nuclear and thirteen non-nuclear autistic children. He was unable to use epidemiological methods, but he had the impression that the prevalence was lower than that found in the European studies. He pointed out that six of the twenty-two children (three from each subgroup) were not of indigenous African origin, five being of mixed race and one a West Indian child adopted by an African family.

The reliability of Lotter's impression must remain in doubt, owing to the problems of case-finding in developing countries with few services for handicapped children. In any case, it is difficult to calculate the effect on prevalence of the high infant and child mortality in such countries.

Wing (1979) found evidence of a higher prevalence in Camberwell of early childhood psychoses among children of immigrant parents, the majority of whom were from the Caribbean. The higher rates were most obvious in the aloof subgroup and the results suggested that vulnerability of immigrants and their children to factors such as pre- and post-natal virus infections, including maternal rubella, might account for the findings.

Questions concerning the effects of special problems such as a bilingual home, or a language and social background different from that of the prevailing culture have been raised, but considerably more work, using epidemiological methods, will have to be carried out before they can be answered.

35

Psychological abnormalities in early childhood psychoses

UTA FRITH

More psychological data exist on childhood autism than on any other psychosis in childhood, and hence this account is almost exclusively based on this subgroup.

The psychological studies of autism highlight the general problems of searching for psychological dysfunctions in any developmental disorder. Early psychological theories of autism considered the children's poor performance in school and on many psychological tests to be a secondary consequence of autistic withdrawal. Many studies of cognitive performance in relation to degree of autistic withdrawal have now shown this view to be untenable (Rutter, 1977). Thus the majority of autistic children (about 55 per cent) must be described as severely mentally retarded (IQ below 50), a further 25 per cent as mildly retarded (IQ 50–69), and a small proportion as of normal or above normal intelligence (Wing, L. *et al.*, 1976). In all autistic children, however, regardless of degree of retardation, there are 'disturbances of affective contact', in other words, an impairment of social interaction.

The reverse of the earlier theory was a tempting alternative: social impairment and withdrawal could be considered a consequence of cognitive deficits. Specific cognitive functions were investigated in the hope that functions that differentiated between autistic and other mentally retarded children could be used to explain autistic withdrawal. This theory was also doomed to fail simply by the existence of children who are apparently unimpaired in many of the cognitive functions studied and yet are clearly autistic in the sense of being socially impaired. A third type of theory, less parsimonious, assumes that several functions can be disturbed independently of each other, so that both a cognitive deficit and a social interaction deficit could be crucially involved in explaining behaviour patterns in childhood autism.

Cognition

The studies of cognitive deficits in autistic children, including perception, memory, thinking, and visuo-motor skills are extensive, and can be confusing if no allowance is made for developmental level of the child. Many presumed abnormalities prove to be perfectly adequate behaviour patterns when account is taken of mental age. A low level in any of the functions does not necessarily imply a specific and diagnostically significant problem. A specific problem exists only where the child performs worse than would be expected on the basis of his general level of development.

At the very severely retarded level, massive cognitive impairments are found (Wing & Gould, 1979), while at the non-retarded level there may be none (Wurst, 1976). In both instances, psychotic and control groups are indistinguishable. Between these two extremes, however, very specific cognitive deficits are present that distinguish autistic and non-autistic children and these can explain a significant amount of psychotic behaviour (Rutter, 1979).

Problems of the severely retarded children have received major emphasis, because this subgroup is the largest. Ornitz and Ritvo (1968a,b) have investigated the frequently reported abnormalities in responses to sensory stimuli, described as either hyper- or hypo-responsiveness. They found dysfunction of the vestibular system and showed that there is a general faulty modulation of sensory input, auditory or visual, leading to perceptual inconstancy. This is correlated with motility disturbances (such as hand-flapping, toe-walking, rocking) which these authors consider to be compensatory behaviour that serves the function of obtaining frequent kinesthetic feedback. This type of feedback may be especially important if there is an impairment of visual perception (Ornitz, 1974).

Another explanation of the abnormal responses to stimuli has been suggested by Lovaas and colleagues (1971) who hypothesized that over-selectivity is a basic feature of psychotic behaviour. Thus, for example, if a light and a tone are presented together, the child might respond to the light but not the tone. This applies to all sensory modalities (Reynolds *et al.*, 1974).

It is likely that abnormal vestibular function and abnormal motility patterns are associated with very severe mental retardation and do not distinguish psychotic from non-psychotic children. This may also apply to other abnormalities of sensory perception, including over-selectivity. There is a general inability to process complex stimuli in severely retarded autistic children, just as with other severely retarded children. However, it is important to note that there are exceptions to this rule. Thus, severely retarded autistic children occasionally reach relatively high levels in some cognitive skills, which would not be expected from their performance in other areas. A case in point is exceptional musical talent that has frequently been reported anecdotally, and the exceptional drawing ability documented in a severely retarded autistic girl (Selfe, 1977). Exceptions of this kind are discussed by Park (1978). The existence of these cases indicates that complex visual and auditory discrimination, memory, and visuo-motor skills, in certain areas at least, can be unimpaired in an otherwise very impaired child. This is also relevant to the observation of graceful spontaneous motor movements in autistic children and their high skill at fitting and assembly tasks. Precise movement programmes are usually not within reach of non-psychotic retarded children. While 'islets of intelligence' can occur also in non-autistic retarded people, dissociated functions have probably been noted more often in autistic children (DeMyer, 1976) than in other children. Such findings emphasize that a distinction should be made between specific cognitive deficits due to specific neurological abnormality and general deficit due to any kind of neurological dysfunction (O'Connor & Hermelin, 1971; O'Connor, 1973).

Investigations of cognitive skills in the less severely retarded autistic child have shown that a specific deficit in perceptual processing exists (Hermelin & O'Connor, 1970). It can legitimately be referred to as 'specific' because it is not found in non-autistic children with comparable degrees of retardation. This deficit is situated at a central, not at a peripheral stage of processing. It can be thought of as an inability to encode stimuli meaningfully. In other words, an autistic child finds it difficult to make sense of what he sees or hears (Hermelin & Frith, 1971).

The extraction of meaning, or more generally, of rules and redundancies in input information is presumed to be a built-in function, improving with development in the normal child. This function was studied in experiments in which children had to remember and reproduce words, sentences, or digits. These stimuli were presented either as a random string or as a structured, that is, redundant, pattern. All children benefited from structure, in that their recall improved. However, the autistic children benefited significantly less. Mildly retarded autistic children could deal with more complex structures than severely retarded ones, but they were less affected by presence or absence of structure than their mental age matched controls.

These experiments also illustrate a dissociation of functions. There were many retarded autistic children with a high capacity for short-term recall. Thus they could reproduce long strings of unstructured material, longer than most retarded children of a comparable developmental level. This memory capacity is very noticeable in the children's echolalic utterances. In the severely retarded autistic children the echoing is remarkably accurate, which is unusual with control children, especially if they are asked to echo nonsense. Findings that confirm these conclusions were obtained by Prior and Chen (1976), Fyffe and Prior (1978), and by Boucher (1978). Long-term recall was studied by Boucher and Warrington (1976) who demonstrated that when information was not immediately available to recall, it could be elicited by appropriate cues.

In contrast to their good rote memory, the autistic children were impaired in their ability to make use of redundancy. This ability enables one to remember meaningful sentences better than nonsense, or words better than strings of letters. One consequence of the normal use of redundancy is marked increase in memory capacity over that for rote memory. Since rote memory capacity of autistic children seems to be superior, one might speculate that they therefore feel less need for making use of redundancy. In any case, there appears to be a problem of extracting rules, or themes, or key features, which are normally used to reconstruct information that cannot be handled because of capacity limitations. Instead of extracting rules, autistic children show a tendency to impose their own rules (Frith, 1970a, b). Furthermore, they adhere strictly and rigidly to these self-imposed rules, which is unusual in other retarded and very young children (Frith, 1972). There may be

a close link between this cognitive dysfunction and the important diagnostic symptoms of stereotypies and routines.

There is thus in the autistic child (regardless of degree of retardation) a specific deficit in the encoding of complex sequential input, whether or not this input is speech. However, the deficit may be even more general and apply also to non-sequential input. This is indicated by studies on the perception of faces (Langdell, 1978). Normally, upright faces are very readily, but inverted faces very poorly, recognized. This is probably due to the integration of all the features into a meaningful whole which becomes meaningless when turned upside down. In autistic children there was no difference in perception between upright and upside-down faces and this would be expected if recognition were based on single details, equally detectable regardless of orientation and of meaningful context. Thus a failure to integrate features into meaningful wholes may be a general characteristic of the input coding deficit. A failure of integration has been suggested by Goldfarb (1961) as the central pathology of childhood schizophrenia (a term used by him to cover all forms of childhood psychosis). Rimland (1965) also postulated that the underlying cognitive dysfunction in infantile autism was an inability to integrate or to relate experiences meaningfully.

Language and communication

Since the presence of language and communication problems is one of the essential features for the diagnosis of early childhood autism, they have been the focus of many theories based on psychological investigations (see Baltaxe & Simmons, 1975, for a review). Language has to be considered as a system of several different but interacting levels. Three levels – phonology, syntax, and semantics – have received much emphasis. However, the fourth level, pragmatics, has often been neglected. Yet it is this level that, in autism, shows severe deficiencies relative to the others, which appear to develop in keeping with each other and may be as low or as high as would be expected from a normal child of a comparable level of development. Pragmatics concerns the use of speech and language in interpersonal communications, encompassing comprehension as well as production. It is easy to confuse semantics and pragmatics. The question that is asked when studying semantics is: what does this utterance mean? and when studying pragmatics: why did this utterance come to be produced?

All investigations of comprehension and use of language and speech in autistic children have revealed serious problems. Many of these can be considered as disorders of language *use* rather than as abnormalities of language processes. This is true of mutism, delayed echolalia, pronoun-reversal, neologisms, metaphorical (idiosyncratic) use of habitual language, habitual thinking aloud, use of 'no' rather than 'yes', inappropriate intonation, and use of stereotyped phrases. These peculiarities appear to be independent of intelligence and are not usually found in any groups other than autistic children. However, there are other examples of language peculiarities reported in retarded autistic children, for example, naming difficulties, reversal of phonemes in words, errors with pronouns (other than reversal) and with function words, abbreviations, and telegrammatic speech, which can all be found at initial stages of normal language development. These are therefore related to a low level of attainment and do not constitute problems specific to autism.

Bloom and Lahey (1978), when defining language disorders in childhood, distinguish between disorders of *form, content,* and *use* and pay special attention to the possible disruption of the interaction between these components of communicative speech. In extreme cases, in characteristically autistic children, there can be a complete dissociation. This manifests itself clearly in stereotypic or echolalic speech without apparent connexion to the context. There may be meaningful content in some echolalic speech, but this may be understood only by those who know the child very well. Thus, for example, a child may say 'be a good boy' when hitting the interviewer (Cunningham, 1968), an expression which was associated with an event in the child's past experience.

A clear dissociation between presence of meaning and lack of communication was shown by Ricks (1975) in autistic children at a pre-verbal level. Ricks studied vocal expressions in situations that involve social interaction (greeting, anticipation, frustration, surprise). Autistic children showed marked abnormalities. Instead of the 'natural' noises that were commonly produced by pre-verbal normal or retarded children and readily understood by any adult listener, he found that the autistic children produced idiosyncratic utterances that only the parents could recognize. The findings could be interpreted in terms of an inborn behaviour pattern that (surprisingly) exists in all normal and many mentally retarded children, but is missing in the psychotic child.

Another pragmatics deficit in pre-verbal children was shown by Curcio (1978). He found that none of the mute autistic children he studied, whatever their level of sensori-motor development, used spontaneous pointing to show objects to adults. Bates (1976) has discussed the importance of early pointing to pragmatic skills and states that these 'protodeclarative' gestures are vital milestones of normal pre-linguistic development. Around the age of 12 months, that is, at a very low level of sensori-motor development, normal children begin to use such gestures that apparently serve no other purpose than to point out something to someone else. Therefore, the absence of such gestures in pre-lingual autistic children of a higher level of sensori-motor development must be considered significant.

Pragmatics deficits are especially clear-cut in the non-retarded autistic child. In an important study of language disorder, Bartak, Rutter and Cox (1975) (see also Bartak *et al.,* 1977; Rutter, 1978) compared dysphasic and autistic boys of normal non-verbal intelligence on a large range of language and communication tasks. The essentially language-less dysphasic children were nevertheless able to communicate. In contrast, the autistic children showed a much lower level of competence with all communicative functions, especially in the use and understanding of gesture.

Performance of autistic children testable on the WISC Verbal Scale has been analysed (Lockyer & Rutter, 1969; Tymchuk *et al.,* 1977; DeMyer, 1976; Rutter, 1979) and the results point to an impairment of language *use* rather than *content* or *form.* The comprehension subtest (consisting of a series of questions such as, 'what do you do if you cut your finger?') consistently shows the lowest scores. In the above example a typical answer given by an autistic child of normal intelligence on standardized tests, was 'bleed' (Wing, 1966). Scores on this test are lower than scores on information ('How many days are there in a week?') or vocabulary ('What is a book?') subtests. This difference can readily be explained by an impairment in pragmatics. In the comprehension subtest one has to understand not only the question (as in the other subtests) but, for a correct answer, one also has to know why it is being asked. Hence the answer 'bleed' is correct semantically, but not pragmatically.

Especially in the more competent and older autistic child, there are noticeable peculiarities of language use. These include literalness, pedantic wording, lack of humour, and narrowness of content (see, for example, Creak, 1972). Baltaxe (1977) has demonstrated pragmatics deficits in autistic adolescents, such as impairment in the speaker–hearer role relationship, in rules governing a dialogue, and in the foregrounding and backgrounding of information. Specific linguistic dysfunctions cannot account for these deficits. The normal speaker is expected to comprehend beyond literal meaning. Knowledge of grammar and referential meaning are not as essential in this respect as are social skills. 'Language' without social context but with complex grammar and meaning is conceivable. Mathematics or music may be examples. It is therefore possible for autistic children to excel in 'languages' not dependent upon social context, provided they possess the necessary cognitive functions for mastering these skills.

Social interaction

The problem that is common to all childhood psychoses is social impairment (Wing, L., 1978). This problem exists at the mildest and most severe degrees of retardation at the youngest as well as at the oldest ages described. Follow-up studies (for a review see Lotter, 1978) confirm that social interaction is abnormal even in the most improved cases of childhood autism. Bartak, Rutter, and Cox (1975) demonstrated that there is a basic failure to develop normal social attachment even in autistic children of normal intelligence, shown by gaze aversion or inappropriate use of eye contact, lack of group play, lack of friends, and disturbed behaviour in social contexts. Many studies have shown that social maturity is poor in autistic children relative to any controls (for example, Bartak & Rutter, 1976).

Nevertheless, the nature of the impairment varies considerably with age, with educational treatment, and with degree of handicap. Wing and Gould (1979) distinguished three forms of impaired social interaction in psychotic children regardless of etiology: namely, *aloof, passive,* and *odd* (see chapter 29). Each of these categories relates to a specific repertoire of cognitive skills. Aloofness is the characteristic form at the lower IQ levels. Odd behaviour (i.e. pestering with idiosyncratic talk) or passivity (not joining voluntarily in group games, but not objecting to involvement if directed by others) are characteristic of the higher levels. These authors showed, in an epidemiological study of a total population of children in one geographical area, that above IQ 70 social impairment is extremely rare, but below IQ 50 it occurs in about half of all the children studied. Since very low IQ can be considered an index of severe brain damage, with increasing extent of damage it is increasingly likely that systems responsible for adequate social functioning are involved in the affected areas. Nevertheless, in half the cases of extensive brain damage, these systems are spared and such children do not show the psychotic behaviour pattern. An important contrast to the psychotic group is Down's syndrome (Wing, L., 1969; 1979) where, with few exceptions, no social impairment is found. The surprising inference is that there must be a brain system for social interaction that is as specific as old theories of instinct would assume. The 'herd instinct', in the layman's sense of the term, probably describes the specific system that is damaged. A biological disturbance of affective contact was of course the main part of Kanner's (1943) first theory of early childhood autism.

Peculiarities that have been described in autistic children in infancy can readily be interpreted as a failure of social interaction patterns: the lack of anticipatory posture, lack of protodeclarative pointing, and idiosyncratic vocalizations in social situations. The development of such patterns in normal children is currently the focus of much research (see Lock, 1978), as is the closely related area of pragmatics (Bates, 1976).

Many observations suggest that, even if the whole system of instinctual social behaviour patterns were missing, the child can still acquire some social skills. With intact intellectual functions there can be considerable compensation, and explicit teaching will improve the ability to handle various social situations. The aspects most resistant to improvement can be deduced from case descriptions of autistic people without intellectual deficit (Asperger, 1944; Kanner *et al.*, 1972). Relationships to peers seem to be most affected, especially courting and mating, to use some other terms from instinct theories. Awkwardness in social situations is always noted as a remnant (Ricks & Wing, 1976). Typical examples are: not following an unspoken code of politeness, 'smugness' resulting from lack of insight into problems of social involvement, poor use and comprehension of mime and gesture. All these examples could readily be seen as pragmatics deficiencies.

An important indicator of social communication skills is eye contact. Kendon (1967) has shown that in normal adult dialogue eye contact is used for very precise functions, but entirely without awareness. For instance, the listening partner will seek eye contact with the speaking partner if he wants to speak. In turn the speaker will look away if he wants to indicate that he still wishes to continue speaking. Eye-gaze avoidance or inappropriately prolonged eye-gaze are well known characteristics of autistic children. They are among the most striking symptoms, probably because the observer normally can rely on their automatic, unconscious, functioning and is perplexed by the dysfunctional use. That eye-gaze has no specific communicative functions in autistic children has been demonstrated by O'Connor and Hermelin (1967). They found that autistic children gazed equally little at objects and faces.

The central importance of social impairment and/or pragmatics deficiencies in childhood autism can be seen especially clearly in biographical accounts. The case of an exceptionally intelligent autistic girl (Park, 1967; Park & Youderian, 1974) shows that sick children can compensate to some extent for their social disabilities, though they rarely overcome them completely. The case of a retarded boy (Lovell, 1978) shows the extraordinary, but typical, pattern of dissociated functions and dysfunctions that makes social interactions unpredictable for the outsider.

Several authors (Wing, L., 1969; Wing *et al.*, 1977; Wing & Gould, 1979; Rutter, 1978) have discussed and provided evidence for the remarkable association between impaired social relationships and lack of imaginative play. It appears that in all retarded autistic children this type of play is absent or very severely impaired. Yet it is found in very young normal, and in most mentally retarded non-psychotic, children provided that the mental age is over 19 months. In view of this critical level which has been held by Piaget (1951) to be the beginning of symbolic functions in normal development, Ricks and Wing (1976) and Hermelin (1978) suggested that there is a deficit in symbolic thought. Some evidence for a deficit in symbolic images is provided by O'Connor and Hermelin's experiments (1978) on coding spatial and temporal stimuli. In these experiments autistic children were compared with children of normal intelligence who had either no vision or no hearing, and with those who had a general cognitive impairment. All three contrast groups were better able to use internalized imagery than autistic children.

However, a social deficit exists already in autistic children at the pre-symbolic level and this deficit alone may prevent the development of imaginative play. Because skills in handling social interactions are apparently innate, one could argue that normal infants relate to toy objects as if they were social objects. The inborn behaviour patterns may be generalized to situations that are not social and give rise to pretend play. Thus psychological motives are attributed not only to other people but also to animals and lifeless objects. The projection of a person into something else is a possible mechanism for this behaviour pattern. Role play can certainly be thought of as projecting one person into another. It is conceivable that a process of projection is true for real social interactions as well as imaginary ones. Given this theory, a single underlying dysfunction in the social instinctual domain would appear to account for the diverse symptoms of social impairment and lack of imaginative play. Due to this dysfunction, psychotic children treat people as objects, while normal children, in play, treat objects as people.

One significant characteristic of autistic children's 'play' is its repetitive nature (Wing, L., 1978). Frith (1972) found that a rigid and repetitive quality distinguished the play products, in this case colour patterns, and tone sequences on a xylophone, of severely retarded autistic children from their severely retarded controls. Similarly, Boucher (1977) found strong perseveration tendencies with autistic children in a different play situation.

Rigid and repetitive behaviour is present in childhood autism by definition. 'Insistence on sameness' is the highly descriptive term used for this symptom. With very severe levels of retardation, simple stereotyped movements can be found, regardless of whether or not there is psychosis. However, at the less severe levels tendencies to stereotyped movements do discriminate psychotic from non-psychotic children. Bartak and Rutter (1976) found that both retarded and normally intelligent autistic children show strong attachments to objects. Both groups generally have great difficulties in adaptation. As one might expect, the more intelligent groups showed more complex routines rather than simple stereotyped movements. It remains to be seen whether insistence on sameness is primary or secondary, being possibly part of cognitive or social dysfunctions. A sound psychological theory of these processes is at present not available.

Summary

Regardless of whether there is a mild or severe degree of mental retardation there are two major psychological dysfunctions in childhood psychosis. First, there is a dysfunction of certain innate social interaction patterns. This abnormality can account for specific social impairments, both verbal and nonverbal communication impairments, and possibly lack of imaginative play. Second, there is a cognitive dysfunction regarding the encoding of stimulus information. The capacity to perceive and to remember unconnected information is better than one would expect at a given level of cognitive development, while the handling of redundant or meaningful structure is worse. In general, there may be a lack of integration of stimulus details into meaningful structures or wholes.

With increased severity of brain damage, a general depression of cognitive functions can be observed. The comparison with appropriate control groups allows one to identify which deficit is simply part of this general depression of functions, and which is specific to psychosis. This distinction (O'Connor, 1977) is essential in delineating subgroups of developmental disorders.

36
The genetics of childhood psychoses

D. R. HANSON
I. I. GOTTESMAN*

Introduction

Establishing whether or not childhood psychoses have an appreciable genetic component in their aetiology presents a difficult challenge to psychiatric geneticists. Childhood psychoses are rare, but, unlike most rare genetic disorders, they do not follow the simple patterns of inheritance. Polygenic models of inheritance are often invoked when 'non-classical' familial clustering suggests genetic aetiology. However, polygenic models are intended for relatively common disorders with general population frequencies of about 1 per cent or more. Virtually no childhood psychotics have children when they grow up, thus hindering pedigree studies and precluding studies of adopted-away offspring of affected individuals. With these limitations in mind, the evidence for and against a genetic contribution to the development of infantile autism and pre-adolescent schizophrenia is reviewed. We will also take a look at the scant literature relating to the genetics of childhood affective psychoses.

Our perspective is guided by modern biological and population genetic theorizing which specifies that genetic traits need not be congenital (witness Huntington's disease), nor need they be continu-

Visiting, Professor, Washington University School of Medicine, 1979. We wish to thank Janet W. Hoffman for secretarial assistance and Professor S.
B. Hoffman for secretarial assistance and Professor S. B. Guze. Preparation of this chapter was aided by a post-doctoral fellowship in behavioral genetics to D. R. H., MH-14647, V. E. Anderson, P. I.

ously present after they are once expressed (witness acute intermittent porphyria), nor does everyone with the same abnormal genotype have the same symptoms (again, AIP) (Gottesman, 1974). Often the expression of a genetic predisposition will be modified by environmental factors. Genetic diseases *are* treatable, sometimes more readily than environmental ones. The fact that genetic theories have mathematical foundations provides the opportunity to make point predictions (Meehl, 1973, 1977, 1978) that allow straightforward confirmation or refutation of ideas about genetic causation.

Patterns of prevalence

Do childhood psychoses occur in relatives of affected individuals more often than in members of the general population? If familial clustering is found, it could be for either genetic or environmental reasons. Genetic influences could be inferred if the distribution of affected cases fitted Mendelian expectations or fitted polygenic models that specify: (1) a clinical range of severity from borderline through severe, (2) severely ill probands have more affected relatives than mildly affected ones, (3) the risks to relatives increase as the number of other affected family members increases, (4) risks drop off sharply as one goes from near relatives (identical twins) to distant ones (cousins), and (5) cases are distributed on both maternal and paternal sides of the family (Falconer, 1965; Curnow and Smith, 1975). Polygenic disorders may be expressed differently, or at different rates in different sexes (Reich *et al.*, 1975; Cloninger *et al.*, 1978). When a disorder occurs more often in males, say, separate population prevalence and familial risk rates should be given for each sex. Unfortunately, this is never done for childhood psychoses even though two to four times as many males are affected.

The difficulties of distinguishing the early childhood psychoses from other mental handicaps and of classifying them into subgroups are discussed in chapter 29. The outcome of evaluating any 'excess' of these psychoses among relatives of affected children will depend upon the diagnostic criteria used, and the rigour with which they are applied (Hanson & Gottesman, 1976).

Families of autistic and schizophrenic-like children

Childhood psychoses tend to begin either in the first two years of life or sometime after the age of

6 or 7 (Rutter, 1974). Onset in the middle years of childhood is exceptionally rare. Furthermore, the symptomatology of the early and late childhood onset groups appears quite different (Hanson & Gottesman, 1976). The notion that there are at least two separate diagnostic groups is supported by the data on the differential prevalences of psychoses in the relatives of childhood psychotics (table 36.1). Children with psychoses that begin in later childhood have parents who have a much higher frequency of adult-type schizophrenia. The sibling rate is also high in Kallmann and Roth's study. Kolvin's sample of later-onset childhood psychosis is too young for the siblings to show adult-type schizophrenia.

Kallman and Roth's (1956) study of pre-adolescent schizophrenics includes 52 pairs of twins in addition to the singleton probands listed in table 36.1. The pairwise concordance rates for pre-adolescent (onset before age 15) schizophrenia are 71 per cent for MZ (monozygotic) and 17 per cent for DZ (dizygotic) twins. Adding 5 additional co-twins who broke down after age 15 increases the MZ and DZ rates to 88 per cent and 17 per cent respectively. The higher concordance rates for MZ v. DZ, plus the high rate of adult schizophrenia in the relatives of the pre-adolescent cases led Kallmann and Roth to the reasonable conclusion that the development of pre-adolescent schizophrenia is influenced by the same genetic factors that predispose to adult onset schizophrenia; the earlier onset was presumed to be due to secondary factors that exacerbate the expression of the predisposition.

Kallmann and Roth's twin data are valuable because they are unique, but they have some puzzling features. There is an excess of same-sex (SS) DZ pairs (SS and opposite-sex [OS] pairs should occur with about equal frequency) as could occur if discordant MZ pairs were mistakenly categorized as DZ. If true, corrected zygosities would decrease MZ concordance rates and reduce the apparent importance of genetic factors. On the other hand, some OS DZ pairs may have been overlooked, making sample evaluation indeterminate (Gottesman & Shields, 1966). Since males are affected more often than females, male-male pairs would have a greater chance of being ascertained.

An additional problem arises from the fact that Kallmann and Roth's survey for pre-adolescent schizophrenics produced 52 pairs of twins but only 50 singletons, unlike the general population ratio of about one pair of twins for every 100 singletons born.

Table 36.1. *Prevalence of selected psychotic conditions in first-degree relatives of children with early- and late-onset psychosis*

Investigator	Age of onset in probands (yrs)	Total number	Parents hospitalized for schizophrenia % affected	Total number	Psychotic sibs % affected
	Early onset				
Kanner (1954)	<2	200	*0*	131	*2.3*
Creak & Ini (1960)	( )[a]	204	*1.7[b]*	234	*0.7*
Meyers & Goldfarb (1962)	<5	84	*2.4[c]*	48	*8.3*
Lotter (1967)	<4½	60	*0[d]*	62	*0[e]*
Rutter & Lockyer (1967)	<5	126	*0*	85	*0[f]*
Kolvin *et al.* (1971)	<3	92	*1.1*	68	*0*
Fish (1977)	<2	70	*5.7*	44	*4.5*
Bender (cited in Fish, 1977)	<2	100	*7.0*	( )	–
	Late onset				
Kallmann & Roth (1956)	7–11	204	*8.9[h]*	234	*7.7*
Kolvin *et al.* (1971)	>5	64	*9.4*	56	*1.8*
Bender (cited in Fish, 1977)	>2	100	*12*	( )[g]	–

[a] Ages not reported but most known to be early onset.

[b] Other psychiatric disorders include one case each: dementia following head injury, anxious depression, anorexia nervosa (schizophrenia?).

[c] Eighteen cases of schizophrenia in 84 parents (21.4 per cent) were reported, but only 2 cases were hospitalized.

[d] Five parents reportedly had been hospitalized for psychiatric care and include 1 case each: recurrent depression, reactive depression, amphetamine psychosis, possible paranoid psychopath, no diagnosis available.

[e] In addition there were reported 1 case of 'depressive psychosis' with IQ = 56, 1 case 'very autistic-like' with IQ = 65, and 1 case with severe personality disorder, possible retardation, but friendly.

[f] Plus 1 questionable case of 'autism'; at age 9 was described as 'somewhat unusual' but 'appeared quite normal and certainly could not be termed psychotic'.

[g] Bender's sibling data were not subdivided by age of onset in proband. Among the 87 siblings of early- plus late-onset probands, 13.8 per cent were diagnosed schizophrenic.

[h] Ten additional cases of 'uncertain schizophrenia' were also reported.

It has been argued that twins are more susceptible to developing schizophrenia, but this is not the case for adult onset schizophrenia (Rosenthal, 1960; Gottesman & Shields, 1972). Twins *are* more at risk for brain injury and severe mental retardation. About 2 per cent of the general population surviving infancy are twins, but more than 3 per cent of institutionalized retardates are twins (Allen & Kallmann, 1962) – a 50 per cent excess. Brain damage may contribute to the early release of schizophrenia and may account, in part,

for the uneven sex ratio. (Males are more susceptible to the effects of birth and pregnancy complications.) Additionally or alternatively, some of the twins called schizophrenic may have been symptomatic cases of various brain syndromes (see Davison & Bagley, 1969; Shaffer, 1977a).

It seems that some late-onset childhood psychoses are genetically related to adult schizophrenia and represent instances where adult-type schizophrenia begins at an unusually early age. Better measures of affected individuals' developmental ages at breakdown are needed in future research to determine whether these cases represent psychoses in late childhood or psychoses in early adolescence, biologically defined. In the meantime our conclusion about the biological homogeneity of schizophrenic-like psychoses in late childhood and adult schizophrenia should be viewed as a challenge to future researchers, not as an established fact.

Turning to the early onset childhood psychoses, we see, with the exception of Bender's and Fish's data, no evidence to link adult schizophrenia with these disorders. Excluding Bender's and Fish's data, for the moment, there is a 0.5 per cent rate of hospitalizable schizophrenia in parents and a 1.5 per cent rate of schizophrenia or schizophrenic-like psychoses in siblings. These values are not significantly different from general population risks for adult schizophrenia; this suggests that early-onset psychoses are not genetically homogeneous with adult schizophrenia.

Fish (1977, 1979), on the basis of her own data and those of Bender, has come to the opposite conclusion. She suggests that different diagnostic criteria for selecting probands led to the discrepant results. She (and Bender) excluded most cases with organic involvement, whereas, she claims, the other investigators' samples contained large proportions of children with organic psychoses. These organic cases would not be of genetic origin and would not be associated with family histories of mental illness. Extending this line of reasoning, we would infer that the other investigators' samples contained almost exclusively organic psychoses; otherwise, the rate of schizophrenia in parents should be above the population base rate. It seems unlikely that the other investigators would systematically exclude cases of early childhood psychoses that were related to adult schizophrenia, so we are left with the conclusion that the vast majority of early childhood psychoses do not share a common aetiology with adult schizophrenia. Bender's and Fish's data require us to withhold final judgement until a cross-national study of family history variables as a function of diagnostic styles provides a resolution of the variation.

Claiming that the majority of early-onset childhood psychoses are genetically different from adult schizophrenia does not preclude other genetic effects. If genetic factors are important, they are not inherited in a simple Mendelian pattern. Consanguinity rates do not appear elevated (Creak & Ini, 1960) as

they are for rare recessive disorders. No biochemical abnormalities suggestive of an inborn error of metabolism have been found (Guthrie & Wyatt, 1975; Ritvo, 1977). If there is a single biochemical abnormality in most such children, it would set a medical precedent. There are no known inborn errors of metabolism that produce such severe psychopathology in children without causing a wide range of other symptoms (cf. Lesch-Nyhan syndrome, Seegmiller, 1972).

Chromosomal abnormalities are not expected, because these children do not show the multiple physical and biochemical abnormalities associated with cytogenetic errors and because maternal age is not increased (Creak & Ini, 1960; Lotter, 1967; Treffert, 1970) as it often is with chromosomal errors such as Down's syndrome. Not surprisingly, no cytogenetic errors have been found (Böök, Nichtern & Gruenberg, 1963; Bender & Sankar, 1968; Judd & Mandel, 1968; Wolraich, Bjostek, Neu & Gardner, 1970).

Two other genetic possibilities deserve consideration – rare mutations and polygenic inheritance. If new mutations were the cause of autism and other early childhood psychoses, we would expect parents and siblings to be unaffected. Fraternal twins should always be discordant, identical twins should always be concordant, and 50 per cent of the children of affected individuals would also be affected. Boys and girls should be affected with equal frequency. As we will see below, the identical twin concordance rate is far from 100 per cent. This fact, combined with the very unequal sex ratio, unseats a simple dominant mutation theory. It is possible that the expression of a dominant gene might be modified by environmental or other genetic (including sex) factors which leads to consideration of multifactorial polygenic transmission.

If a polygenic disorder results in a genetic lethal (i.e., the condition results in virtually no offspring being born to affected individuals), we would expect parents of affected children to be free of the disorder though there may be something distinctive about them because they possess a subthreshold 'dose' of the deleterious genes. Siblings, including DZ twins, however, should have an increased risk, and the risk to MZ twins should be even higher. As we have seen, most studies report only population base rates of psychoses among the parents of early onset psychotic children; no one has, for example, reported classic autism in the parent of an autistic child, though Van

Krevelen (1971) has described Asperger's syndrome, a condition that may be related to autism (see chapter 29), in the father of a typically autistic child. The early and often cited claims that most parents of early onset psychotics are 'emotional refrigerators' or have other forms of deviant personalities could not be replicated (Creak & Ini, 1960; Kolvin, Garside & Kidd, 1971; Cox, Rutter, Newman & Bartak, 1975; Wing, L., 1976). These recent studies indicate that the vast majority of the parents are quite normal. When parents of psychotic children do exhibit an unusual trait, it may well be in response to their child's abnormality (Hirsch & Leff, 1975; Schopler & Loftin, 1969a,b). We find no convincing evidence from parent data to support a polygenic hypothesis.

Seven studies report ten cases of psychoses among 574 (1.7 per cent) siblings of early-onset child psychotics. In no study were the diagnoses of the secondary cases confirmed by independent diagnosticians nor were standard diagnostic schemes used nor are case histories given – a reflection of the state of the art when these projects were completed. Thus we find no adequately documented (by current standards) cases of infantile autism among the siblings of autistic children, though some of these siblings do appear to have major behavioural disturbances. We would expect, by chance, that about 2–5 per cent of the sibs would have some form of severe psychopathology such as mental retardation, personality disorder, hyperactivity, etc. Counting all ten cases of possible psychoses among the siblings does suggest familial clustering compatible with polygenic theorizing. However, not all of these ten cases are autistic, and we would have to consider this 1.7 per cent rate to be an inflated upper limit.

The last line of genetic evidence comes from twin studies. The numerous single case reports of twins affected with autism have been reviewed by Rutter (1967), and Hanson and Gottesman (1976). Collections of such single case studies are unsuitable for genetic analysis because of strong reporting biases favoring MZ cases, especially concordant pairs. This seems to be true for autistic twins; about 14 pairs of MZ v. only about 4 DZ pairs have been recorded. We expect general population rates of one MZ for every two or more DZ pairs. Zygosity determination was often casually reported.

The only systematic study of autistic twins has been conducted by Folstein and Rutter (1977) who found 4 of 11 MZ pairs concordant and none of 10 DZ. (The statistical significance of this finding [Fisher Exact Test] has a $p = 0.055$.) These data in isolation are consistent with a polygenic theory, but interpretation is made difficult by the high rate of early developmental (including pre-natal) trauma in most of the affected cases. Twin data on congenital malformations provide a useful precedent for an other-than-genetic explanation. The MZ concordance rate for congenital malformations of any kind is 34 per cent compared to 0.7 per cent in DZs (Myrianthopoulos, 1976), very much like the 36 per cent v. 0 per cent rates found for autism. The higher concordance of MZ twins for congenital malformations could arise if there is an inherited vulnerability to congenital malformation or it could arise because of some special feature of the MZ in-utero environment (see Bulmer, 1970). The fact that the rate of congenital malformations in twins, especially MZ twins, is much higher than the rate in singletons supports the latter interpretation. Whether or not twins in general, and especially MZ twins, are more susceptible to autism becomes an important but difficult question to answer. In samples of SS pairs (Folstein and Rutter did not study OS pairs) there should be slightly more DZ than MZ pairs. Folstein and Rutter found the opposite trend, but the numbers of pairs is small enough for this result to be within chance expectations. We saw earlier that there was a 50 per cent overrepresentation of twins among institutionalized retardates. If twinning has a similar effect on the occurrence of autism and, for the sake of illustration, the true population prevalence of autism was 1 per 10 000, then the rate would be 1.5 per 10 000 among twins. Such an increase would not be detectable with a sample the size of Folstein and Rutter's.

In conclusion, the twin data are consistent with a polygenic interpretation, but they are also consistent with a pre-natal or perinatal brain trauma theory. The disorder is too rare to allow assembly of large enough twin samples to perform statistical-genetic analyses.

If not genetic factors, then what causes early childhood psychoses?

We find little firm evidence to support the idea that genetic factors are important in the development of psychotic conditions that begin within the first few years of life. Shortcomings in the data make it impossible to rule out genetic causation. However, it seems far more parsimonious to postulate biological, probably pre-natal or perinatal brain trauma given the ample evidence implicating CNS pathology including increase in birth and pregnancy complications (Lobascher, Kingerlee & Gubbay, 1970; Kolvin, Ounsted & Roth, 1971; Finegan & Quarrington, 1979), increased frequency of epilepsy, EEG abnormalities and other neurological signs (Rutter et al., 1967; Creak & Pampiglione, 1969; Kolvin, Ounsted & Roth, 1971; Gubbay, Lobascher & Kingerlee, 1970; Schain & Yannet, 1960), perceptual abnormalities (Ornitz & Ritvo, 1968a,b; Creak, 1961), the presence of prenatal CNS viral infection (Chess, 1971, 1977; Stubbs, 1978; Desmond et al., 1970), retrolental fibroplasia (Rimland, 1965), metabolic disturbance (Hackney, 1967; Knobloch & Pasamanick, 1975), degenerative disease (Creak, 1963; Heller, 1954; Corbett et al., 1977), and abnormal evoked EEG responses (Student & Sohmer, 1978). The demonstration of enlarged left temporal ventrical horns in 15 of 17 autistic-like children is the most direct evidence to date implicating organic dysfunction in general and language hemisphere pathology in particular (Hauser, DeLong & Rosman, 1975). See chapters 31, 37 and 38 for more extended discussion.

Some of the facts that lead us to be sceptical of genetic explanations (mostly normal parents and sibs) for early childhood psychosis also make us doubt the many psychodynamic explanations of such conditions. It is true that parents do not treat all their children alike, but we cannot accept the psychogenic view as useful until we see evidence explaining how normal parents, through subtle means, can produce gross psychopathology in newborns while other children in the family remain normal. We cannot help wondering what kind of psychodynamic interpretation would be applied to the fact that little boys with Lesch-Nyhan syndrome invariably gnaw their fingers if given the chance. Fortunately, the knowledge that the cause of this rare childhood psychosis is an X-linked inherited hypoxanthine guanine phosphoribosyl transferase deficiency precludes dynamic interpretations. New advances in foetoscopy, radiology (e.g., emission tomography scans) and in EEG techniques may lead to similar biological definitions for early onset childhood psychoses.

Childhood affective psychoses

No one disputes that depressive symptomatology is found in many normal children (MacFarlane et al., 1962) as well as in childhood disorders. However, the existence of 'pure' affective psychoses in childhood is still debated (Lefkowitz & Burton, 1978; Welner, 1978; Anon, 1979). Mounting evidence from clinical and pharmacological reports supports the notion that childhood affective psychoses (both depressive and manic) do exist. No direct behavioural genetic analyses of childhood affective psychoses have been done, but the gleanings available suggest a biological, probably genetic, connection between adult and childhood affective disorders.

A series of case histories (Brumback & Weinberg, 1977; Frommer, 1968; White & O'Shanick, 1977; Bowdan, 1977; Warneke, 1975) and investigations of the effects of lithium on childhood behavioural disorders (Graham & Rafaelsen, 1972; DeLong, 1978a; Greenhill et al., 1973) show that lithium treatment resulted in marked improvement of manic-like behaviours in some children. Notably, many of the children who respond have a positive family history for adult affective disorder. Two hyperkinetic (? hypomanic) children of lithium-responding manic-depressive parents improved on lithium (Dyson & Barcai, 1970). Unselected samples of hyperactive children do not improve on lithium, suggesting genotype-drug specificity. Severely depressed children appeared to respond to tricyclic antidepressants (Jørgensen, 1979; Puig-Antich et al., 1977); and again, pharmacological intervention appeared to work best in cases that had a positive family history of affective disorder. Finally, children of affectively disturbed parents appear to have a high rate of adult-like affective symptoms (Welner et al., 1977; McKnew et al., 1979). Taken as a whole, the literature presents a psychopharmacogenetic suggestion that there is a commonality between some psychotic or near-psychotic affective syndromes in children and the more common adult forms. However, most of the drug response reports lack methodological rigour, and detailed epidemiological and family studies of affective disorders in relatives of child probands have yet to be done.

Conclusions

The contrasts between parents' hopeful expectations for normal children versus the realities of rearing psychotic children are numbing. The magnitude of the psychopathology far outweighs the rarity of the disorders and enormous energies are applied to the questions of aetiology. Yet, the origins of childhood psychoses that lack clear organic brain pathology elude us. The distinction between early- and late-onset childhood psychoses seems to be a forward step that could lead to better pharmacological treatment of the later-onset group by calling on the accumulated understanding of the pharmacological treatment of adult schizophrenia. Likewise, the treatment of childhood affective disorders could draw on the experience gained with adults if the adult and child disorders were proven to be the same. If it should turn out to be true that schizophrenia never starts before the biological initiation of puberty, we would have a valuable clue to genetic regulatory mechanisms (Hanson & Gottesman, 1979) that govern the expression of the schizophrenic diathesis. At present, the early-onset cases appear to be largely due to exogenous disruptors of CNS development. Specific treatments for already affected individuals may be possible (Shaffer, 1977b) and the hope for prevention (as with Rh incompatibility) may be an attainable goal.

37
Molecular pathology in the early childhood psychoses

J. GERALD YOUNG
DONALD J. COHEN
BENNETT A. SHAYWITZ*

Introduction

Biochemical research on the childhood psychoses was initiated as a series of empirical studies which applied findings and technical advances from other fields. Single reports appeared in the literature, and findings were not followed up or replicated or theoretically co-ordinated with other reports. None of the biochemical results had any clear aetiological significance, or undisputed status as a biological correlate of a disorder; however, several findings form the core of ongoing research and can be placed within the organizing framework of neurochemical investigation. This section describes promising lines of investigation centred on neurotransmitter metabolism, giving particular attention to the best-studied neurotransmitters in the neuropsychiatric disorders, indoleamines (serotonin and related compounds) and catecholamines (dopamine, norepinephrine, and epinephrine) (Young & Cohen, 1979). Reviews of earlier biochemical research on the childhood psychoses are available (Ritvo, 1977; Ritvo, Rabin, Yuwiler, Freeman & Geller, 1978), and these numerous unrelated reports will not be summarized. Other recent studies of critical components of metabolism have failed to detect abnormalities. For example, such blood components as plasma and red cell folate, vita-

* Supported by the William T. Grant Foundation, Children's Clinical Research Center grant RR00125, Mr. Leonard Berger, the Solomon R. & Rebecca D. Baker Foundation, Inc., and grants no NS 12384 and AA 03599.

min B_{12}, ceruloplasmin, electrolytes, calcium, and phosphorus have been determined as occurring in normal levels in autism. Folate, protein, and cells in the spinal fluid are within the normal range; spinal fluid immunoglobulins, an indicator of viral activity, are present in normal amounts (Young, Caparulo, Shaywitz, Johnson & Cohen, 1977).

Blood measures of indoleamine metabolism
Clinical studies of whole blood serotonin

Abnormal levels of blood serotonin (5-hydroxytryptamine, 5-HT) have been reported in several neurological and psychiatric disorders of childhood, including Down's syndrome, phenylketonuria, severe mental retardation, and childhood autsim (Hanley, Stahl & Freedman, 1977). While the cause and physiological significance of these findings are obscure, they have been consistently replicated and their association with serious childhood disorders is clear. Neither a reduction nor an elevation in blood serotonin has been established as a marker for a neuropsychiatric diagnosis or a genetic trait.

Hyperserotonaemia is characteristic of a subgroup of autistic and severely retarded children, appears to be persistent into adulthood, and may be associated with an increase in seizures and aggressiveness and diminished intellectual function. The cause and effects of hyperserotonaemia in autism remain unknown. Blood serotonin is carried almost entirely in blood platelets, with very little free in plasma, and the total concentration decreases over childhood and adolescence. As there is a similar decrease in blood platelet count, altered levels of serotonin might be secondary to a change in platelet count. Although there is a modest elevation in platelet count in childhood autism, the elevated blood serotonin concentration is 'real' in the sense that the serotonin per platelet level is increased (Young, Belendiuk, Freedman, Sternstein & Cohen, 1982a). Increased serotonin release from platelets of autistic children has been reported, but this finding is disputed. The presence of a serotonin-degrading enzyme in platelets (monoamine oxidase, MAO) suggested that impaired enzyme function might play a causal role in hyperserotonaemia. Platelet MAO activity is normal in children with autism (Cohen, Young & Roth, 1977) and is not related to the blood serotonin level when they are measured simultaneously (Young et al., 1982a). Mean platelet MAO activity is increased in male patients with psychiatric disorders during

childhood and adolescence (Young, Cohen, Waldo, Feiz & Toth, 1980a), so further studies of this enzyme will be of interest. The elevation of blood serotonin appears not to be the result of circadian rhythm or diet, and an attempt to affect behaviour in autistic children by lowering serotonin levels through the administration of levo-dopa led to little change in blood serotonin level, platelet count, or behavior. Platelet transport of other amines is not altered (Ritvo, 1977; Ritvo et al., 1978).

Laboratory measurement of blood serotonin

Differences in assay procedure are an important source of inconsistent findings in studies of the physiological mechanism underlying hyperserotonaemia. Blood 5-HT levels cannot be directly compared across laboratories because of variations in methods, and each laboratory must establish its own normative data. In addition, whole blood serotonin levels have been expressed in several ways: per millilitre whole blood, per platelet, and per milligramme of platelet protein (Young et al., 1982a).

Sources of variance include number of platelets in a sample and heterogeneity in platelet size, density, ultrastructure, metabolism, and age. Larger platelets of greater density are probably younger and metabolically more optimal, glycolytic enzymes and MAO are more active, and these platelets have a higher concentration of serotonin-containing granules (Karpatkin, Khan & Freedman, 1978). These heavier platelets are more likely to be 'lost' in most centrifugation procedures currently used for studying platelet function. New work on blood serotonin assay methods must be done before differences can be interpreted.

Diagnostic controversy: the autistic phenotype and hyperserotonaemia

A bias in mean blood serotonin levels for an autistic group might occur because of the overlap in clinical features of autistic and severely retarded children. Since abnormal blood serotonin levels have been repeatedly demonstrated in retarded children (reduced levels in Down's syndrome and phenylketonuria, and elevated levels in a sizable percentage of other severely retarded children), hyperserotonaemia in autistic subject groups could be related to diagnostic criteria. The use of less specific clinical criteria for the diagnosis of autism might lead to the selection of a group with a disproportionately large number of severely retarded children who have other contributing pathophysiological factors. A group of autistic subjects chosen according to strict diagnostic criteria applied after extensive clinical and metabolic evaluation, and followed closely over an extended time-period, might contain a smaller number of children with hyperserotonaemia (Young *et al.*, 1982a).

Comparisons of groups which differ in the strictness of diagnostic criteria for autism show no difference in either mean blood 5-HT levels or percentage of hyperserotonaemic subjects within the groups; the small number of phenotypically autistic children whose diagnosis is changed from primary childhood autism to an alternative classification contribute an insignificant bias. Hyperserotonaemia is clearly associated with a subgroup of children with meticulously diagnosed primary childhood autism and is not only a manifestation of other confounding features, such as severe mental retardation (Young *et al.*, 1982a).

The percentage of autistic children with hyperserotonaemia is approximately 40 in most studies, higher than in other subject groups, including patients with neuropsychiatric syndromes. The highest absolute values in these studies were from autistic children, with the occasional exception of a parent of an autistic child who had a very high blood serotonin level (Young *et al.*, 1982a).

Familial studies of blood serotonin levels

Blood serotonin levels of members of the same family tend to cluster, although occasional families have a wide distribution of 5-HT levels.

There appears to be a correlation of moderate strength between an autistic child and the mother's 5-HT level (Young *et al.*, 1982a). Results from familial studies suggest that careful family study is needed to clarify the genetic contribution to blood serotonin levels.

Urinary and blood measures of catecholamine metabolism

Urinary free catecholamines and MHPG

Urinary catecholamines and their metabolites have been of limited interest in psychiatric research because they primarily reflect peripheral sympathetic activity. The only exception to this appears to be urinary 3-methoxy-4-hydroxyphenethyleneglycol (MHPG), largely the product of central noradrenergic metabolism (Maas, Hattox, Greene & Landis, 1979). Peripheral catecholamines and MHPG may, however, provide useful indices of psychological state,

particularly alterations in arousal, activation, or stimulus readiness. Considerable psychological and observational evidence has suggested that autistic and similar children may have dysfunctions in the regulation of arousal and in the deployment of attention.

Disturbances in attention and arousal, although reflecting a central deficit, can be monitored through cardiovascular indices of sympathetic function (Cohen & Johnson, 1977) and might be correlated with peripheral fluid concentrations of norepinephrine, the sympathetic neurotransmitter.

Urinary studies in normal (mean age = 11.2 years) and autistic boys (mean age = 10.2 years) showed a significant reduction in both mean MHPG and mean free catecholamine excretion in the autistic group compared with the normal group (Young, Cohen, Brown & Caparulo, 1978; Young, Cohen, Caparulo, Brown & Maas, 1979). The urinary free catecholamines predominantly reflect noradrenergic activity.

New evidence suggests that norepinephrine and MHPG in peripheral fluids may reflect CNS noradrenergic activity irrespective of its actual derivation from brain or peripheral sympathetic nervous system. The locus coeruleus controls sympathetic function through descending noradrenergic pathways to the sympathetic lateral columns of the spinal cord. This implies that peripherally derived norepinephrine and its metabolite, MHPG, may be associated with the prevailing level of central noradrenergic activity. Several lines of behavioural and metabolic evidence from animal studies support the hypothesis that activity of the locus coeruleus is associated with response to stressful conditions (Young *et al.*, 1978).

Studies of cardiovascular correlates of attention have indicated that autistic children have higher pulse rates, higher mean blood-pressure, higher mean blood-flow, and lower peripheral vascular resistance than normal children and adults. This pattern may be conceptualized as a state of sensory rejection associated with higher levels of arousal or defense against environmental stimulation. Reduced urinary catecholamines may reflect an adaptive response to persistently elevated anxiety and the children's attempts defensively to ward off further stimulation, through dampening and reversing an initial increase in noradrenergic activity. Alternatively, the children might be hypothesized to have a developmental inability to integrate a full and co-ordinated physiological response to stress (Young *et al.*, 1978, 1979).

Serum DBH activity

Dopamine-beta-hydroxylase is a critical synthetic enzyme in the noradrenergic pathway and has been investigated to determine if there is an abnormality at this point of norepinephrine synthesis in autism. Studies have been inconsistent, with reports of normal, reduced, and elevated levels. Our studies of DBH activity did not show abnormal DBH activity in autistic children, and the wide variation in enzyme activity, largely genetically based, makes comparison across diagnostic groups hazardous (Young, Kyprie, Ross & Cohen, 1980b). The usual increase in DBH activity with age does not occur in the autistic children, indicating possible noradrenergic impairment (Young, Kyprie, Ross & Cohen, 1980b). Serum DBH activity and blood serotonin level are not related (Young *et al.*, 1982a).

Cerebrospinal fluid measures of indoleamine and catecholamine metabolism

The probenecid method

The most direct method for studying biogenic amine metabolism in children involves sampling of cerebrospinal fluid for the major metabolites of dopamine (homovanillic acid, HVA), serotonin (5-hydroxyindoleacetic acid, 5-HIAA), and norepinephrine (MHPG). HVA and 5-HIAA are actively excreted into the CSF. When membrane transport is inhibited by administration of probenecid, the egress of these acid metabolites from the CSF is inhibited, and their concentrations increasingly reflect parent amine turnover in the brain during a specified period of time.

Interpretation of metabolite data without actual measurement of CSF probenecid is hazardous because the levels of CSF metabolites are highly related to the levels of probenecid achieved in the spinal fluid (Cohen, Shaywitz, Johnson & Bowers, 1974).

CSF metabolites in the childhood psychoses

Without probenecid loading, the concentrations of the two major metabolites of dopamine and serotonin (HVA and 5-HIAA) in autistic children are low, closely clustered, and within the range roughly defined for adults: HVA (mean ± S.E. = 65 ng/ml ± 7.7) and 5-HIAA (mean ± S.E. = 41.2 ng/ml ± 4.2) (Cohen, Caparulo, Shaywitz & Bowers, 1977).

Following 10–12 hours of oral probenecid administration, the accumulations of the amine metabolites increase significantly (HVA, 184.2 ± 28.8 ng/ml, and 5-HIAA, 90.5 ± 12.0 ng/ml). The major

difference between autistic and other diagnostic groups studied to date is a reduced level of CSF 5-HIAA accumulation in the autistic children as compared with the age- and sex-comparable, nonautistic, early-onset psychotic children. This finding may be related to differences in the severity of disorders, since the autistic children were more pervasively afflicted.

The functional relations between HVA and 5-HIAA may differ between diagnostic groups, reflecting differences in the balance between the parent neurotransmitter systems. To assess this relation, a ratio of 5-HIAA/HVA may be constructed both for individuals (within a group) and for diagnostic groups. This ratio may be especially important in the light of the different roles played by serotonergic and dopaminergic mechanisms in the organization of brain behavior. For example, the serotonergic midbrain raphe system may subserve sensory modulating or gating functions, while the dopaminergic system appears to be involved in motor activation and arousal. As will be discussed, the ratio of the metabolites of these two systems may be related to aspects of behavioural disorganization. Most studies of adult schizophrenia and depressed patients with the probenecid method have reported a ratio of 5-HIAA/HVA between 0.5 and 0.7, although several studies report values on both sides of this range. For autistic children, the 5-HIAA/HVA ratio is at the lower end of the adult range. This may reflect, in part, the relatively higher HVA levels observed in child patients and a negative relation between CSF dopamine metabolites and age (Cohen *et al.*, 1980).

Since CSF metabolite concentrations span such a considerable range within the autistic and nonautistic early childhood psychosis groups, the detection of between-group differences is quite difficult. Thus, alternative strategies have (a) delineated subpopulations within diagnostic groups and (b) correlated metabolites with explicit dimensions of behaviour, within and across diagnostic groups. In studies of childhood psychosis, amine metabolites have been correlated with dimensions such as language comprehension and expression, activity, movement abnormalities, and social relatedness, using rating scales completed by clinicians, parents, and teachers. One subgroup within the autistic population was found to have especially elevated levels of CSF HVA, both absolutely and in comparison with 5-HIAA (as reflected in 5-HIAA/HVA ratios). This subgroup was behaviourally distinguished by the greatest degree of stereotypic, repetitive behavior (flapping, twirling, finger-flicking, and the like) and locomotor activity, and was over all the most severely afflicted group.

Correlations between CSF metabolites and ratings of behavioural dimensions have suggested hypotheses about serotonin and dopamine metabolites and the organization of behaviour. For example, for ten autistic children, HVA/P was negatively correlated with behavioural ratings of social responsiveness and attention; the ratio of 5-HIAA/HVA was also very highly correlated with these behavioural ratings. Autistic children with higher functional competence had higher levels of 5-HIAA and lower levels of CSF HVA. For 33 neuropsychiatrically handicapped children who were intensively rated by clinically involved and also independent observers, social responsiveness and attention were positively related to 5-HIAA and 5-HIAA/log probenecid. Thus, increased serotonin turnover, as assessed by measurement of metabolite concentration following probenecid, was associated with less impairment in social and attentional functioning in autistic and neuropsychiatrically disturbed children (Cohen *et al.*, 1980).

CSF amine metabolites in a monozygotic twinship concordant for childhood autism were consistent with this generalization based on statistical correlations between behaviour and metabolite concentrations. In this twinship, one twin was more hyperactive and showed considerably more motoric stereotypy. Both with and without probenecid administration, the CSF HVA concentrations were higher in this active twin than in the less active twin. Both children were treated with haloperidol. The more stereotypic, hyperactive child tolerated a larger dose before displaying toxicity, a pharmacological effect that can be interpreted as consistent with relatively greater dopaminergic activity and the finding of increased CSF HVA.

In summary, findings concerning CSF metabolites in the serious, early-onset neuropsychiatric disorders of childhood are similar in type to those found in adult psychiatric disorders, such as schizophrenia. There is great variability within each diagnostic syndrome, and there are no major differences among groups. However, there are suggestions of relations between CSF metabolites and aspects of behavioural impairment (such as attention): following probenecid administration, more disorganized children appear to have relatively lower concentrations of CSF 5-HIAA and higher concentrations of CSF HVA.

Peripheral and central measures of serotonin metabolism

Spinal fluid specimens have not yet been obtained from children at the same time as blood serotonin levels, but the stability of blood serotonin and CSF 5-HIAA in an individual for long periods suggested that their relation could be examined in a preliminary way.

Since increased blood serotonin has been associated with more severe retardation and general impairment, and decreased CSF 5-HIAA has been related to a lower level of global function in autistic, atypical and Tourette syndrome children, it was anticipated that the relationship between the two might be negative. However, a positive association was found between blood serotonin and CSF 5-HIAA (Young *et al.*, 1982a).

While several mechanisms at the molecular level might be postulated, the most conservative way of explaining the data in this small number of subjects would be to suggest that these findings reflect the aetiological heterogeneity of autism and help explain why there have not been significant differences in levels of CSF 5-HIAA among the contrast groups in prior studies. The 'autistic' group might be a composite of two or more subgroups.

Response to medication

Response to medication can be a sensitive tool for biological differentiation of diagnostic groups. The tranquillizers (phenothiazines and butyrophenones) have been the most useful class of drugs for the childhood psychoses, although they are far from uniformly successful in all children and for all symptoms. Their action as dopamine receptor blocking agents suggests that a principal mode of their ameliorative action is reduction of the increased dopaminergic activity which has been suggested on the basis of clinical and biochemical studies. The minor tranquillizers, thought to act principally through gamma-amino-butyric acid neuronal systems, have little specific effect on psychotic children. On the other hand, agents which enhance dopaminergic function, such as the amphetamines, generally lead to marked exacerbation of the clinical symptoms of autistic children, increasing their stereotypy, activity, and anxiety; in contrast, amphetamine can ameliorate the hyperactivity and behavioural disturbances of children with attention deficit disorders, presumably by facilitating the processes involved in selective attention. Similarly, clonidine, a partial noradrenergic agonist which reduces noradrenergic function at low doses, aggravated the symptoms in two autistic children to whom it was administered. This might be related to noradrenergic dysfunction implied by the reduction in urinary free catecholamines and MHPG, with a further decrement in noradrenergic activity aggravating the symptoms.

New pharmacological methods give greater precision to determination of the molecular mechanisms of drugs. For example, receptors for some neurotransmitters are located on both membranes of the synaptic space; pre-synaptic receptors play an important regulatory role at the nerve ending as one of several feedback inhibition systems. When transmitter levels in the synaptic space increase, activation of the pre-synaptic receptor causes a reduction in transmitter release. Some drugs, such as clonidine, have a selective effect at the pre-synaptic receptor when given in a low dose. This causes a reduction in noradrenergic neuronal activity, while having little effect at post-synaptic receptors. Higher doses have different clinical effects because of post-synaptic receptor activation. Similarly, low doses of amphetamine decrease the activity of dopaminergic neurons, reflected in reduced plasma HVA and activity on single cell recordings, by stimulating pre-synaptic dipaminergic autoreceptors. This phenomenon might explain the clinical observation that low doses of amphetamine and methylphenidate, which usually worsen the clinical status of psychotic children, can transiently improve their attention and behaviour. The range of effects elicited by a medication are the resultant of activities on various neuronal systems and at both pre- and post-synaptic sites. These processes are being investigated by simultaneous measurement of plasma levels of drugs and endogenous biogenic amine metabolities. In turn, careful manipulation of drug levels is one of several new methods for altering and stressing metabolic systems in order to clarify molecular dysfunction.

Development of monoamine neuronal systems during childhood

Normal ontogeny

Another perspective in neurochemical research relevant to autism is examination of the development and functional balance of neurotransmitter neuronal systems in childhood and adolescence. Concepts

guiding these studies are that (1) while levels of a compound in a fluid may be within the normal range established for adults, they may be unusual for a given period in childhood because of developmental changes; and (2) while levels of a compound may appear to be within a normal range for that age, an abnormal developmental profile of neuronal systems in a specific diagnostic group may be most visible when the relative functional interaction among systems is examined and found to be atypical when compared to contrast and normal groups. Biochemical studies of childhood autism have required establishment of normal ontogeny of neurotransmitter neuronal systems through a composite assessment of transmitters, enzymes, and metabolites in body fluids in relation to age, and the delineation of over-all functional relations among these systems (Young, Cohen, Anderson & Shaywitz, 1982b). Data is this area are still preliminary.

Schematic developmental profiles of NE-related compounds in human physiological fluids suggest increasing noradrenergic function with age, and there is evidence implying simultaneous, but opposite, changes in thyroid function in males. Similar data suggest decreasing dopaminergic activity and stable or decreasing serotonergic activity with development through childhood and adolescence (Young *et al.*, 1982b). These ontogenetic profiles imply a changing balance among the systems and might lead to recognizable functional results. For example, it would appear that the gradually decreasing activity of the dopaminergic system is reflected in diminishing activity levels during childhood, as modulated by the effects of other neuronal systems.

Pathology of neurotransmitter ontogeny

As profiles of neurotransmitter maturation in various tissues and body fluids are established with more assurance, it will be possible to investigate the relation of abnormal developmental sequences at the molecular level to familiar clinical pathology. Pilot work along these lines suggests how this perspective might be applied. While serum DBH activity and thyroid function in autistic children appear to be within the normal range, preliminary studies of age-related changes in these measures suggest the possibility that their maturation might differ. Normally, serum DBH activity tends to increase with age across childhood and adolescence; this developmental change was not observed in autistic patients, but large variance in serum DBH activity might have masked this phenomenon (Young *et al.*, 1980b).

Another finding in studies of autistic patients illustrates this approach. Thyroid hormone is known to interact with catecholamines. Estimated free thyroxine (EFT) in plasma decreases with age in males, yet in a group of 44 autistic patients, this age-related change did not occur. On the other hand, there was a greater than normal age-related decrease in EFT in another diagnostic group, Tourette's syndrome of chronic multiple tics (Young, Holliday, Lowe & Cohen, 1982c). These preliminary findings indicate the impact of alterations in the development of the endocrine system on neuronal function.

Overview

Metabolic studies of the childhood psychoses are in general agreement that there appears to be a preponderance of dopaminergic activity which is relatively less compensated by serotonergic and noradrenergic function when compared to normal and other disturbed groups of children. The degree of imbalance varies across subgroups of the childhood psychoses, being most pronounced in childhood autism. Many other neuronal systems should be considered to be potentially involved in this pathology, and the evidence to date does not give any indication of which molecular or anatomical site is the primary pathophysiological locus. The clinical heterogeneity of the childhood psychoses probably will be paralleled by a diversity of aetiologies (Cohen *et. al.*, 1978; Fish & Ritvo, 1979). The principal finding, which has not yet been clearly related to this general theoretical synthesis, is the elevated blood serotonin in a subgroup of autistic children. The metabolic implications of hyperserotonaemia, if any, have not been clarified. Although abnormal indoleamine metabolism has long been associated with the childhood psychoses, substantial evidence is now being accumulated which indicates alterations in catecholamine neuronal function. The complex interactions of these systems, the profiles of their development, and their response to pharmacological intervention will be primary targets for future research.

38

Causes and pathology of early childhood psychoses

I. KOLVIN

In the majority of the studies reported here, the subjects are referred to by the authors as 'autistic'. The criteria for case selection vary. Some authors use a narrow definition of autism based on Kanner's publications, whereas others cover a wider group, but they are all concerned with children in whom the psychosis began before five and, in the great majority, before three years of age (Kolvin, 1971; Kolvin, Ounsted, Humphrey & McNay, 1971).

Social and psychological factors

In the past, it was commonly assumed that the fundamental determinants of psychiatric abnormalities in childhood were parental personality, attitudes and emotional disturbance, so it was to be expected that research workers seeking explanations for autism would initially investigate such factors.

Studies of children referred to particular clinical services have usually reported that the parents of classically autistic children come predominantly from the upper social strata and are of above average intelligence (Creak & Ini, 1960; Kolvin, 1971; Kolvin, Ounsted, Richardson & Garside, 1971; Rutter & Lockyer, 1967). Only a few groups of workers (e.g. Ritvo et al., 1971; Schopler, Andrews & Strupp, 1979) have to date published studies of autistic children in which the findings on the parents were out of step with those of the other major research groups. The first epidemiological study of autism (Lotter, 1967) and the largest in scale found a tendency to higher social class, especially among the parents of the most typically autistic children.

As discussed in chapter 34 some recent evidence (Wing, 1980b) has failed to confirm these findings, and more detailed investigation is needed to examine the relationship of social class to various subgroups among children with autism and other early childhood psychoses. However, as most studies have reported a social-class bias in the former, it is not surprising that this has been used to support the hypothesis of an environmental origin for childhood autism. The earlier descriptions of social formality and lack of overtly expressed warmth in the mothers (Kanner, 1943; 1949) and in fathers (Eisenberg, 1957) led to the concept of 'refrigerator parents', who were said to have obsessive and cold personalities, rather than to these features being seen as relatively common characteristics of the public manners of the middle and upper classes.

Unfortunately, these early theoretical explanations were considered to have been proved without checking the validity of the basic premise. A plethora of similar theories has been advanced, mainly stemming from clinical practice, most of which are unacceptable on the grounds of being based on heterogeneous, biased, or unduly small series; similarly, reliable and objective techniques have not been used to accumulate empirical data upon which a theory could be based (Kolvin, Garside & Kidd, 1971). Not only were some of the theories that were developed incapable of generating testable hypotheses, some theorists did not even attend to the two axiomatic methodological steps of demonstrating a correlation between child and parent variables and of carrying out experimental or observational studies in an attempt to validate a cause–effect relationship. In addition, most theorists did not consider the possibility that the syndrome might have a multifactorial basis.

Modern Anglo-American research has not confirmed the parental personality stereotype, irrespective of whether it has been based on self-rating schedules such as the Maudsley Personality Inventory (Kolvin, Garside & Kidd, 1971), assessments of parental warmth based on clinical interview (Creak & Ini, 1960), parent attitude scales (Pitfield & Oppenheim, 1964), objective tests of thought disorder (Schopler & Loftin, 1969a, b), or combinations of clinical assessment and objectively rated interviews (DeMyer *et al.*, 1972b). The last-mentioned did not identify any unusual rearing or attitudinal patterns

in parents of autistic children with regard to warmth in nurturing, acceptance of their infants, or degree of general stimulation. They found that child-care practices of parents of autistic children were similar to those of the parents of matched normal children. Finally, there is the study of Cox, Rutter, Newman, and Bartak (1975), who used objective clinical interviews plus parental self-rating inventories. These researchers reported that mothers showed somewhat less warmth to their autistic than to their non-autistic children, but interpreted it as difficulty in interacting with an unresponsive child, especially since the difference was small and half the mothers were rated as very warm to their autistic children.

Thus, there is no evidence that autism is secondary to abnormal parental personalities, nor unusual child-rearing practices. As pointed out by Rutter (1972b), there is also no evidence of a link with extremely depriving circumstances. Ferster (1961) suggested that autism was due to faulty conditioning, but none of the relevant findings have supported this view. Wing (1966) notes that it would be difficult to imagine how any of these extreme environmental experiences could give rise to the complex but specific patterns of impairments in such diverse areas as cognitive, perceptual, motor, and autonomic functioning. Bartak, Rutter, and Cox (1975) studied autistic children of normal intelligence in whom no overt neurological disorder could be identified. Even in this group they found evidence of cognitive disorder and concluded that 'it is most unlikely that the condition is primarily psychogenic' (Cox, Rutter, Newman & Bartak, 1975). The sum total of these studies and reviews provides strong refutation of a psychogenic hypothesis. In addition, there is suggestive evidence (Bell, 1968, 1971; Cox, Rutter, Newman & Bartak, 1975) that some of the parental social reactions may be secondary to the autism and that social isolation, when present in mothers of autistic children, appears to follow the onset of the disorder (Kolvin, Garside & Kidd, 1971).

Biological factors
Gross organic causes
Current research suggests that early childhood psychosis may be the final common behavioural expression of a wide variety of organic-cum-developmental influences. The evidence for this is impressively extensive. First, presumptive evidence of cerebral injury has been obtained from studies of perinatal complications, with particularly high rates being

reported in clinical studies (Gittelman & Birch, 1967; Gubbay, Lobascher & Kingerlee, 1970; Lobascher, Kingerlee & Gubbay, 1970; Kolvin, Ounsted & Roth, 1971; Knobloch & Pasamanick, 1966; Folstein & Rutter, 1977) and also, but to a less marked degree, in population studies (Lotter, 1967; Treffert, 1970). Other evidence of neurological involvement comes from DeMyer and colleagues (1972b), who reported reduced alertness in infancy and more overt signs of brain damage.

Second, in about half of the cases in two major hospital series, evidence of cerebral dysfunction was found (Rutter & Lockyer, 1967; Kolvin, Ounsted & Roth, 1971). In the course of time, autistic children and adolescents develop epileptic fits far more frequently than might be expected by chance (Rutter, 1970; Kolvin, Ounsted & Roth, 1971; DeMyer *et al.*, 1973). Early childhood psychosis can also be associated with previous episodes of infantile spasms (Kolvin, Ounsted & Roth, 1971; Taft & Cohen, 1971). The association is discussed in chapter 31.

Third, certain identifiable organic conditions appear to have a close relationship with the behavioural abnormalities characteristic of early childhood psychosis. Chess (1971) reported that, in a series of 243 children of mothers who had had rubella in pregnancy, 10 children had classic autism (a rate of 412 per 10,000) and 8 had a 'partial autistic syndrome' (329 per 10,000). These rates are more than one hundred times greater than would be expected in the general population (see chapter 34). Not all of these rubella children had visual impairments. Early childhood psychosis can also be found in children with congenital blindness, or partial sight, combined with brain damage due, for example, to retrolental fibroplasia (Keeler, 1958; Freedman, 1971).

Encephalitis or encephalopathy from causes other than maternal rubella have been reported as occurring during the first two or three years of life in some children with early childhood psychosis (Greenbaum & Lurie, 1948; Wing & Gould, 1979). The pattern of behaviour has also been described in untreated phenylketonuria (Jervis, 1963), tuberose sclerosis (Critchley & Earl, 1932; Earl, 1934; Creak, 1963; Lotter, 1974), and cerebral lipoidosis (Creak, 1963). In some reported cases, the diagnosis of the neurological condition was not made until after death (Creak, 1963; Lotter, 1974). Darby (1976) summarized the results of all the cases of childhood autism and psychosis where post-mortem examination of the brain had been carried out; several cerebral pathologies were found.

It is of interest that Down's syndrome is comparatively rarely associated with early childhood psychosis (Wing, 1969, 1971; Wakabayashi, 1979; Wing & Gould, 1979).

It has been suggested that, in at least some cases, autism has a genetic basis. The evidence for and against this is discussed in chapter 39.

Biochemical, metabolic, or allergic theories of aetiology have been put forward but remain not proven. Possible lines of investigation in this field are discussed in chapter 37.

Localization of the brain pathology
So far we have little idea of the nature of the specific brain dysfunction. The diversity of EEG and seizure patterns, which range from focal epilepsy to the widespread disorganization of hypsarrhythmia (Rutter & Lockyer, 1967; Kolvin, Ounsted & Roth, 1971; Taft & Cohen, 1971), appears to argue against a single underlying homogeneous pathological mechanism. On the basis of knowledge available at the time he was writing, Rutter (1974) found it impossible to suggest a site for the lesion and favoured the hypothesis of a non-specific syndrome of biological impairment. Wing and Wing (1971), on the other hand, attempting to account for the complex clinical picture, argued that multiple neurological deficits do not necessarily imply multiple lesions. 'A number of different brain functions could be affected by, for example, a single genetic or biochemical abnormality, or anatomical proximity could make different centres vulnerable to the same lesion.' On this hypothesis, any condition that produces abnormality or delayed maturation of the relevant brain areas could, theoretically, lead to the impairments found in childhood autism or other early childhood psychoses.

There are a variety of views as to which brain areas have to be involved to produce the characteristic behaviour. Crawley (1971) considered that the problem might be in the association areas. The pattern of deficiencies in language and symbolic processes, with better retention of visuo-spatial skills, has led some workers to suggest that the lesion or dysfunction underlying childhood autism affects the dominant hemisphere of the brain (Hermelin, 1966; Barry & James, 1978). One group of workers (Hauser, DeLong & Rosman, 1975) reported enlargement of the temporal horn of the lateral ventricle with atrophy of the adjacent area of the left medial temporal lobe. But there is doubt about the methodology and the homogeneity of the sample. It has been suggested that the subjects were highly selected with heavy loadings of neurological disorder (Lancet, 1976).

Ross and Mesulam (1979) and Sackeim and Gur (1978) produced evidence that the non-dominant hemisphere is concerned in the comprehension and expression of emotion in non-verbal ways. Impairment of non-verbal as well as verbal communication is characteristic of autism and other early childhood psychoses. If the involvement of the non-dominant hemisphere in non-verbal communication is confirmed, this would suggest that the problems in such conditions are probably not confined to the dominant hemisphere alone. The lesion or dysfunction must be capable of impairing all aspects of language and communication, as well as explaining the other features of the clinical picture.

Damasio and Maurer (1978) considered the possibility of dysfunction of a single and yet widely based system consisting of the bilateral neural structures of the mesolimbic cortex. They postulated that autism might be the result of macroscopic or microscopic changes in the above-mentioned target areas or structure influencing them. On the basis of this hypothesis, the broadly homogeneous functional aberration of autism might be the result of very different types of structural disorganization. Unfortunately, this theory is so far-ranging that it would be difficult to test. Other workers have suggested subcortical dysfunction, which directly or indirectly affects the reticular activating system involving either under- or over-arousal (Hutt, Hutt, Lee & Ounsted, 1964; 1965) or an imbalance between these systems (Des Lauriers & Carlson, 1969). The empirical evidence advanced in support of these conflicting hypotheses is rather questionable (Hermelin & O'Connor, 1968).

Cognitive deficits

The nature of the cognitive deficits is discussed in chapter 35. They are so marked, so characteristic and, beyond a certain point, so unresponsive to environmental modification, that it is tempting to suggest a common pathological origin. However, none of the theories so far put forward is able to explain all the abnormalities of language, perceptual, motor and autonomic function and there is, as yet, no direct evidence of a necessary and sufficient pathology.

Section 9

CHAPTERS 39 AND 40

Treatment and management

39
Medical management of psychotic children

D. M. RICKS

The various ways in which a doctor can help the psychotic child and his family include counselling the child's parents, helping him to learn skills which at least enable his parents to run a more or less normal household, and to stop or reduce behaviour which prevents this. For a detailed description of the problems experienced by the parents, see DeMyer (1979). In addition he may occasionally be called upon to advise whether such a child is at any time ill or in pain. This is usually because the parents are faced with a hitherto unexpected behaviour, or behaviour which is not only atypical in pattern but also in timing, for example, after meals or in the middle of the night, so that it seems more sinister than the array of bizarre activities to which they have already become accustomed. Finally, he will need to acquaint himself with various local agencies and support groups run for the parents' benefit. These facets of a medical role will be discussed in order.

Counselling parents
Counselling parents may have two phases. Initially feelings will run high about why this tragedy has happened at all – why particularly to them – so that the emphasis of questioning will be on aetiology. Later, although this will continue to intrude into their private feelings and discussions with each other, and it is to be hoped, with the doctor, it will gradually be superseded by a practical concern about how to improve the child's behaviour. Indeed, part of the

initial misery and self-recrimination afflicting parents with handicapped children of all kinds is generated by a sense of helplessness. Equipping parents with some course of action can be very supportive, not least in reducing this understandable preoccupation with the origins of the tragedy. The first phase of questioning – *why* does he behave like this? – is extremely important and will be dealt with first in this section. The second phase – counselling parents in their efforts to help the child – will be discussed later.

Doctors need to appreciate their limitations in advising on daily care and training. On the whole, this is better undertaken by educationalists, therapists, and psychologists, providing they work in close co-operation with parents. Although the doctor's responsibility is clear in establishing a diagnosis, assessing and investigating disabilities as they affect the child's functioning, and advising on medication, he can cause himself undue anxiety and undermine the efforts of others if he feels obliged to monitor too closely the child's progress. This will inevitably be patchy and those directly involved will need flexibility in their programmes and scope for trial and error if they are to become confident, expert or consistent enough in their handling. Being available for advice, offering expert explanations about problem behaviour, and sharing responsibility for tackling it can be best achieved by facilitating the efforts of others, rather than by directing them. It is important never to lose sight of the fact that one's patient is the parent's child.

Confronted by a psychotic child, what impresses the doctor is the unique combination of exasperation and despair that pervades the family. Realization by parents that they have any form of highly abnormal child unleashes a whole series of reactions needing urgent help which may present quite acutely. These are discussed in volume 4, chapter 2. An apparently normal babyhood, often devoid of any alerting episode of cerebral insult, followed by average motor achievements, but emotional inaccessibility, lends an additional dimension to the family's tragedy in the case of the psychotic child. The second year may have been increasingly worrying and bewildering to his parents as behaviour becomes more and more bizarre, with protracted episodes of unshared content or totally self-contained misery, unresponsive to coaxing or affection and punctuated by apparently causeless outbursts of screaming with fury or fear. Each mood may be accompanied by a repertoire of strange behaviour described in earlier chapters. This has set the family scene at the time when the doctor usually becomes first involved.

The child, often normal and even attractive in appearance, has a disturbing and immediately apparent abnormal facial response. He is active and nimble with a dexterity quite sufficient for self-help; he may readily vocalize, humming in tune; in short he has all the practical skills that could fulfil his parents' enjoyment of him. His alert gaze is fleeting and impersonal though he may look long and intently at any object which absorbs him. His attention is selective, quickly picking up convenient routine or anticipating unwelcome change which he resists furiously. His manipulative skills are put to his own often inconvenient use, such as dismantling furniture or piling crockery, yet not to hold a spoon or to fasten buttons. Because of the autistic language disability the specifity of his verbal comprehension will be totally perplexing. If he can listen to spoken TV advertisements, why not to his mother's voice? Why, if he knows a particular door is a door does he not understand, or have to be laboriously taught, about other doors in the house? It is quite bewildering to be confronted by a child who cannot generalize his understanding, however rudimentary, of the use of objects and what they are called – the more so because this capacity, even in the retarded, is one everyone takes for granted and does not question.

It is here that the doctor's role can be supportive, since the parents bring not only their distress but also their exasperation at the utter incomprehensibility of the child's symptoms – and, quite often, their growing conviction that these are contrived. The doctor must encourage the parents to express their sadness and exasperation and in particular to be frank about their reason for thinking the child's behaviour is deliberate and provocative. Some of it will be, and a great deal of relief will be gained by disentangling and correcting the deliberate misbehaviour and identifying what is produced by the child's disabilities. The family need to be helped carefully over several sessions to appreciate what it means to their child to have difficulty in focusing attention in some situations, or recognizing constraints, or accepting delay, or breaking routine or, in particular, being unable to comprehend language except with highly specific connotations (Churchill, 1978; Ricks & Wing, 1975). To help the parents and involved staff towards a close empathy with the child and a clearer understanding of the disordered world he experiences is a major component of medical management. Without such an understanding, parents cannot be helped to cope with feelings that the child generates or to participate constructively in his management.

Medical investigations

In almost all but the mildest cases, psychotic children will be a sufficient source of concern to be referred to their doctor before school age. Some will be seen by the family GP, perhaps via the health visitor, or by the local authority medical officer. They may then be referred to the local paediatrician and such children often receive their first comprehensive review in a paediatric assessment clinic; from here they may be referred to a centre for handicapped children or child psychiatric clinic. Which avenue of referral the child takes will depend on whether the local district services adopt assessment procedures advocated by the Court Report (1976) or the National Development Group (1977). To some extent, this influences whether the child is seen primarily as a developmental or a psychiatric problem.

However it occurs, initial assessment will need to involve the family. Investigation of the child's impairments needs time and appropriate surroundings. Observing the child for several sessions, preferably in his own home, or at least in an environment with which he has become familiar, will help reveal the extent of his impairments, his skills and apparent triggers for his behaviour disturbance. The extent of his disability and disturbance will be evident enough in any formal clinic. A careful history and close sympathetic questioning of parents and siblings will reveal skills and idiosyncrasies which may well be invaluable in formulating an educational programme. As far as practicable, the child should be observed by specialized staff since simply detecting responses and learning difficulties in these bizarre children needs experience. From an initial appraisal of impairments, further investigations may be indicated (Corbett, 1976): blood and urine samples may be needed to test for biochemical or chromosome disorders. When the child is more settled and co-operative a careful physical examination may reveal skin lesions which may suggest, for example, epiloia, when one remembers that the more obvious facial adenoma sebaceum may appear quite late (after five years) or hardly at all.

It is in exploring the child's attention defects that special tests may be most helpful, though to safeguard the child, (and the relevant hospital departments) care should be taken to base suspicions of, for instance, hearing defect, on controlled observation. In psychotic children the distinction between not hearing and not listening or between not seeing and not looking is very difficult to establish. Positive responses to single tests, for example, if a child clearly turns to a sound or moves some distance to pick up a small object, are immensely valuable. Hence the value of assessment in familiar surroundings where the child feels more confident. What he cannot do is obvious enough; what he can do is what matters. However, special tests for vision and hearing may be valuable not only to establish defect conclusively, but to reveal its quality and extent, for example, high tone hearing loss or severe short sight, so that teaching and everyday handling can compensate appropriately. For hearing tests, apparent conditioning to a response of language and sound (Bricker, Bricker & Larsen, 1968) may be feasible with sufficient co-operation, while some procedures under light anaesthesia are valuable if co-operation is absent. These include transtympanic cochleography, sound evoked response, and crossed acoustic reflex audiometry. Such tests confirm or refute the passage of nerve impulses to the CNS. Transtympanic recording has the occasional added advantage of revealing a gluey condition of the middle ear which can then be treated. It must always be borne in mind that fluctuating, occasionally severe, hearing loss, in a young retarded child at critical language learning phases, may disrupt his behaviour to a level that may provoke serious and progressive interaction problems within the family, leading to behaviour disorder indistinguishable from childhood psychosis.

An equally painstaking investigation of vision might pay dividends, particularly in the young child. Ophthalmological examination of psychotic children can be a sore trial to clinic staff, though in some cases such children will fix on a light (indeed will rivet their attention on it) in a dark room, if sensible steps are taken to reassure them. In such a case, refraction is feasible so that gross refractive error can be more effectively excluded than under anaesthesia. At a later examination a more accurate refraction can be attempted with ophthalmoplegic drops and a search made for lens opacities or retinal pathology, which may affect the child's prognosis, modify his teaching programme or indicate genetic counselling. It is surprising how effectively the mobile retarded child can adapt to poor vision. It seems that refractive error must be gross and more or less symmetrical – otherwise a strabismus would alert to its presence – to be a previously unrecognized and serious contribution to the child's behaviour problems. If serious visual or auditory defect is detected, a trial of wearing spectacles or a deaf aid will need to be discussed at length with parents and teaching staff.

The value of EEG recording in the management of such children must be weighed carefully (Pond, 1963), not least because their investigation is no mean task. A record showing rhythms normal for the age tends to encourage staff and parents' efforts and reassure them about the prognosis, though the evidence for this confidence is slight. More significantly, cerebral dysrhythmia, sharp waves or wave/spike, may be revealed by an EEG in a child with no clinical evidence of minor fits. These may be masked in the episodic stereotyped behaviour of these children. Such dysrhythmias, if frequent or prolonged, can further disrupt the child's fragile attention, yet can be remedied by anticonvulsants. Serial EEG records can be of value, particularly in an inexplicable disturbed episode when a change of drugs may be indicated by a changed or deteriorated record. Such series may reveal a deteriorating pattern of shifting localized disturbance – as in epiloia – or be the first indication of organic aetiology, as with infantile spasms (see chapter 31).

The doctor should explore in as much detail as needed the manner in which clinical disorders impair the learning and social response of psychotic children. Any pathology needs to be explained, not only giving the probable reasons as to why the child behaves as he does, but suggesting what practical steps can be taken to help him. For example, it is helpful to know that auditory attention may need to be prompted with an alerting vocal signal before a simple message is conveyed, or preceded by capturing visual interest with face-to-face gaze, and so on. Experienced teachers and psychologists will develop these tactics and incorporate them into self-help and social training, but it is of value to them and a reassurance to parents if the doctor explains adequately why these steps are necessary with their child.

Behaviour disturbance

In addition to his contribution to helping to improve the skills of the psychotic child the doctor is frequently called on to advise on behaviour disturbance. For much of the time, this will be a recurrent and obvious theme: the child's disorder conflicting with the parents' normal requirements for a reasonably ordered life. This may be inadvertently aggravated by the parents themselves. Periodically, however, much more serious acute episodes of disturbance may arise calling for urgent medical advice. Psychotic children are capable, on occasions, of quite alarming levels of disturbance requiring the doctor to disentangle the cause, if any, and to advise what steps should be taken.

An occasional reason for these disturbed episodes, all too easily overlooked, is that the child may be in pain or acute discomfort. Their reactions to injury may be quite unlike that of a normal child and may be indistinguishable from fear or anger. When this occurs, with no obvious sign of cause or without any apparent precipitating event in a child virtually impossible to examine, it is often understandably missed. Common causes are carious teeth or dental abscess (often producing nocturnal outbursts or distress after meals), a foreign body in the ear, a sting or burn, or minor crushing, particularly to the fingers. Examining the child sufficiently to exclude such minor trauma can on occasions be rewarding. An equally 'trivial' cause with similarly alarming repercussions can be the loss of a prized possession carried around by the child. This can be a quite small everyday object like a hair grip, a cork or a sock. If it is twiddled or carried conspicuously its loss will be noted, but it is always sensible to enquire of parents or familiar staff whether they can call anything to mind which the child may be missing. Its return can be quite spectacularly beneficial.

Apart from such incidental accidents, two forms of acute disturbance may present in psychotic children, the first environmental in origin, the other probably not. They need distinguishing because, although they produce similar clinical states, the effective management of one may be different from the other and their confusion can be disastrous.

On some occasions an episode of serious disturbance may be the result of prolonged and accumulating pressure on the child, perhaps due to the efforts of his parents struggling to cope with him, and failing to do so, often as the result of some additional domestic problem. A characteristic history is of frequent outbursts of temper reaching a crescendo after a period of two to three weeks, perhaps associated with some increased inconvenience, such as moving house, or illness of another family member. The psychotic child becomes more continually restless than usual, looks agitated, often with repetitive crying, may be more than usually intolerant of breaks in routine, and may more avidly seek favourite but forbidden pleasures, for example, in the garden or refrigerator. The most demoralizing feature as the days pass is attacks of screaming when directly involved with his parents at crucial times in the household's day such as dressing, taking meals, going to the lavatory, or being put to bed. Events which were previously prized episodes of stable predictable response become the focus of disturbance. During this period tranquillizers or sedatives may have been prescribed, which can increase agitation and add nocturnal disturbance or disrupted sleep rhythms. Such an episode can be effectively remedied by removing the child from home temporarily. A request for this will often be the major reason for a medical referral. The child needs prompt transfer to an appropriate accepting setting with experienced staff. On transfer staff should be advised to allow the child to give full rein to his restless activity, his drugs should be reduced and stopped, he should be encouraged, but not compelled, to participate in the unit's daily activities, and above all his handling by a single member or not more than a small group, of staff for dressing and bathing and at meal-times should be calm, kindly and unfussed, with a minimum of verbal embroidery. Great benefit to the child can quickly result from this change from an anxiety-ridden situation to one which is anxiety-free, unrestricted, yet domestically containing with little verbal pressure. This allows breathing space for the family and the agencies involved to try to rectify the home situation to which the child can return.

Such an episode, clearly situational in origin, contrasts with the second type of episodic disturbance. This usually has a shorter history, developing over a few days or a week, arising with no detectable change in the child's life-style, but often on enquiry seeming to be a repetition of previous episodes. The child's disturbance, typical for him, often has a physiological flavour. Screaming may be more protracted and accompanied by head-banging or self-mutilation; bouts of restless activity may alternate with rocking or masturbation; appetite may increase and the child may forage vigorously, or the child may stop eating altogether; frequently such episodes are accompanied by sharply increased drinking; sleep disturbance is common. The apparent organic nature of these episodes, their periodicity, the fact that often they run a similar course for any given child with a rapid onset and decline apparently independent of circumstances suggests some internally generated disorder, possibly biochemical. Various syndromes have been described suggesting such a cause (Jervis, 1963; Nyhan, Olivier & Lesch, 1965; Sass, Itabashi & Dexter, 1965; Creak, 1963). The fact that a majority of such children are in long-stay hospitals and may require virtually permanent sedation may, in some

cases, mask the periodicity of such disturbance. Certainly, if psychotropic drugs are used in such an episode, the dose needs to be adequate. Psychotic children are often resistant to ordinary levels of medication.

A disturbing feature of the management of such episodes is that they often cannot be controlled by medication, or by behaviour modification, or by involving the child in a more intensive and diverting daily programme, or by any change in their daily life. If such episodes are the result of temporary change in the child's awareness or sensitivity to external stimuli through, for example, alternations in synaptic chemistry, such imperviousness is to be expected. Quite often, if allowed to do so, the child himself will seek out the situation most therapeutic for him and for a period may quieten only if he is allowed to secrete himself in a place of his choosing which may be dark, quiet or cool. Modifying the child's routine to respect this, combined with gentle enabling rather than persuading him at meal-times etc., may be the only effective therapeutic programme. If it is, this apparently passive management often requires the doctor to reassure parents and staff about its justification. In long-term settings with staff shortages and the need to fit the child into an accepted regime he may unfortunately, but quite understandably, be sedated and the episode prolonged. In his own home or community settings there is likely, equally understandably, to be an anxious emphasis on active remedies, which may be of no avail or intensify the disturbance. Simply by supporting, or indeed advising daily management, which, for a period, respects the child's need for reduced stimulation, the doctor may not only benefit the child, but support staff and parent morale, since it is one thing to allow self-seclusion as a last resort, but quite different to see it as a constructive remedy on the child's behalf.

Sleeplessness is a particularly difficult problem. The child may keep the whole family awake every night because of his screaming. If nothing else works, the doctor may prescribe a sedative as a temporary measure but it is then essential to ensure that the dose is adequate, since the sedation threshold may be increased and inadequate doses can make the behaviour disturbance worse.

The supervention of other psychiatric disorders, in particular the affective psychoses, has been mentioned in chapter 30. The commonest problem is depression, especially in adolescence and early adult life. It is important for the doctor to be aware of the possibility since the patient does not complain of symptoms and the language impairment makes clinical examination difficult. Patients with fair language skills may, however, describe typical depressive delusions, guilt and self-reproach. The depressed mood is indicated by weeping; anorexia, loss of weight and early waking can be observed. Antidepressant medication is often effective.

Supporting parents and care-staff

Finally, a highly significant component of medical management is the doctor's role in helping parents cope with the everyday demands of their psychotic child. With their more direct involvement, teachers or care staff will, of course, play a major part in day-to-day discussions resolving differences and complaints to support the family in their efforts. These are discussed in chapter 40. The doctor, perhaps seen by the parents as a key team member or in his role as psychiatrist, will have a crucial responsibility. When parents are reaching the end of their tether, when they realize their own weariness or exasperation are making things worse, when they find themselves disagreeing with school practice, when they concern themselves with future arrangements, then the doctor, perhaps to his own discomfort, may find himself regarded as an arbiter or someone who should independently know what is 'right' for the family. In many of these situations he will be well advised to accept a 'catalyst' role within the group, drawing together with the parents all involved with the child's care. Occasional open discussions of this nature are invaluable provided they are frank. The doctors may find that a personal capacity for constructive compromise, maintaining the consensus best for the child, is the most valuable professional resource they can cultivate. Successful, consistent management of a psychotic child by any group of people is a demanding experience and no doctor should feel that his support and, if required, guidance of such a group is a peripheral responsibility. It may be his major one. With poor empathy for the group and its efforts, he can actually make things worse.

At a more individual level, parents may confide anxieties about their own lack of success compared with, for instance, school staff. Most doctors realize the obstacles to 'successful' management which confront parents in their efforts simply because it is their child. Although the impact of such personal involvement is acknowledged, too few doctors really appreciate how abnormal are the practices often required for effective help with such children. The degree to which they are not only different but totally contrasted to the ways in which a parent may respond to a normal child in a similar situation are discussed elsewhere (see volume 4, chapter 1). Parents' responses, by which normal children are guided, coaxed, or reprimanded into acceptable patterns of behaviour, are spontaneous and largely intuitive. They are therefore the way in which most of us would immediately behave with the psychotic child. To realize that they are inappropriate, and therefore to check them and modify them drastically, is enormously demanding of any parent. Indeed so much so that many do not achieve it. Those that do may find it personally distressing as 'unnatural'. For the doctor to be seen to appreciate this, to recognize the efforts entailed and to reassure parents that such efforts testify to their normality rather than to neurosis or inadequacy, can make all the difference between coping and failing within the family. Even if successful in this therapy, the doctor must accept that his personal rapport and advice may be less reassuring for the struggling parents than direct contact with others who have struggled similarly. A national society for parents and professional workers concerned with autistic children and adults has been formed (address given below) and there may be a local society in the child's locality. The doctor should equip himself with information about them and discover whether play groups or schools have similar parent support services either through experienced delegated parents or staff such as educational welfare workers. In providing this service, close liaison with the family's social worker, whether from the child guidance clinic or the Social Service area team, will be imperative; in addition to counselling and support such professionals can help the family acquire their due financial benefits and grants for aid.

A number of books can be recommended to parents. Some are accounts by mothers of their own autistic children (Hundley, 1971; Junker, 1964; Lovell, 1978; Park, 1967), while others give practical advice on management and teaching (Everard, 1976; Jeffree & McConkey, 1976; Jeffree, McConkey & Hewson, 1977; Schopler, Reichler & Lansing, 1979b; Wing, L., 1976, 1980a). Professional workers would find it salutary to read Eberhardy (1967) and Kysar (1968) who describe the distress produced when parents are assumed to have caused autism in their children.

Details of books, pamphlets and of the services available for autistic children can be obtained from the National Society for Autistic Children, 1A Golders Green Road, London NW11 8EA.

40
Education and management of psychotic children

PATRICIA HOWLIN

Introduction

The prognosis for children suffering from early childhood psychosis is poor. Only 11 of the 96 autistic children followed up by Kanner in 1973 were able to lead a relatively independent life, and similar findings have been reported by Rutter and Lockyer (1967), DeMyer and colleagues (1973) and Lotter (1974). The gloomy outlook, even for relatively intelligent children, has led to a search for treatment techniques which might avert the tragedy, eventually faced by many parents, of seeing their child placed in a subnormality hospital or long-stay institution.

In the past, extravagant claims have been made for the effects of physical stimulation programmes (Delacato, 1974), or of various drugs, diets, and vitamins (see Cambell, 1973). Unfortunately, none of these claims has been supported by convincing experimental evidence. The most effective treatment, at present, seems to be the use of structured educational and management programmes at home and at school. Even these techniques, although valuable in producing improvements in skills and behaviour, cannot be considered as 'cures' for autism, and the majority of autistic people will remain handicapped throughout their lives. Nevertheless, with appropriate schooling and practical help at home many difficulties may be ameliorated.

The effectiveness of early schooling

Early studies of autistic children (Rutter & Lockyer, 1967; Kanner, 1973) indicated that there was a relationship between schooling and eventual outcome. Even with minimal schooling (often as little as two years) autistic children made appreciable educational and social gains (Rutter & Lockyer, 1967) and it was suggested that with adequate education the prognosis in autism might be rather more favourable. Further follow-up studies (Mittler, Gillies & Jukes, 1966; DeMyer *et al.*, 1973; Lotter, 1974) tended to confirm the view that prognosis and amount of education were related. However, the relationship is not a straightforward one and is complicated by the child's intellectual level. Thus, the more intelligent children are most likely to receive extended education, whilst more retarded children tend to be placed in subnormality units at an earlier age. The effects of education also differ according to the child's intelligence. Few children with an IQ below 40 are likely to gain any useful scholastic skills, no matter how much schooling they receive, although with appropriate teaching they may gain other skills. Children with an IQ above 50, on the other hand, can be expected to make relatively good progress in arithmetic, reading, and writing (Rutter & Bartak, 1973). Unfortunately, the benefits of a good education do not necessarily guarantee later employment. Thus, whereas both Kanner (1973) and Lotter (1974) found that only children who had received appropriate schooling subsequently found outside employment, only a tiny minority, even of the most highly educated children, actually obtained independent jobs.

Types of educational management

Although the long-term effects of early education remain somewhat unclear and rather disappointing, there is some information on the type of educational management which is likely to prove effective, at least in the short term. Schopler and his colleagues (1971) found that the behaviour of autistic children improved considerably in a structured setting. Bartak and Rutter (1973) in a systematic comparison of different educational systems, also found that a structured teaching programme, adapted to the child's specific cognitive ability, such as that described by Elgar (1966) resulted not only in greater educational gains, but in improved social behaviour in the classroom. Children in more permissive school environments made significantly less progress in all of these areas. However, social behaviour in the children's own homes improved to an equal extent whichever type of school they attended.

Home-based treatment

A structured programme has also been found to be effective in the home-based treatment of autistic children (Howlin *et al.*, 1973; Hemsley *et al.*, 1978). In a controlled study of the effects of different approaches to treatment it was found that giving parents direct training at home in the management of behaviour problems and in the development of specific skills resulted in considerable improvements. Behavioural problems declined, social, constructional, and linguistic abilities increased, and the interaction between children and parents also improved. Children in the control families who were not involved in structured management programmes failed to show such improvements.

The use of behavioural techniques

In recent years numerous single case studies have demonstrated the effectiveness of behaviour modification techniques in the treatment of a wide range of autistic problems, from delays in language and social development to disruptive behaviour such as tantrums, rituals and obsessions (Lovaas, Schaeffer & Simmons, 1965; Lovaas, 1977; Brawley *et al.*, 1969; Nordquist & Wahler, 1973; Marchant, Howlin, Yule & Rutter, 1974).

Controlled group studies have also shown behavioural techniques to be more effective than other therapies (for example, play therapy: Ney, Palvesky & Markely, 1971) and more effective than the traditional type of out-patient treatment (Hemsley *et al.*, 1978). Briefly, behavioural techniques involve consistent reinforcement for appropriate behaviour, whilst undesirable behaviours are reduced by withdrawing attention or other positive consequences for the child. Behavioural management is essentially an individually oriented approach. Careful observation of the child prior to intervention is needed to assess the factors which appear to be maintaining inappropriate behaviours, and to identify potential reinforcers which can be used to increase desirable behaviours. Detailed assessments of the child's level of functioning are also necessary to ensure that training programmes are adapted to the individual child's skills and deficits. (See Gelfand & Hartmann, 1975, for a useful introduction to behaviour therapy with children.)

Improving skills

Language and communication problems. In varying severity, these occur in all autistic children. For children lacking in even the simplest comprehension skills the combination of reinforcement principles with techniques such as physical prompts, or visual cues (which can be gradually reduced) may be used to teach the child to associate the spoken word with particular objects, people, or actions. Later, children may be taught to imitate sounds and subsequently to chain these sounds together to produce words and, eventually, phrases. In the case of children who use echolalic utterances or stereotyped speech, the *consistent* use of reinforcement for appropriate speech, whilst inappropriate utterances are consistently corrected or, possibly, ignored, frequently results in a rapid decrease in inappropriate speech. Lovaas (1966, 1977) and Sloane and MacAulay (1968) have given a full description of these techniques.

For children who fail to develop spoken language, alternative forms of communication, for example by gesture, pictures, or writing, may be taught. Far from hindering the development of spoken language, these alternative forms of training frequently result in improvements in verbal skills (De Villiers & Naughton, 1974; Fulwiler & Fouts, 1976; Deich & Hodges, 1977).

Play and imitation. Imitative behaviours are almost invariably impoverished in autistic children. However, by the use of physical prompts and by using activities which are interesting to the child and appropriate to his level of development, rudimentary imitative behaviours (such as clapping or waving, or building simple brick towers or 'Lego' models) may be developed. Similar techniques may also be used to teach the child how to 'play' with, or at least manipulate, dolls, cars, or other toys. Gradually, as the child begins to show simple, spontaneous, imitative or play behaviour, physical prompts may be withdrawn and the complexity of these activities increased (Howlin *et al.*, 1973).

Self-help skills. Skills such as dressing, toileting, feeding, are often delayed in autistic children. Again behavioural techniques, such as prompting and reinforcement, may be used effectively. Yule and Carr (1979) give details of suggested programmes for training children in these skills.

Increasing other skills. The development of specific skills, such as constructional abilities and, later,

reading and writing, is also best taught in a gradual, step-by-step fashion. At first the child's existing skills should be used to encourage his co-operation in simple, relatively low-level tasks (e.g. picture matching or jigsaws). Eventually both the complexity of such tasks should be increased to develop pre-number and pre-reading skills, as well as the amount of time the child will spend on them. The use of these techniques in teaching programmes is fully discussed in Everard (1976).

Decreasing behaviour problems

Social withdrawal. Social withdrawal is frequently a problem in the younger autistic child and is often best dealt with by deliberate, but gentle, intrusion into the child's favourite solitary activities, until he learns to tolerate, and eventually enjoy, adult intervention (Rutter & Sussenwein, 1971; Hemsley & Howlin, 1976).

Disruptive behaviour. Sometimes as children learn to understand and communicate more effectively and learn to develop simple social and constructional skills, disruptive behaviours, such as tantrums or 'hyperactivity' tend to disappear or improve without active intervention. However, in many cases, more direct methods of treatment will still be needed. Consistent reward and encouragement for desirable behaviours (particularly those which are incompatible with the problem behaviours) together with systematic withdrawal of attention or other positive consequences for disruptive activities is generally effective in reducing behaviours such as tantrums, aggression, or destructiveness (Hemsley *et al.*, 1978, Hemsley & Howlin, 1976).

Phobias. Severe phobias are frequent in autism and may range from those that are fairly common even in normal children, such as being frightened of dogs or birds or aeroplanes, to those that are totally inexplicable, perhaps of a particular corner of a radiator, or a certain programme on the radio. In-vivo desensitization techniques, such as those used with normal children, are often rapidly effective in reducing the phobia without causing distress to the child or to his parents (Howlin *et al.*, 1973).

Rituals and obsessions. Obsessional behaviours, rigid attachments to objects, rituals, and resistance to change, are also typical of autistic children and can severely disrupt family life. In such cases a 'graded change' approach, in which children are encouraged to accept minor alterations in their environment or daily routine, has been successfully used. Gradually the amount of change the child is required to tolerate is increased until obsessional and ritualistic behaviours are reduced to a minimum, without distress either to the child or his parents (Marchant, Howlin, Yule & Rutter, 1974).

Self-injury. This is rarely a problem in more intelligent autistic children, but is associated with severe mental subnormality (Bartak & Rutter, 1976; Schroeder, Schroeder, Smith & Dalldorf, 1978). If it is relatively mild, and used mainly to gain attention, it can usually be reduced by systematic withdrawal of attention, together with rewards for alternative behaviours. However, if it is not used as an attention-seeking device, but as a form of self-stimulation, it is a much more intransigent and distressing problem, and may even become a danger to life (Baumeister & Rollings, 1976). Reinforcement of incompatible behaviour often has only transitory effects (Lovaas, Schaeffer & Simmons, 1965). Although more substantial claims have been made for the use of punishment techniques, including severe electric shock (Lichstein & Schreibmann, 1976), the effects are rarely permanent enough to justify such procedures (Frankel & Simmons, 1976). A combination of milder corrective techniques, such as 'over-correction' (Azrin, Kaplan & Foxx, 1973) combined with reinforcement for alternative behaviours has been claimed to be more successful (Measel & Alfieri, 1976). However, the reduction of self-injury is a notoriously difficult task, and for treatment to be effective careful analysis needs to be made of the factors causing and maintaining such behaviour (Maisto, Baumeister & Maisto, 1979).

Problems of education and management

Although the effectiveness of a structured approach to the education and management of autistic children is now well documented, there remain many problems still to be solved.

Problems of generalization. The failure of autistic children to generalize skills learned in one setting to other situations or to other people has been noted in a number of investigations (Frith, 1972; Hermelin, 1972; Koegel & Rincover, 1974; Rincover & Koegel, 1975). Many early studies of behavioural intervention had only limited effects, in that improvements made by the child in a hospital or clinic setting did not persist when the child returned home (Browning, 1971;

Lovaas, Koegel, Simmons & Long, 1973). Only if parents are actively involved in treatment are gains likely to be more permanent. Thus, wherever possible, all those concerned with the child's care should be involved in treatment. A close liaison between teachers and parents is desirable at all times (Hemsley & Howlin, 1976), and in cases where in-patient care is necessary, parents and hospital staff should work closely together. Management programmes can also be adapted to make optimal use of the special skills shown by social workers (Rutter & Sussenwein, 1971) or by occupational therapists, nurses, and others (Murphy *et al.*, 1977).

Individual differences in response to treatment. Autistic children, although handicapped, are nevertheless individuals in their own right, and the problems they show, and their response to treatment can vary considerably. The study by Hemsley and her colleagues (1978), for example, indicated that while all children benefited from programmes designed to improve behaviours, as long as these were adapted to suit the individual child and his home circumstances, fewer children benefited from programmes to develop complex language skills. Verbal training programmes, although successful in many cases, had little effect on children who were severely limited in their production of sounds, their comprehension of speech, and their imaginative ability (Howlin, 1980; Rutter, 1980). For such children, placing the emphasis on comprehension training or alternative, non-verbal, means of communication proved far more valuable.

The treatment and management of autistic children is a demanding and exhausting task and it seems that some children are more likely to benefit from certain programmes than others. If it were possible to predict, in advance, which children were most likely to profit from a particular form of training, much frustration and possible heartbreak might be avoided. In order to do this, however, more controlled studies and reports on the characteristics of children who do *and do not* respond to treatment are needed.

The age at which intervention should begin. The work of Ricks and Wing (1975) and Rutter and his colleagues (1971) on the nature of autism has suggested that it is the cognitive and linguistic impairment which is central to the disorder. Behavioural problems are regarded as being secondary to these so that it might be possible to avoid them if treatment is begun early enough (Rutter, 1974). Unfortunately, intervention studies with very young children are still few in number and, although the work by Hemsley and colleagues (1978) reported rapid improvements in the youngest children in their study, Goldfarb (1974) found a negative correlation between outcome and the age at which intervention began. It is possible, of course, that the age of taking children into treatment is related to severity of impairment and more work is needed on this topic. However, in the absence of conclusive data it would seem advisable, both for the parents' and the children's sake, to begin intervention at as early an age as possible.

Counselling and other techniques

Although this chapter has stressed the value of behaviourally oriented techniques, there remains much to be known about the relative importance of various other aspects of treatment. Whereas a few American studies (Lovaas, 1977) pursue a strictly operant approach to treatment, most other studies involving parents (Hemsley *et al.*, 1978; Schopler & Reichler, 1971) offer much broader help.

The stresses created by a handicapped child can be considerable and counselling of relatives to deal with feelings of guilt or despair or with family and marital difficulties needs to be used in conjunction with behavioural methods. Medical treatment for problems such as depression may be required. Practical advice about schooling, holiday placements, or baby-sitting arrangements is frequently necessary. As yet we do not know the extent to which help in these other areas affects outcome. Simply having someone to discuss problems with and to give suggestions about how to occupy the child constructively may,

for some families, be as important as the use of operant reinforcement techniques. Identifying salient treatment variables remains an outstanding task.

Long-term effects

Finally, to return to the discussion of prognosis, there is the question of how far early intervention at home or school affects eventual outcome. The study of Hemsley and colleagues (1978) showed that the effects of home-based treatment were maintained over eighteen months, but, unfortunately, neither this, nor any other treatment study, has yet followed up children through adolescence or early adulthood. Even for those few who cope well at home and school, the demands of holding down a regular job or leading a relatively independent life frequently prove overwhelming. The social and work problems faced by autistic adolescents still need more detailed investigation and specialized management and training programmes (such as those now offered in some adolescent units) need to be further developed. Because the types of problems shown by autistic children tend to alter with age, it is unlikely that a relatively brief period of intervention in early childhood will generalize to later life. If the outcome is to be improved, skilled and carefully structured management programmes, extending well into adulthood, will probably be required. This is true also of the majority of autistic people who will never be able to hold down a job. Attention paid to decreasing undesirable behaviours and increasing skills improves the quality of life, even in a sheltered environment.

References

Abe, K. (1963) Season fluctuation of psychiatric admissions, based on the data for seven prefectures in Japan for a seven-year period 1955–61, with a review of the literature. *Folia psychiat. neurol. jap.*, **17**, 101–12

Abrams, R. & Taylor, M.A.T. (1976) Mania and schizo-affective disorder, manic type: a comparison. *Am. J. Psychiat.*, **133**, 1445–7

— (1977) Catatonia: Prediction of response to somatic treatments. *Am. J. Psychiat.*, **134**, 78–80

Achtè, K. A. (1967) On the experience gained during the first year of operation of the Haaga Rehabilitation Institute. *Institute of Occupational Health*. No. 66

Ackner, B. (1954) Depersonalization. I. Aetiology and phenomenology. *J. ment. Sci.*, **100**, 838–53

Ackner, B., Harris, A. & Oldham, A. J. (1957) Insulin treatment of schizophrenia. *Lancet*, **ii**, 607–11

Ackner, B. & Oldham, A J. (1972) Insulin treatment of schizophrenia – a three year follow-up of a controlled study. *Lancet*, **ii**, 504–6

Adelstein, A. M., Downham, D. Y., Stein, S. & Susser, M. W. (1968) The epidemiology of mental illness in an English city. *Soc. Psychiat.*, **3**, 47–59

Akiskal, H. S., Djenderedjian, A. H., Rosenthal, R. H. & Khani, M. K. (1977) Cyclothymic disorder: Validating criteria for inclusion in the bipolar affective group. *Am. J. Psychiat.*, **134**, 1227–33

Akiskal, H. S. & McKinney, W. T., Jr. (1975) Overview of recent research in depression: Integration of ten conceptual models into a comprehensive clinical frame. *Arch. gen. Psychiat.*, **32**, 285–305

Akiskal, H. S., Rosenthal, R. H., Rosenthal, T. L., Kashganian, M., Khani, M. K. & Puzantian, V. R. (1979) Differentiation of primary affective illness from situational, symptomatic, and secondary depressions. *Arch. gen. Psychiat.*, **36**, 635–43

Alarcon, R. de & Carney, M. W. P. (1969) Severe depressive mood changes following slow release intramuscular fluphenazine injection. *Brit. med. J.*, **3**, 564–7

Allen, G. & Kallmann, F. J. (1962) Etiology of mental subnormality in twins. In: *Expanding Goals of Genetics in Psychiatry*, ed. Kallmann, F. J. New York: Grune & Stratton

Allers, R. (1920) Über psychogene Störungen in sprachfremder Umgebung. Der Verfolgungswahn der sprachlich Isolierten. *Z. ges. Neurol. Psychiat.*, **60**, 281

Alpern, G. D. (1967) Measurement of untestable autistic children. *J. abnorm. Psychol.*, **73**, 478–96

Altschule, M. (1976) Historical perspective – evolution of the concept of schizophrenia. In *The Biology of the Schizophrenic Process*, ed. Wolf, S. & Berle, B. B., pp. 1–15. New York: Plenum Press

Altshuler, K. Z. & Sarlin, M. B. (1962) Deafness and schizophrenia: interaction of communication stress, maturation lag and schizophrenic risk. In *Expanding Goals of Genetics in Psychiatry*, ed. Kallmann, F. J., pp. 52–62. New York: Grune & Stratton

Ambelas, A. (1979) Psychological stressful events in the precipitation of manic episodes. *Brit. J. Psychiat.*, **135**, 15–21

American Psychiatric Association (1952) *Diagnostic and Statistical Manual of Mental Disorders*. 3rd ed. (1980) Washington: American Psychiatric Association

Anastasi, A. (1968) *Psychology Testing*. 3rd ed. New York: Macmillan

Andreason, N. (1979) *Cluster Analysis and the Classification of Depression*. Presented at American College of Neuropharmacology, Puerto Rico, December, 1979

Andreason, N. J. C. & Powers, P. S. (1974) Overinclusive thinking in mania and schizophrenia. *Brit. J. Psychiat.*, **125**, 452–56

Andrews, G. & Tennant, C. (1978) Being upset and becoming ill: an appraisal of the relation between life events and physical illness. *Med. J. Aust.*, **1**, 324–7

Angrist, B., Gershon, S., Sathananthan, G., Walker, R. W., Lopez-Ramos, B., Mandel, L. R. & Vandenheuvel, W. J. A. (1976) Dimethyltryptamine levels in blood of schizophrenic patients and control subjects. *Psychoparmacol.*, **47**, 29–32

Angst, J. (1966) Zur Ätiologie und Nosologie endogener depressiver psychosen. *Monographien aus der Neurologie und Psychiatrie*, No. 112, pp. 1–118. Berlin: Springer

— (1980) Verlauf unipolar depressiver, bipolar manisch-depressiver und schizoaffektiver Erkrankungen und Psychosen. Ergebnisse einer prospektiven Studie. *Fortschr. Neurol. Psychiat. Grenzgeb.*, **48**, 3–30

Angst, J., Baastrup, P., Grof. P., Hippius, H., Poldinger, W. & Weis, P. (1973) The course of monopolar and bipolar psychoses. *Psychiat. Neurol. Neurochirurg.*, **76**, 489–500

Anon. (1979) Manic states in affective disorders of childhood and adolescence. *Brit. med. J.*, **1**, 214–15.

Anthony, E. J. (1958a) An etiological approach to the diagnosis of psychosis in childhood. *Rev. Psychiat. infant.*, **25**, 89–96

— (1958b) An experimental approach to the psychopathology of childhood autism. *Brit. J. med. Psychol.*, **21**, 211–25

Anthony E. J. & Scott P. D. (1960) Manic-depressive psychosis in childhood. *J. child Psychol. Psychiat.*, **1**, 53–72

Anton, G. (1899) Über die Selbstwahrnehmung der Herderkrankungen des Gehirns durch den Kranken bei Rindenblindheit und Rindentaubheit. *Arch. Psychiat. Nervenkr.*, **32**, 86

Asarnow, R. F., Steffy, R. A., MacCrimmon, D. J. & Cleghorn, J. M. (1977) An attentional assessment of foster children at risk for schizophrenia. *J. abnorm. Psychol.*, **86**, 267–75

Åsberg, M., Thóren, P., Träskman, L., Bertilsson, L. & Ringberger, N. (1976) Serotonin depression – a biochemical subgroup within the affective disorders. *Science*, **191**, 478

Ashcroft, G. W., Blackburn, I. M., Eccleston, D., Glen, A. I. M., Hartley, W., Kinlock, N. E., Lonorgan, M., Murray, L. G. & Pullar, I. A. (1973a) Changes on recovery in the concentration of tryptophan and the biogenic amine metabolites in the cerebrospinal fluid of patients with affective illness. *Psychol. Med.*, **3**, 319–25

Ashcroft, G. W., Crawford, T. B. B., Cundall, R. L., Davidson, D. L., Dobson, J., Dow, R. C., Eccleston, D., Loose, R. W. & Pullar, I. A. (1973b) 5-Hydroxytryptamine metabolism in affective illness. The effect of tryptophan administration. *Psychol. Med.*, **3**, 326–32

Ashcroft, G. W., Crawford, T. B. B., Eccleston, D., Sharman, D. F., MacDougall, E. J., Stanton, J. B. & Binns, J. F. (1966) 5-Hydroxyindole compounds in the cerebrospinal fluid of patients with psychiatric or neurological disease. *Lancet*, **ii**, 1049

Ashcroft, G. W., Dow, R. C., Yates, C. M. & Pullar, I. A. (1974) Significance of lumbar c.s.f. metabolic measurements in affective illness. *Proc. Vlth. Int. Congress Pharmacol.*, ed. Tuomisto, J. & Paasonen, M. K. **3**, 277–84

Ashcroft, G. W., Eccleston, D., Murray, I. G., Glen, A. I. M., Crawford, T. B. B., Pullar, I. A., Shields, P. J., Walter, D. S., Blackburn, I. M., Connechan, P. J. & Walter, D. A. (1972) Modified amine hypothesis for the aetiology of affective illness. *Lancet*, **i**, 573–7

Asni, C., Leopold, M., Duvoisin, R. & Schwartz, A. (1977) A survey of tardive dyskinesia in psychiatric outpatients. *Am. J. Psychiat.*, **134**, 1367–70

Asperger, H. (1944) Die autistischen Psychopathen im Kindesalter. *Arch. Psychiat. Nervenkr.*, **117**, 76–137

Astrup, C., Fossum, A. & Holmboe, R. (1959) A follow-up study of 270 patients with acute affective psychoses. *Acta psychiat. neurol. scand.*, Supp. 135.

Astrup, C. & Noreik, K. (1966) *Functional Psychoses – Diagnostic and Prognostic Models*. Springfield, Illinois: Charles C. Thomas

Ayd, F. J. (1978) Intravenous haloperidol therapy. In *Internat. Drug Therapy Newsletter*. Baltimore, USA: Ayd Publications

Aylward, M. (1973) Plasma tryptophan levels and mental depression in postmenopausal subjects. Effects of oral piperazine-oestrone sulphate. *I. R. C. S. med. J.*, **1**, 30

Azrin, N. H., Kaplan, S. J. & Foxx, R. M. (1973) Autism-reversal: eliminating stereotyped self-stimulation in retarded individuals. *Am. J. ment. Defic.*, **78**, 241–8

Babigian, H. M. (1975) Schizophrenia: epidemiology. In *Comprehensive Textbook of Psychiatry*, ed. Freedman, A. M., Kaplan, K. I. & Sadock, B. J., 2nd ed., vol. I. Baltimore: Williams & Wilkins

Baer, L., Durell, J., Bunney, W. E., Murphy, D., Levy, B. S., Greenspan, K. Cardon, P. V. (1970) Sodium balance and distribution in lithium carbonate therapy. *Arch. gen. Psychiat.*, **22**, 40–44

Bagley, C. (1973) Occupational class and symptoms of depression. *Soc. Sci. Med.*, **7**, 327–39

Bagley, C. (1973) Social policy and the prevention of suicidal behaviour. *Brit. J. soc. Work*, **3**, 473–95

Baldwin, J. A. (1979) Schizophrenia and physical disease. *Psychol. Med.*, **9**, 611–18

Baltaxe, C. A. M. (1977) Pragmatic deficits in the language of autistic adolescents. *J. pediat. Psychol.* **2**, 176–80

Baltaxe, C. A. M. & Simmons, J. Q. (1975) Language in childhood psychosis: a review. *J. Speech Hear. Disord.*, **40**, 439–58

Bancroft, J. H. J., Skrimshire, A. M., Reynolds, F., Simkin, S. & Smith, J. (1975) Self-poisoning and self-injury in the Oxford area: epidemiological aspects 1969–73. *Brit. J. Prev. soc. Med.*, **19**, 170–77

Bancroft, J., Skrimshire, A., Casson, J., Harvard-Watts, O. & Reynolds, F. (1977) People who deliberately poison or injure themselves: their problems and their contacts with helping agencies. *Psychol. Med.*, **7**, 289–303

Bannister, D. (1968) The logical requirements of research into schizophrenia. *Brit. J. Psychiat.*, **114**, 181–8

Barker, D. J. P. & Rose, G. (1976) *Epidemiology in Medical Practice*. London: Churchill Livingstone

Baron, M. (1977) Linkage between an X-chromosome marker (deutan color blindness) and bipolar affective illness. *Arch. gen. Psychiat.*, **34**, 721–5

Barraclough, B. M. (1972) Suicide prevention, recurrent affective disorder and Lithium. *Brit. J. Psychiat.*, **121**, 391–2

— (1973) Differences between national suicide rates. *Brit. J. Psychiat.*, **122**, 95–6

Barraclough, B., Bunch, J., Nelson, B. & Sainsbury, P. (1974) A hundred cases of suicide: clinical aspects. *Brit. J. Psychiat.*, **125**, 355–73

Barraclough, B., Nelson, B., Bunch, J. & Sainsbury, P. (1971) Suicide and barbiturates prescribing. *J. R. Coll. gen. Pract.*, **21**, 645–53

Barraclough, B. M. & Pallis, D. J. (1975) Depression followed by suicide: a comparison of depressed suicides with living depressives. *Psychol.* **5**, 55–61

Barry, R. J. & James, A. C. (1978) Handedness in autistics, retardates and normals of a wide age range. *J. Autism child. Schiz.*, **8**, 315–24

Bartak, L. & Rutter, M. (1973) Special educational treatment of autistic children: a comparative study: I. Design of study and characteristics of units. *J. child Psychol. Psychiat.*, **14**, 161–79

— (1976) Differences between mentally retarded and normally intelligent autistic children. *J. Autism child. Schiz.*, **6**, 109–20

Bartak, L., Rutter, M. & Cox, A. (1975) A comparative study of infantile autism and specific developmental receptive language disorder: I. The children. *Brit. J. Psychiat.*, **126**, 127–45

— (1977) A comparative study of infantile autism and specific developmental receptive language disorder III: Discriminant function analysis. *J. Autism child. Schiz.* **6**, 297–302

Barton, R. (1959) *Institutional Neurosis*. Bristol: Wright

Bates, E. (1976) *Language and Context: The Acquisition of Pragmatics*. New York: Academic Press

Bateson, G., Jackson, D., Haley, J. & Weakland, J. (1956) Toward a theory of schizophrenia. *Behav. Sci.*, **1**, 251

Batt, J. C. (1948) Homicidal incidence in the depressive psychoses. *J. ment. Sci.*, **94**, 782–92

Bauman, E. (1971) Schizophrenic short-term memory: A deficit in subjective organization. *Can. J. Behav. Sci.*, **3**, 55–65

Bauman, E. & Murray, D. J. (1968) Recognition versus recall in schizophrenia. *Can. J. Psychol.* **22**, 18–25

Baumeister, A. A. & Rollings, J. P. (1976) Self injurious behavior. In *International Review of Research in Mental Retardation*, vol. 8. New York: Academic Press

Bayley, N. (1969) *Bayley Scales of Infant Development*. New York: The Psychological Corporation

Bebbington, P. E. (1978) The epidemiology of depressive disorder. *Culture, Med. Psychiat.*, **3**, 297–341

Beck, A. T. (1976) *Cognitive Therapy and the Emotional Disorders*. New York: International Universities Press

Becker, R. E. & Shaskan, E. G. (1977) Platelet monoamine oxidase activity in schizophrenic patients. *Am. J. Psychiat.*, **134**, 512–17

Beckman, L., Perris, C., Standman, E. & Wahlby, L. (1978) HLA antigens and affective disorders. *Hum. Hered.*, **28**, 96–9

Beigel A. & Murphy, D. L. (1971) Unipolar and bipolar affective illness: differences in clinical characteristics accompanying depression. *Arch. gen. Psychiat.*, **24**, 215–20

Belknap, I. (1956) *Human Problems of a State Mental Hospital*. New York: McGraw Hill

Bell, R. Q. (1968) A reinterpretation of the direction of effects in studies of socialisation. *Psychol. Rev.*, **75**, 81–95

— (1971) Stimulus control of parent or caretaker behaviour by offspring. *Dev. Psychol.*, **4**, 63–72

Bellissimo, A. & Steffy, R. A. (1975) Redundancy-associated deficit in schizophrenic reaction time performance. *J. abnorm. Psychol.*, **80**, 299–307

Bender, L. (1947) Childhood schizophrenia: clinical study of 100 schizophrenic children. *Amer. J. Ortho-psychiat.*, **17**, 40–56

— (1961) The brain and child behaviour. *Arch. gen. Psychiat.*, **4**, 531–47

Bender, L. & Sankar, D. V. S. (1968) Chromosome damage not found in leukocytes of children treated with LSD-25. *Science*, **159**, 749

Bennahum, D., Troup, G., Rada, R., Kellner, R. & Kyner, W. (1976) The histocompatibility antigens of schizophrenic and manic-depressive patients. Unpublished data cited in Gershon *et al.*, Genetic studies and biologic strategies in the affective disorders. *Prog. med. Genet.*, **2**, 101–64

Bennett, D. H. (1975) Techniques of industrial therapy, ergotherapy and recreative methods. In *Psychiatrie der Gegenwart*, vol. III, ed. Kisker, K. P., Meyer, J. -E., Müller, C. & Strömgren, E. Heidelberg: Springer

— (1978) Social forms of psychiatric treatment. In *Schizophrenia: Towards a New Synthesis*, ed. Wing, J. K., chap. 9, pp. 211–31. London: Academic Press

Bennett, J. P., Enna, S. J., Bylund, D. B., Gillin, J. C., Wyatt, R. J. & Snyder, S. H. (1979) Neurotransmitter receptors in frontal cortex of schizophrenics. *Arch. gen. Psychiat.*, **36**, 927–34

Berger, M. (1970) The third revision of the Stanford-Binet (form L–M): some methodological limitations and their practical implication. *Bull. Brit. psychol. Soc.*, **23**, 17–26

Berger, M. & Yule, W. (1972) Cognitive assessment in young children with language delay. In *The Child with Delayed Speech. Clin. dev. Med.* no. 43, ed. Rutter, M. & Martin, J. A. M., pp. 120–35. London: Heinemann

Berner, P. (1972) Paranoide Syndrome. In *Psychiatrie der Gegenwart*, II/1, ed. Kisker, P. K., Meyer, J.-E., Müller, C. & Strömgren, E., pp. 175–6. Berlin: Springer Verlag.

Bernhardson, G. & Gunne, L.-M. (1972) Forty-six cases of psychosis in cannabis abusers. *Int. J. Addict.*, **7**, 9–16

Bernstein, A. S. (1964) The galvanic skin response orienting response among chronic schizophrenics. *Psychonomic Sci.*, **1**, 391–2

— (1970) Phasic electrodermal orienting response in chronic schizophrenics. *J. abnorm. Psychol.*, **75**, 145–56

Bernstein, S. & Kaufman, M. R. (1960) A psychological analysis of apparent depression following Rauwolfin Therapy. *J. Mt. Sinai Hosp.*, **27**, 525–30

Bertelson, A., Harvald, B. & Hauge, M. (1977) A Danish twin study of manic-depressive disorders. *Brit. J. Psychiat.*, **130**, 330–51

Bhrolcháin, M., Brown, G. W. & Harris, T. (1979) Psychotic and neurotic depression: 2. clinical characteristics. *Brit. J. Psychiat.*, **134**, 94–107

Bird, E. D., Spokes, E. G. S. & Iversen, L. L. (1979) Increased dopamine concentration in limbic areas of brain from patients dying with schizophrenia. *Brain*, **102**, 347–60

Birley, J. L. T. & Brown, G. W. (1970) Crises and life changes preceding the onset and relapse of acute schizophrenia: clinical aspects. *Brit. J. Psychiat.*, **116**, 327–33

Birtchnell, J. (1970) Depression in relation to early and recent parent death. *Brit. J. Psychiat.*, **116**, 299–306

— (1972) Birth order and mental illness – a control study. *Soc. Psychiat.*, **7**, 167

Birtchnell, J. & Grad de Alarcon, J. (1971) Depression and attempted suicide: a study of 91 cases seen in a casualty department. *Brit. J. Psychiat.*, **118**, 289–96

Blackburn, I. M. (1975) Mental and psychomotor speed in depression and mania. *Brit. J. Psychiat.*, **126**, 329–35

Bleuler, E. (1908) Die Prognose der Dementia praecox (Schizophreniegruppe). *Allg. Z. Psychiat. Psychischgerichtl. Med.*, **56**, 436

— (1911) *Dementia praecox oder Gruppe der Schizophrenien*. Wien: Deuticke. (English translation, 1950: *Dementia praecox or the groups of schizophrenias*. New York: International Universities Press)

Bleuler, M. (1972) *Die schizophrenen Geistesstörungen im Lichte langjähriger Kranken- und Familiengeschichten*. Stuttgart: G. Thieme (Trans. Clemens, S. M., 1978: *The Schizophrenic Disorders: Long-term Patient and Family Studies*. New Haven: Yale University Press)

— (1978) The long-term course of schizophrenic psychoses. In *The Nature of Schizophrenia*, ed. Wynne, L. C., Cromwell, R. L. & Matthysse, S. New York: Wiley

Bloom, L. & Lahey, M. (1978) *Language Development and Language Disorders*. New York: Wiley

Bockoven, J. S. (1956) Moral treatment in American psychiatry. *J. nerv. ment. Dis.*, **124**, 167–94 and 292–321

Bonhoff, G. & Lewrenz, H. (1954) Über Weckamine (Pervitin und Benzedrin). Berlin, Göttingen & Heidelberg: Springer

Böök, J. A. (1953) A genetic and neuropsychiatric investigation of a North Swedish population. *Acta. genet.*, **4**, 345–414

Böök, J. A., Nichtern, G. & Gruenberg, F. (1963) Cytogenetical investigations in childhood schizophrenia. *Acta psychiat. scand.*, **39**, 309–23

Böök, J. A., Wetterbergh, L., Modrzewska, K. & Unge, C. (1978) Schizophrenia in a north Swedish population 1900–75. *Clin. Genet.*, **13**, 110

Boucher, J. (1976) Articulation in early childhood autism. *J. Autism child. Schizophrenia*, **6**, 297–302

— (1977) Alternation and sequencing behaviour and response to novelty in autistic children. *J. child Psychol. Psychiat.*, **18**, 67–72

— (1978) Echoic memory capacity in autistic children. *J. child Psychol. Psychiat.*, **19**, 161–6

Boucher, J. & Warrington, E. K., (1976) Memory deficits in early infantile autism: some similarities to the amnesic syndrome. *Brit. J. Psychol.*, **67**, 73–87

Bourne, H. R., Bunney, W. E., Coburn, R. W., Davis, J. M., Davis, J. N., Shaw, D. M. & Coppen, A. (1968) Noradrenaline, 5-hydroxytryptamine and 5-hydroxyindolacetic acid in the hind brains of suicidal patients. *Lancet*, **ii**, 805

Bowdan, N. D. (1977) Hyperactivity or affective illness. *Am. J. Psychiat.*, **134**, 329

Bowers, M. B. (1974) Central dopamine turnover in schizophrenic syndromes. *Arch. gen. Psychiat.*, **31**, 50–54

Bowers, M. & Astrachan, B. (1967) Depression in acute schizophrenic patients. *Am. J. Psychiat.*, **123**, 976–9

Bowers, M. B., Heninger, G. R. & Gerbode, F. (1969) Cerebrospinal fluid 5-hydroxyindolacetic acid and homovanillic acid in psychiatric patients. *Int. J. Neuropharmacol.*, **8**, 255

Brask, B. H. (1967) On behovet for hospitalspladser til psykotiske børn. *Ugeskrift for Laeger*, **129**, 1559–70

— (1972) A prevalence investigation of childhood psychoses. In *Nordic Symposium on the Comprehensive Care of Psychotic Children*, pp. 145–55. Oslo: Barnepsykiatrist Forening

Bratfos, C. & Haug, J. O. (1968) The course of manic depressive psychoses: A follow-up investigation of 215 patients. *Acta psychiat. scand.*, **44**, 89–112

Brawley, E. R., Harris, F. R., Allen, K. E., Fleming, R. S. & Peterson, R. F. (1969) Behavior modification of an autistic child. *Behav. Sci.*, **14**, 87–97

Breakey, W. R. & Goodell, H. (1972) Thought disorder in mania and schizophrenia evaluated by Bannister's grid test for schizophrenic thought disorder. *Brit. J. Psychiat.*, **120**, 391–5

Brenner, M. H. (1973) *Mental Illness and the Economy*. Cambridge, Mass.: Harvard University Press

Brezinova, V. & Kendell, R. E. (1977) Smooth pursuit eye movements of schizophrenics and normal people under stress. *Brit. J. Psychiat.*, **130**, 59–63

Bricker, D., Bricker, W. A. & Larsen, L. A. (1968) *Operant Audiometry for Difficult to Test Children*. Papers and Reports, vol. 5, No. 19. Nashville, Tennessee: Institute on Mental Retardation and Intellectual Development

Bridges, P. K. & Bartlett, J. R. (1977) Psychosurgery: yesterday and today. *Brit. J. Psychiat.*, **131**, 249–60

Brill, N. O., Crumpton, E., Eiduson, S., Grayson, H., Hellman, L. I. & Richards, R. A. (1959) Relative effectiveness of various components of electroconvulsive therapy. *Arch. Neurol. Psychiat.*, **81**, 627–35

Brimer, M. A. & Dunn, L. M. (1966) *English Picture Vocabulary Test*, 2nd ed. Windsor: National Foundation for Educational Research

Briscoe, C. W. & Smith, M. D. (1973) Depression and marital turmoil. *Arch. gen. Psychiat.*, **29**, 812–17

Broadbent, D. E. (1958) *Perception and Communication*. London: Pergamon Press

Brockington, I. F., Kendell, R. E., Kellett, J. M., Curry, J. H. & Wainwright, S. (1978a) Trial of lithium, chlorpromazine and amitryptyline in schizo-affective patients. *Brit. J. Psychiat.*, **133**, 662–8

Brockington, I. F., Kendell, R. E. & Leff, J. P. (1978b) Definitions of schizophrenia: concordance and prediction of outcome. *Psychol. Med.*, **8**, 387–98

Brockington, I. F. & Leff, J. P. (1979) Schizo-affective psychosis: definitions and incidence. *Psychol. Med.*, **9**, 91–9

Brodwall, O. (1947) The course of the manic depressive psychosis. *Acta psychiat. neurol. scand.*, **22**, 195–210

Broen, W. E. & Storms, L. H. (1966) Lawful disorganization: The process underlying a schizophrenic syndrome. *Psychol. Rev.*, **74**, 265–79

Brown, G. W. (1959) Social factors influencing length of hospital stay of schizophrenic patients. *Brit. med. J.*, **2**, 1300–2

Brown, G. W., Bhrolcháin, M. & Harris, T. O. (1975) Social class and psychiatric disturbance among women in an urban population. *Sociology*, **9**, 225–54

Brown, G. W. & Birley, J. L. T. (1968) Crisis and life changes and the onset of schizophrenia. *J. Health hum. Behav.*, **9**, 203–14

Brown, G. W., Birley, J. L. T. & Wing, J. K. (1972) Influence of family life on the course of schizophrenic disorders: a replication. *Brit. J. Psychiat.*, **121**, 241–58

Brown, G. W., Bone. M., Dalison, B. & Wing, J. K. (1966) *Schizophrenia and Social Care*. Maudsley Monograph No. 17. London: Oxford University Press

Brown, G. W., Davidson, S., Harris, T., Maclean, U., Pollock, S. & Prudo, R. (1977) Psychiatric disorder in London and N. Uist. *Soc. Sci. Med.*, **11**, 367–77

Brown, G. W. & Harris, T. O. (1978) *Social Origins of Depression: A Study of Psychiatric Disorder in Women*. London: Tavistock Publications

Brown, G. W., Monck, E., Carstairs, G. M. & Wing, J. K. (1962) Influences of family life on the course of schizophrenic illness. *Brit. J. prev. soc. Med.*, **16**, 55–68

Brown, G. W. & Rutter, M. (1966) The measurement of family activities and relationships: a methodological study. *Hum. Relations*, **19**, 241–63

Brown, W. A., Johnston, R. & Mayfield, D. (1979) The 24-hour Dexamethasone Suppression Test in a clinical setting: relationship to diagnosis, symptoms, and response to treatment. *Am. J. Psychiat.*, **136**, 543–7

Browning, R. M. (1971) Treatment effects of a total behavior modification program with five autistic children. *Behav. Res. Ther.*, **9**, 319–28

Brumback, R. A. & Weinberg, W. A. (1977) Mania in childhood. II. Therapeutic trial of lithium carbonate and further description of manic-depressive illness in children. *Am. J. Dis. Children*, **131**, 1122–6

Bucher, K. & Elston, R. C. (1980a) The transmission of manic-depressive illness. I. Theory, description of the model, and summary of results. *J. Psychiat. Res.* **16**, 53–63

Bucher, K. & Elston, R. C., Helzer, J. & Winokur, G. (1980b) The transmission of manic-depressive illness. II. Segregation analysis of three sets of family data. *J. Psychiat. Res.* **16**, 65–70

Buchsbaum, M. S. & Haier, P. J. (1978) Biological homogeneity, symptom heterogeneity and the diagnosis of schizophrenia. *Schiz. Bull.*, **4**, 473–75

Buchsbaum, M. S., Murphy, D. L., Coursey, R. D., Lahe, C. R. & Zeigler, M. G. (1978) Platelet monoamine oxidase, plasma dopamine-beta-hydroxylase and attention in a "biochemical high risk" sample. *J. psychiat. Res.*, **14**, 215–24

Buck, C. & Simpson, H. (1978) Season of birth among the sibs of schizophrenics. *Brit. J. Psychiat.*, **133**, 358–60

Bulmer, M. G. (1970) *The Biology of Twinning in Man*. Oxford: Clarendon Press

Bunch, J., Barraclough, B., Nelson, B. & Sainsbury, P. (1971) Suicide following bereavement of parents. *Soc. Psychiat.*, **6**, 193–9

Bunney, W. E., Fawcett, J. A., Davis, J. M. & Gifford, S. (1969) Further evaluation of urinary 17-hydroxycorticosteroids in suicidal patients. *Arch. gen. Psychiat.* **21**, 138–50

Bunney, W. E., Mason, J. W. & Hanbury, D. A. (1965) Correlation between behavioural variables and urinary 17-hydroxycorticosteroids in depressed patients. *Psychosom. Med.*, **27**, 299–308

Burgemeister, B. B., Hollander Blum, L. & Lorge, I. (1972) *Columbia Mental Maturity Scale*. 3rd ed. New York: Harcourt Brace Jovanovich

Burke, L., Deykin, E., Jacobson, S. & Haley, S. (1967) The depressed woman returns. *Arch. gen. Psychiat.* **16**, 548–53

Butcher, H. J. (1968) *Human Intelligence – Its Nature and Assessment*. London: Methuen

Butler, P. W. P. & Besser, G. M. (1968) Pituitary-adrenal function in severe depressive illness. *Lancet*, **ii**, 1234–6

Butterworth, A. T. (1962) Inhibition of extrapyramidal side effects of haloperidol through the joint use of imipramine-type drugs. *Psychosomatics*, **13**, 328–32

Cade, J. P. (1964) A significant elevation of plasma magnesium levels in schizophrenia and depressive states. *Med. J. Aust.*, **1**, 195–200

Cadoret, R. (1978) Evidence for genetic inheritance of primary affective disorder in adoptees. *Am. J. Psychiat.*, **135**, 463–6

Caffey, E. M., Diamond, L. S., Frank, T. V., Grasberger, J. C., Herman, L., Klett, C. J. & Rothstein, R. (1964) Discontinuation or reduction of chemotherapy in chronic schizophrenics. *J. chron. Dis.*, **17**, 347–58

Cairns, H. S. & Cairns, C. E. (1976) *Psycholinguistics: A Cognitive View of Language*. New York: Holt, Rinehart & Winston

Cambell, M. (1973) Biological interventions in psychoses of childhood. *J. Autism child. Schiz.*, **3**, 347–73

Cantwell, D., Howlin, P. & Rutter, M. (1977) The analysis of language level and language function: a methodological study. *Brit. J. Disord. Commun.*, **12**, 119–35

Carenzi, A., Gillin, J. C., Guidotti, A., Schwartz, M. A., Trabucchi, M. & Wyatt, R. J. (1975) Dopamine-sensitive adenyl cyclase in human caudate nucleus. A study in control subjects and schizophrenic patients. *Arch. gen. Psychiat.*, **32**, 1056–9

Carlson, G. A., Davenport, Y. B. & Jamison, K. (1977) A comparison of outcome in adolescent and late-onset bipolar manic depressive illness. *Am. J. Psychiat.* **134**, 919–22

Carlson, G. A. & Goodwin, F. K. (1973) The stages of mania. *Arch. gen. Psychiat.* **28**, 221–8

Carlson, G. A., Kotin, J., Davenport, Y. B. & Adland, M. (1974) Follow-up of 53 bipolar manic-depressive patients. *Brit. J. Psychiat.* **124**, 134–9

Carney, M. W. P., Roth, M. & Garside, R. F. (1965) The diagnosis of depressive syndromes and the prediction of E.C.T. response. *Brit. J. Psychiat.* **111**, 659–74

Carothers, J. C. (1947) A study of mental derangement in Africans. *J. ment. Sci.*, **93**, 548–97

Carpenter, M. D. (1976) Sensitivity to syntactic structure: Good versus poor premorbid schizophrenics. *J. abnorm. Psychol.*, **85**, 41–50

Carpenter, W. T., Fink, E. G., Narasimhachari, N. & Himwich, H. E. (1975) A test of the transmethylation hypothesis in acute schizophrenic patients. *Am. J. Psychiat.*, **132**, 1067–71

Carr, J. (1976) The severely retarded autistic child. In *Early Childhood Autism*, ed. Wing, L. 2nd ed., pp. 247–70. Oxford: Pergamon Press

Carroll, B. J., Curtis, G. C. & Mendels, J. (1976) Neuroendocrine regulation in depression. I. Limbic system adrenocortical dysfunction. *Arch. gen. Psychiat.*, **33**, 1039–44

— (1976) Neuroendocrine regulation in depression. II. Discrimination of depressed from non-depressed patients. *Arch. gen. Psychiat.*, **33**, 1051–8

Carroll, B. J. & Davies, B. (1970) Clinical associations of 11-hydroxycorticosteroid suppression and non-suppression in severe depressive illnesses. *Brit. med. J.*, **1**, 780–91

Carroll, B. J., Greder, J. F., Rubin, R. T., Haskett, E., Feinberg, M.

& Schteingart, D. (1978) Neurotransmitter mechanism of neuroendocrine disturbance in depression. *Acta endocrinol.*, Supp. 220, 14

Carroll, B. J., Stevern, L., Pope, R. A. & Davies, B. (1969) Sodium transfer from plasma to CSF in severe depressive illness. *Arch. gen. Psychiat.*, **21**, 77–81

Casey, J. F., Hollister, C. J., Klett, C. J., Lasky, J. J. & Caffey, E. M. (1961) Combined drug therapy of chronic schizophrenics. Controlled evaluation of placebo dextroamphetamine, Trimipramine, isocarboxazid and trifluoperazine added to maintenance doses of chlorpromazine. *Am. J. Psychiat.*, **117**, 997–1003

Caspar, R. C., Davis, J. M., Pandey, G. N., Garver, D. L. & DeKirmenjian, H. (1977) Neuroendocrine and amine studies in affective illness. *Psychoneuroendocrinology*, **2**, 105–14

Chapman, J. (1966) The early symptoms of schizophrenia. *Brit. J. Psychiat.*, **112**, 225–51

Charington, M. (1970) Parkinsonism, L-Dopa and mental depression. *J. Am. geriat. Soc.*, **18**, 513

Checkley. S. A. (1979) Corticosteroid and growth hormone responses to methylamphetamine in depressive illness. *Psychol. Med.*, **9**, 107–16

Checkley, S. A., Murray, R. M., Oon, M. C. H., Rodnight, R. & Birley, J. L. T. (1980). A longitudinal study of the excretion of N,N-dimethyltryptamine in patients with psychotic illness. *Brit. J. Psychiat.*, **137**, 236–9

Checkley, S., Oon, M. C. H., Rodnight, R., Murphy, M. P., Williams, R. S. & Birley, J. L. T. (1979) Urinary excretion of dimethyltryptamine in liver disease. *Am. J. Psychiat.*, **136**, 439–41

Chen, C.-N. (1979) Sleep, depression and antidepressants. *Brit. J. Psychiat.*, **135**, 385–402

Chess, S. (1971) Autism in children with congenital rubella. *J. Autism child. Schiz.*, **1**, 33–47

— (1977) Follow-up report on autism in congenital rubella. *J. Autism child. Schiz.*, **7**, 69–81

Chess, S., Korn, S. H. & Fernandez, P. B. (1971) *Psychiatric Disorders of Children with Congenital Rubella*. New York: Brunner/Mazel

Childers, R. T. (1961) Comparison of four regimes in newly admitted female schizophrenics. *Am. J. Psychiat.*, **120**, 1010–11

Chomsky, N. (1957) *Syntactic Structures*. The Hague: Mouton

— (1965) *Aspects of the Theory of Syntax*. Cambridge, Mass.: MIT Press

Churchill, D. W. (1971) Effects of success and failure in psychotic children. *Arch. gen. Psychiat.*, **25**, 182–97

— (1972) The relation of infantile autism and early childhood schizophrenia to developmental language disorders of childhood. *J. Autism child. Schiz.*, **2**, 182–97

— (1978) *Language of Autistic Children*. New York: Wiley

Clark, H. H. (1971) The importance of linguistics for the study of speech hesitations. In *The Perception of Language*, ed. Horton & Jenkins. Columbus, Ohio: Charles Merrill

Clark, P. & Rutter, M. (1977) Compliance and resistance in autistic children. *J. Autism child. Schiz.*, **7**, 33–48

Clarke, A. M. & Clarke, A. D. B. (1976a) (Ed.) *Early Experience: Myth and Evidence*. London: Open Books

— (1976b) Formerly isolated children. In *Early Experience: Myth and Evidence*, ed. Clarke, A. M. & Clarke, A. D. B., pp. 27–34. London: Open Books

Clayton, P. J., Halikas, J. A. & Maurice, W. L. (1972) The depression of widowhood. *Brit. J. Psychiat.*, **120**, 71–8

Clayton, P. J., Rodin, L. & Winokur, G. (1968) Family history studies. III. Schizoaffective disorder, clinical and genetic factors including a one to two year follow-up. *Compr. Psychiatry*, **9**, 31–49

Clérambault, G. de (1942) Automatisme mental et psychoses hallucinatoires chroniques. *Oeuvre Psychiat.*, pp. 455–656. Paris: Le François

Cloninger, C. R., Christiansen, K. O., Reich, T. & Gottesman, I. (1978) Implications of sex differences in prevalences of antisocial personality, alcoholism, and criminality for familial transmission. *Arch. Gen. Psychiat.*, **35**, 941–51

Cloninger, C. R., Rice, J. & Reich, T. (1979a) Multifactorial inheritance with cultural transmission and assortative mating. II. A general model of combined polygenic and cultural inheritance. *Am. J. Hum. Genet.*, **31**, 176–98

— (1979b) Multifactorial inheritance with cultural transmission and assortative mating. III. Family structure and the analysis of separation experiments. *Am. J. hum. Genet.*, **31**, 366–88

Cloninger, C. R., Reich, T. & Wetzel, R. (1979c) Alcoholism and the affective disorders: familial association and genetic models. In *Alcoholism and the Affective Disorders*, ed. Goodwin, D. & Erickson, C., pp. 57–86. New York: Spectrum Press

Cobb, S. (1976) Social support as a moderator of life stress. *Psychosom. Med.*, **38**, 300–14

Cochrane, N. & Nielson, M. (1977) Depressive illness: the role of aggression further considered. *Psychol. Med.*, **7**, 283–8

Cochrane, R. (1977) Mental illness in immigrants to England and Wales: an analysis of mental hospital admissions 1971. *Soc. Psychiat.*, **12**, 25–35

Cohen, B. D. & Camhi, J. (1967) Schizophrenic performance in a work-communication task. *J. abnorm. Psychol.*, **72**, 240–6

Cohen, B. D., Nachmani, G. & Rosenberg, S. (1974) Referent communication disturbances in acute schizophrenia. *J. abnorm. Psychol.*, **83**, 1–13

Cohen, D. J., Caparulo, B. K., Gold, J. R., Waldo, M. C., Shaywitz, B. A., Ruttenberg, B. A. & Rimland, B. (1978) Agreement in diagnosis: clinical assessment and behavior rating scales for pervasively disturbed children. *J. Am. Acad. child Psychiat.*, **17**, 589–603

Cohen, D. J., Caparulo, B. K., Shaywitz, B. A. & Bowers, M. B., Jr. (1977) Dopamine and serotonin metabolism in neuropsychiatrically disturbed children. *Arch. gen. Psychiat.*, **34**, 545–50

Cohen, D. J. & Johnson, W. T. (1977) Cardiosvascular correlates of attention in normal and psychiatrically disturbed children. *Arch. gen. Psychiat.*, **34**, 561–7

Cohen, D. J., Shaywitz, B. A., Johnson, W. T. & Bowers, M. B., Jr. (1974) Biogenic amines in autistic and atypical children: Cerebrospinal fluid measures of homovanillic acid and 5-hydroxyindoleacetic acid. *Arch. Gen. Psychiat.*, **31**, 845–53

Cohen, D. J., Shaywitz, B. A., Young, J. G. & Bowers, M. B., Jr. (1980) Cerebrospinal fluid monoamine metabolites in neuropsychiatric disorders of childhood. In *Neurobiology of Cerebrospinal Fluid*, ed. Wood, J. New York: Plenum Publishing

Cohen, D. J., Young, J. G. & Roth, J. A. (1977) Platelet monoamine oxidase in early childhood autism. *Arch. gen. Psychiat.*, **34**, 534–7

Cole, J., Klerman, C. L. & Goldberg, S. C. (1964) Phenothiazine treatment of acute schizophrenia. *Arch. gen. Psychiat.*, **10**, 246–61

Collins, A. D. & Dundas, J. (1967) A double-blind trial of amitryptyline/perphenazine, perphenazine and placebo in chronic withdrawn inert schizophrenia. *Brit. J. Psychiat.*, **113**, 1425–9

Collomb, H. (1957) Introduction à la psychiatrie tropicale. *Médecine Trop.*, **17**, 542

Comstock, G. W. & Helsing, K. J. (1976) Symptoms of depression in two communities. *Psychol. Med.*, **6**, 551–63

Connell, P. H. (1958) *Amphetamine Psychosis*. Maudsley Monograph, No. 5, London: Chapman & Hall

Cooper, A. F., Garside, R. F. & Kay, D. W. K. (1976) A comparison of deaf and non-deaf patients with paranoid and affective psychoses. *Brit. J. Psychiat.*, **129**, 532–8

Cooper, B. (1961) Social class and prognosis in schizophrenia. *Brit. J. prev. soc. Med.*, **15**, 17–41

— (1978) Epidemiology. In *Schizophrenia, Towards a New Synthesis*, ed. Wing, J. K., pp. 31–52. London: Academic Press

Cooper, B. & Morgan, H. G. (1973) *Epidemiological Psychiatry*. Springfield, Illinois: Charles C. Thomas

Cooper, J. E., Kendell, R. E., Gurland, B. J., Sharpe, L., Copeland, J. R. M. & Simon, R. (1972). *Psychiatric Diagnosis in New York and London*. Maudsley Monograph, No. 20. London: Oxford University Press

Cooper, J. E. & Sartorius, N. (1977) Cultural and temporal variations in schizophrenia: a speculation on the importance of industrialization. *Brit. J. Psychiat.*, **130**, 50–55

Copas, J. B., Freeman-Browne, D. L. & Robin, A. A. (1971) Danger periods for suicide in patients under treatment. *Psychol. Med.*, **1**, 400–4

Coppen, A. J. (1960) Abnormality of the blood – cerebrospinal fluid barrier of patients suffering from depressive illness. *J. Neurol. Neurosurg. Psychiat.*, **23**, 156–61

— (1974) Serotonin in the affective disorders. In *Factors in Depression*, ed. Kline, N. S. New York: Raven Press

Coppen, A., Brookshank, B. W. L. & Peet, M. (1972a) Tryptophan concentration in the cerebrospinal fluid of depressive patients. *Lancet*, i, 1393

Coppen, A., Eccleston, E. G. & Peet, M. (1972b) Total and free tryptophan concentration in plasma of depressive patients. *Lancet*, ii, 1415–16

Coppen, A. & Ghose, K. (1978) Peripheral L-adrenoceptor and central dopamine receptor activity in depressive patients. *Psychopharmacol.* **59**, 171–7

Coppen, A., Noguera, R., Bailey, J., Burns, B. H., Swami, M. S., Hare, E. H., Gardner, R. & Maggs, R. (1971) Prophylactic lithium in affective disorder. *Lancet*, ii, 275–9

Coppen, A. & Peet, M. (1979) The long term management of patients with affective disorders. In *Psychopharmacology of Affective Disorders*, ed. Paykel, E. S. & Coppen, A., pp. 248–56. Oxford: Oxford University Press

Coppen, A. & Shaw, D. M. (1963) Mineral metabolism and melancholia. *Brit. med. J.*, **2**, 1439–44

Coppen, A., Shaw, D. M. & Costain, R. (1966) Mineral metabolism in mania. *Brit. med. J.*, **1**, 71–5

Coppen, A., Shaw, D. M. & Farrell, J. P. (1963) Potentiation of the antidepressive effect of mono-amine oxidase inhibitors by tryptophan. *Lancet* i, 79–81

Coppen, A., Shaw, D. M., Herzberg, B. & Maggs, P. (1967) Tryptophan in the treatment of depression. *Lancet*, ii. 1178–80

Coppen, A., Shaw, D. M. & Mangoni, H. (1962) Total exchangeable sodium in depressive illness. *Brit. med. J.*, **2**, 295–8

Coppen, A., Swade, C. & Wood, K. (1980) Lithium restores abnormal platelet 5HT transport in patients with affective disorders. *Brit. J. Psychiat.* **136**, 235–8

Coppen, A. & Wood, K. (1978) Tryptophan and depressive illness. *Psychol. Med.*, **8**, 49–57

Corbett, J. (1976) Medical management. In *Early Childhood Autism*, ed. Wing, L., 2nd ed., pp. 271–86. Oxford: Pergamon Press

Corbett, J. A., Harris, E. & Robinson, R. (1975) Epilepsy. In *Mental Retardation and Developmental Disabilities, An Annual Review*, ed. Morris, J., vol. VII, pp. 79–111. New York: Brunner/Mazel

Corbett, J., Harris, R., Taylor, E. & Trimble, M. (1977) Progressive disintegrative psychosis of childhood. *J. child Psychol. Psychiat.*, **18**, 211–19

Corbett, L., Christian, S. J., Morin, R. D., Benington, F. & Smythies, J. R. (1978) Hallucinogenic N-methylated indolealkylamines in the cerebrospinal fluid of psychiatric and control populations. *Brit. J. Psychiat.*, **132**, 139–44

Corsellis, J. A. N. (1962) *Mental Illness and the Ageing Brain*. Maudsley Monograph No. 9. London: Oxford University Press

— (1976) Psychoses of obscure pathology. In *Greenfield's Neuropathology*, ed. Blackwood, W. and Corsellis, J. A. N., 3rd ed., pp. 903–15. London: Edward Arnold

Cottman, S. B. & Mezey, A. G. (1976) Community care and the prognosis of schizophrenia. *Acta psychiat. scand.*, **53**, 95–104

Court, D. (Chairman) (1976) *Fit for the Future*, vol. 1, Cmd. 6684. London: HMSO

Cox, A., Rutter, M., Newman, S. and Bartak, L. (1975) A comparative study of infantile autism and specific developmental receptive language disorder. II. Parental characteristics. *Brit. J. Psychiat.*, **126**, 146–59

Crane, G. (1978) Tardive dyskinesia and related neurological disorders. In *Handbook of Psychopharmacology*. Vol. 10. *Neuroleptics and Schizophrenia*, ed. Iversen, L. L. & Iversen, S. D. New York: Plenum Press

Crawley, C. A. (1971) Infantile autism – an hypothesis. *J. Ir. med. Assoc.*, **64**, 335–45

Creak, E. M. (Chairman) (1961) Schizophrenic syndrome in childhood: progress report of a working party (April, 1961). *Cerebr. Palsy Bull.*, **3**, 501–4

— (1963) Childhood psychosis: a review of 100 cases. *Brit. J. Psychiat.*, **109**, 84–9

— (1972) Reflections on communication and autistic children. *J. Autism child. Schiz.*, **2**, 1–8

Creak, E. M. & Ini, S. (1960) Families of psychotic children. *J. child Psychol. Psychiat.*, **1**, 156–75

Creak, E. M. & Pampiglione, G. (1969) Clinical and EEG studies on a group of 35 psychotic children. *Dev. Med. child Neurol.*, **11**, 218–26

Creer, C. (1978) Social work with patients and their families. In *Schizophrenia: Towards a New Synthesis*, ed. Wing, J. K. London: Academic Press

Creer, C. & Wing, J. K. (1974) *Schizophrenia at Home*. London: National Schizophrenia Fellowship

— (1975) Living with a schizophrenic patient. *Brit. J. hosp. Med.*, **14**, 73–82

Creese, I., Burt, D. R. & Snyder, S. H. (1976) Dopamine receptors and average clinical dose. *Science*, **194**, 546

— (1978) Biochemical actions of neuroleptic drugs. Focus on the dopamine receptor. In *Handbook of Psychopharmacology*. Vol. 10. *Neuroleptics and Schizophrenia*, ed. Iversen, L. L. & Iversen, S. D. New York: Plenum Press

Critchley, M. & Earl, C. J. C. (1932) Tuberose sclerosis and allied conditions. *Brain*, **55**, 311–46

Crocetti, G. M., Lemkau, P. V., Kulcar, Z. & Kesic, B. (1971) Selected aspects of the epidemiology of psychoses in Croatia, Yugoslavia: III. Cluster sample and the results of the pilot survey. *Am. J. Epidem.*, **94**, 126–34

Cronholm, B. & Ottoson, J. O. (1960) Experimental studies of the therapeutic action of electroconvulsive therapy in endogenous depression. *Acta psychiat. scand.*, Sup. 145, **35**, 69–96

Cross, A. J., Crow, T. J. & Owen, F. (1979) Gamma-aminobutyric acid in the brain in schizophrenia. *Lancet*, **i**, 560–61

Crow, T. J. (1978) Viral causes of psychiatric disease. *Postgrad. Med. J.*, **54**, 763–7

Crow, T. J., Baker, H. F., Cross, A. J., Joseph, M. H., Lofthouse, R., Longden, A., Owen, F., Riley, G. J., Glover, V. & Killpack, W. S. (1979) Monoamine mechananisms in chronic schizophrenia: postmortem neurochemical findings. *Brit. J. Psychiat.*, **134**, 249–56

Crow, T. J., Deakin J. F. W., Johnstone, E. C. & Longen, A. (1976) Dopamine and schizophrenia. *Lancet*, **ii**, 563–6

Crow, T. J., Ferrier, I. N., Johnstone, E., Macmillan, J. F., Owens, D. G. C., Parry, R. P. & Tyrell, D. A. J. (1979) Characteristics of patients with schizophrenia or neurological disorder and virus-like agent in cerebrospinal fluid. *Lancet*, **i**, 842–4

Crowe, R. R. & Smouse, P. E. (1977) The genetic implications of age-dependent penetrance in manic-depressive illness. *J. psychiat. Res.*, **13**, 273–85

Crowley, T. J., Hoehn, M. M., Rutledge, C. O., Stallings, M. A., Heaton, R. K., Sundell, S. & Stillson, D. (1978) Dopamine excretion and vulnerability to drug-induced Parkinsonism. *Arch. gen. Psychiat.*, **35**, 97–104

Cunningham, M. (1968) A comparison of the language of psychotic and non-psychotic children who are mentally retarded. *J. child Psychol. Psychiat.*, **9**, 229–44

Curcio, F. (1978) Sensorimotor functioning and communication in mute autistic children. *J. Autism child. Schiz.*, **8**, 281–92

Curnow, R. N. & Smith, C. (1975) Multifactorial models of familial disease in man. *J. R. Stat. Soc.*, A, **138**, 131–56

Curran, W. J. & Harding, T. W. (1978) *The Law and Mental Health: Harmonizing Objectives*. Geneva: WHO

Cutting, J. (1979) Memory in functional psychosis. *J. Neurol., Neurosurg. Psychiat.*, **42**, 1031–7

— (1980) Physical illness psychosis. *Brit. J. Psychiat.*, **136**, 109–19

DaFonseca, A. F. (1963) Affective equivalents. *Brit. J. Psychiat.*, **109**, 464–9

Dalén, P. (1965) Family history, the electroencephalogram and perinatal factors in manic conditions. *Acta psychiat. scand.*, **41**, 527–63

— (1968) Month of birth and schizophrenia. *Acta psychiat. scand.*, Sup. 203, 55–60

— (1975) *Season of Birth: a Study of Schizophrenia and other Mental Disorders*. Amsterdam: North Holland

— (1977) Maternal age and incidence of schizophrenia in Ireland. *Brit. J. Psychiat.*, **131**, 301–5

Damasio, A. R. & Maurer, R. G. (1978) A neurological model for childhood autism. *Arch. Neurol.*, **35**, 777–86

Danneel, R. & Faust, V. (1979) Affective psychosis and month of birth. *Fortschr. Neurol. Psychiat.*, **47**, 47–50

Darby, J. K. (1976) Neuropathologic aspects of psychosis in children. *J. Autism child. Schiz.*, **6**, 339–52

Davidson, G. S. & Neale, J. M. (1974) The effects of signal-noise similarity on visual information processing of schizophrenics. *J. abnorm. Psychol.*, **83**, 683–6

Davis, J. M. (1965) The efficacy of tranquillising and antidepressant drugs. *Arch. gen. Psychiat.*, **13**, 552–72

— (1975) Overview: Maintenance therapy in psychiatry. I. Schizophrenia. *Am. J. Psychiat.*, **132**, 1237–45

— (1976a) Comparative doses and costs of antipsychotic medication. *Arch. gen. Psychiat.*, **33**, 858–61

— (1976b) Recent developments in the drug treatment of schizophrenia. *Am. J. Psychiat.*, **133**, 208–14

Davis, J. M. & Garver, D. L. (1978) Neuroleptics: clinical use in psychiatry. *Handbook of Psychopharmacology*. Vol. 10. *Neuroleptics and Schizophrenia*, ed. Iversen, L. L. & Iversen, S. D. New York: Plenum Press

Davis, R. E. (1979) Manic-depressive variant syndrome of childhood. *Am. J. Psychiat.* **136**, 702–05

Davison, K. (1964) Episodic depersonalization: observations on seven patients. *Brit. J. Psychiat.*, **110**, 505–13

Davison, K. & Bagley, C. R. (1969) Schizophrenia-like psychoses associated with organic disorders of the central nervous system: a review of the literature. In *Current Problems in Neuro-psychiatry*, ed. Herring, R. N. Brit. J. Psychiat. special publication No. 4. Ashford, Kent: Headley

Dear, M., Clark, G. & Clark, S. (1979) Economic cycles and mental health care policy: An examination of the macro-social context for social service planning. *Soc. Sci. Med.* **13**, 43–53

Deich, R. & Hodges, P. (1977) *Language without Speech*. London: Souvenir Press

Delacato, C. H. (1974) *The Ultimate Stranger: The Autistic Child*. New York: Doubleday

Delay, J. & Deniker, P. (1952) Le traitement des psychoses par une méthode neurolytique détirée de l'hibernothérapie. *Congrès de Médecins, Aliénistes et Neurologistes de France*, ed. Ossa, P. C., pp. 497–502. Paris and Luxembourg: Maisson Editeurs Libraires de l'Académie de Médecine

D'Elia, G., von Knorring, L. & Perris, C. (1974) Non-psychotic depressive disorders: A ten year follow-up. *Acta psychiat. scand.*, Supp. **255**, 173–86

DeLong, G. R. (1978a) Lithium carbonate treatment of select behavior disorders in children suggesting manic-depressive illness. *Pediatrics*, **93**, 689–94

— (1978b) A neuropsychological interpretation of infantile autism. In *Autism: A Reappraisal of Concepts and Treatment*, ed. Rutter, M. & Schopler, E., pp. 207–18. New York: Plenum Press

Deming, W. E. (1968) A recursion formula for the proportion of persons having a first admission as schizophrenic. *Behav. Sci.*, **13**, 467–76

DeMyer, M. K. (1976) Motor, perceptual-motor and intellectual disabilities of autistic children. In *Early Childhood Autism*, ed. Wing, L., 2nd ed. pp. 169–96 Oxford: Pergamon Press

— (1979) *Parents and Children in Autism*. Washington: Winston

DeMyer, M. K., Alpern, G. C., Barton, S., DeMyer, W. E., Churchill, D. W., Hingten, J. M., Bryson, C. Q., Pontius, W. & Kimberlin, C. (1972b) Imitation in autistic, early schizophrenic and non-psychotic subnormal children. *J. Autism and child. Schiz.*, **2**, 264–87

DeMyer, M. K., Barton, S. & Norton, J. (1972) A comparison of adaptive verbal and motor profiles of psychotic and non-psychotic subnormal children. *J. Autism child. Schiz.*, **2**, 359–77

DeMyer, M. K., Barton, S., Alpern, G. D., Kimberlin, C., Allen, J., Yang, E. & Steele, R. (1974) The measured intelligence of autistic children. *J. Autism child. Schiz.*, **4**, 42–60

DeMyer, M. K., Barton, S., DeMyer, W. E., Norton, J., Allen, J. & Steele, R. (1973) Prognosis in autism: a follow-up study. *J. Autism child. Schiz.*, **3**, 199–246

DeMyer, M. K., Pontius, W., Norton, J., Barton, S., Allen, J. & Steele, R. (1972b) Parental practices and innate activity in autistic and brain-damaged infants. *J. Autism child. Schiz.*, **2**, 49–66

Denham, J. & Adamson, L. (1971) The contribution of fluphenazine decanoate in the prevention of readmission of schizophrenic patients. *Acta psychiat. scand.*, **47**, 420–30

Denker, S. J., Maln, V., Roos, B. E. & Werdinius, B. (1966) Acid monoamine metabolites of cerebrospinal fluid in mental depression and mania. *J. Neurochem.*, **13**, 1545

Department of Health and Social Security (1977) *In-patient Statistics from the Mental Health Enquiry for England, 1974*. Statistical and research report series No. 17, Table A2.2, p. 22. London: HMSO

Department of Mental Hygiene (1949) *Annual Report*. New York State, Albany, N.Y.

de Sanctis, S. (1906) Sopra alcune varietà della demenza precoce. *Riv. sperim. Freniat. Med. leg.*, **32**, 141–65

— (1908) Dementia praecocissima catatonica oder Katatonie des früheren Kindersalters? *Folia neurobiol.*, **2**, 9–12

Des Lauriers, A. M. & Carlson, C. F. (1969) *Your Child is Asleep*. Illinois: Dorsey

Desmond, M. M., Wilson, G. S., Verniaud, W. M., Melrick, J. L. & Rawls, W. F. (1970) The early growth and development of infants with congenital rubella. In *Advances in Teratology*, vol. IV, ed. Woollam, D. H. M. New York: Academic Press

Detre, T., Himmelhoch, J., Swartzburg, M., Anderson, C. M., Byck, R. & Kupfer, D. J. (1972) Hypersomnia and manic-depressive disease. *Am. J. Psychiat.*, **128**, 1303–5

De Villiers, J. G. & Naughton, J. M. (1974) Teaching a symbol language to autistic children. *J. consult. clin. Psychol.*, **42**, 111–7

Deykin, E. Y. & MacMahon, B. (1979) The incidence of seizures among children with autistic symptoms. *Am. J. Psychiat.*, **136**, 1310–12

Deykin, E. Y., Weissman, M. M. & Klerman, G. L. (1971) Treatment of depressed women. *Brit. J. soc. Work*, **1**, 277–91

Diem, O. (1903) Die einfach demente Form der Dementia praecox. *Arch. Psychiat. Nervenkr.*, **37**, 111

Dohan, F. C. (1978) Schizophrenia: are some food-derived polypeptides pathogenic? Coeliac disease as a model. In *The Biological Basis of Schizophrenia*, ed. Hemmings, G. & Hemmings, W. A., p. 167. Lancaster: MTP Press

Dohrenwend, B. S. & Dohrenwend, B. P. (1974) *Stressful Life Events: Their Nature and Effects*. New York: Wiley

Doll, E. A. (1953) *The Measurement of Social Competence. A Manual for the Vineland Social Maturity Scale*. Washington: Educational Test Bureau

Domino, E. F. (1975) The indole hallucinogen model: Is it worth pursuing? In *Predictability in Psychopharmacology: preclinical and clinical correlations*, ed. Sudilovsky, A., Gershon, S. & Beer, B., pp. 247–68. New York: Raven Press

Domino, E. F. & Davis, J. M. (1975) (Eds.) *Neurotransmitter Balances Regulating Behavior*. Ann Arbor: Edwards

Dorpat, T. L. & Boswell, J. W. (1963) An evaluation of suicide intent in suicide attempts. *Compr. Psychiat.*, **4**, 117–25

Dorpat, T. & Ripley, H. S. (1960) A study of suicide in the Seattle area. *Compr. Psychiat.*, **1**, 349–59

Douglas, J. D. (1967) *The Social Meaning of Suicide.* Princeton: University Press

Dunaif, S. L. & Hoch, P. H. (1955) Pseudopsychopathic schizophrenia. In *Psychiatry and the Law*, ed. Hoch, P. H. & Zubin, J., p. 169. New York & London: Grune & Stratton

Dunham, H. W. (1965) *Community and Psychiatry: an Epidemiological Analysis.* Detroit: Wayne State University Press

— (1971) Sociocultural studies of schizophrenia. *Arch. gen. Psychiat.*, **24**, 206–14

— (1976) Society, culture and mental disorder. *Arch. gen. Psychiat.*, **33**, 147–56

Dunham, H. W., Phillips, S. & Srinivasan, B. (1966) A research note on diagnosed mental illness and social class. *Am. sociol. Rev.*, **31**, 223–7

Dunham, H. W. & Weinberg, S. K. (1960) *Culture of the State Mental Hospital.* Detroit: Wayne State University Press

Dunn, L. M. (1959) *Peabody Picture Vocabulary Test.* Minneapolis: American Guidance Services

Dunner, D. L., Fleiss, J. & Fieve, R. (1976) The course of development of mania in patients with recurrent depression. *Am. J. Psychiat.*, **133**, 905–8

Dunner, D. L., Igel, G. J. & Fieve, R. R. (1978) Social adjustment in primary affective disorder. *Am. J. Psychiat.*, **135**, 1412–13

Durkheim, E. (1897) *Le Suicide: étude de sociologie.* Paris: Alcan (Trans. Spaulding, J. A. & Simpson, G., 1952. London: Routledge)

Dyson, W. & Barcai, A. (1970) Treatment of children of lithium-responding parents. *Curr. Ther. Res.*, **12**, 286–90

Earl, C. J. C. (1934) The primitive catatonic psychosis of idiocy. *Brit. J. med. Psychol.*, **14**, 230–53

Early, D. (1965) Domestic resettlement and economic rehabilitation. In: *Psychiatric Hospital Care*, ed. Freeman, H. London: Bailliere, Tindall & Cassell

Eastwood, M. R. & Peacocke, J. (1976) Seasonal patterns of suicide, depression and electroconvulsive therapy. *Brit. J. Psychiat.*, **129**, 472–5

Eaton, J. W. & Weil, R. J. (1955) *Culture and Mental Disorders.* Glencoe, Illinois: Free Press

Eberhardy, F. (1967) The view from the couch. *J. child Psychol. Psychiat.*, **8**, 257–63

Edwards, C. & Carter, J. (1979) Day services and the mentally ill. In *Social Care for the Mentally Disabled*, eds. Wing, J. K. & Olsen, R. London: Oxford University Press

Eggers, C. (1978) Course and prognosis of childhood schizophrenia. *J. Autism child. Schiz.* **8**, 21–36

Einarson, L. & Strömgren, E. (1961) *Diffuse Progressive Leucoencephalopathy (Diffuse Cerebral Sclerosis) and its Relationship to Amaurotic Idiocy.* Aarhus: Universitetsforlaget; København: Ejnar Munksgaard

Eisenberg, L. (1957) The course of childhood schizophrenia. *Arch. Neurol. Psychiat.*, **78**, 69–83

Ekblom, B. & Frisk, M. (1961) On changes in the death-risk in mental hospitals in Finland during the years 1920–1955. *Acta psychiat. neurol. scand.*, **36**, 300–24

Elgar, S. (1966) Teaching autistic children. In *Early Childhood Autism: Clinical, Educational and Social Aspects*, ed. Wing, J. K. Oxford: Pergamon Press

Elston, R. C. (1973) Ascertainment and age of onset in pedigree analysis. *Hum. Hered.*, **23**, 105–12

Elston, R. C. & Campbell, M. A. (1970) Schizophrenia: Evidence for the major gene hypothesis. *Behav. Genet.*, *New York*, **1**, 3–10

Elston, R. C., Namboodiri, K. K., Spence, M. A. & Rainer, J. D. (1978) A genetic study of schizophrenia pedigrees. II. One-locus hypothesis. *Neuropsychobiology, Basel*, **4**, 193–206

Elston, R. C. & Stewart, J. (1971) A general model for the genetic analysis of pedigree data. *Hum. Hered.*, **21**, 523–42

Emerey, A. E. H. (1976) *Methodology in Medical Genetics.* Edinburgh: Churchill Livingstone

Endicott, J. & Spitzer, R. L. (1978) A diagnostic interview: the schedule for affective disorders and schizophrenia. *Arch. gen. Psychiat.*, **35**, 837–77

Endicott, J. & Spitzer, R. (1979) Use of the research diagnostic criteria and the schedule for affective disorders and schizophrenia to study affective disorders. *Am. J. Psychiat.*, **136**, 52–6

Erdelyi, E., Elliott, G. R., Wyatt, R. J. and Barchas J. P. (1978) S-Adenosylmethionine-dependent N-methyltransferase activity in autopsied brain parts of chronic schizophrenics and controls. *Am. J. Psychiat.*, **135**, 725–8

Erlenmeyer-Kimling, L., Cornblatt, B. & Fleiss, J. (1979) High-risk research in schizophrenia. *Psychiat. Ann.*, *New York*, **9**, 79–111

Erlenmeyer-Kimling, L. & Paradowski, W. (1966) Selection and schizophrenia. *Am. Naturalist* (Tempe, Arizona), **100**, 651–65

Essen Möller, E. (1956) Individual traits and morbidity in a Swedish rural population. *Acta psychiat. neurol. scand.*, Supp. 100

Essen Möller, E. & Hagnell, O. (1961) The frequency and risk of depression within a rural population group in Scania. In *Depression. Acta psychiat. scand.*, Supp. 162

Ettigi, P. G. & Brown, G. GM. (1977) Psychoneuroendocrinology of affective disorders: An overview. *Am. J. Psychiat.*, **134**, 493–501

Everard, M. P. (1976) (Ed.) *An Approach to Teaching Autistic Children.* Oxford: Pergamon Press

Ey, H. (1954) Étude 21: Manie. In *Études Psychiatriques*, vol. 3, pp. 47–116. Paris: Desclée de Brouwer

Ey, H., Bernard, P. & Brisset, Ch. (1974) Acute delusional psychoses. In *Themes and Variations in European Psychiatry*, ed. Hirsch, S. R. & Shepherd, M. p. 395. Bristol: Wright

Fabian, A. A. & Donohue, J. F. (1956) Maternal depression: A challenging child guidance problem. *Am. J. Orthopsychiat.*, **26**, 400–405

Faden, R. & Faden, A. (1977) False belief and the refusal of medical treatment. *J. med. Ethics*, **3**, 133–6

Falconer, D. S. (1965) The inheritance of liability to certain diseases estimated from the incidence among relatives. *Ann. hum. Genet.* **29**, 51–76

Falconer, M. A. (1971) Genetic and related aetiological factors in temporal lobe epilepsy. A review. *Epilepsia*, **12**, 13–31

Falloon, I. R. H., Lindley, P., McDonald, R. & Marks, I. M. (1977) Social skills training of out-patient groups. *Brit. J. Psychiat.*, **131**, 599–609

Falloon, I., Watt, D. C. & Shepherd, M. (1978) A comparative controlled trial of pimozide and fluphenazine decanoate in continuation therapy of schizophrenia. *Psychol. Med.*, **8**, 59–70

Falret, J. (1854) *Leçons Cliniques de Médecine Mentale.* Paris: Baillière

Faragalla, F. F. & Flach, F. F. (1970) Studies of mineral metabolism in mental depression 1. The effects of imipramine and electric convulsive therapy on calcium balance and kinetics. *J. ment. Dis.*, **151**, 120–9

Farberow, N. L. & McEvoy, T. C. (1966) Suicide among patients with diagnosis of anxiety reaction or depressive reaction in general medical and surgical hospitals. *Abnorm. Psychol.* **71**, 287–99

Faris, R. E. L. & Dunham, H. W. (1939) *Mental Disorders in Urban Areas.* Chicago: Hafner

Farley, I. J., Price, K. S., McCullough, E., Deck, J. N., Hordynski, W. & Hornykiewicz, O. (1978) Norepinephrine in chronic paranoid schizophrenia: above normal levels in limbic forebrain. *Science*, **200**, 456–8

Feighner, J. P., Robins, E., Guze, S. B., Woodruff, R. A., Winokur, G. & Munoz, R. (1972) Diagnostic criteria for use in psychiatric research. *Arch. gen. Psychiat.* **26**, 57–63

Fernando, S. J. M. (1966) Depressive illness in Jews and non-Jews. *Brit. J. Psychiat.*, **112**, 991–6

Ferreira, A. J. & Winter, W. D. (1965) Family interaction and decision making. *Arch. gen. Psychiat.*, **13**, 214–23

Ferster, C. B. (1961) Positive reinforcement and behavioural deficits of autistic children. *Child Devel.*, **32**, 437–56

Fieve, R. R. & Dunner, D. L. (1975) Unipolar and bipolar affective states. In *The Nature and Treatment of Depression*, ed. Flach F. F. & Draghi, S. C., pp. 145–60. New York: Wiley

Fieve, R., Mendelwicz, J. & Fleiss, J. (1973) Manic-depressive illness: Linkage with the Xg blood group. *Am. J. Psychiat.* **130**, 1355–9

Fieve, R. R., Mendelwicz, J., Rainer, J. & Fleiss, J. (1975) A dominant X-linked factor in manic-depressive illness: studies with color blindness. In *Genetic Research in Psychiatry*, ed. Fieve, R. R., Rosenthal, D. & Brill, H. Baltimore: Johns Hopkins University Press

Finegan, J. & Quarrington, B. (1979) Pre-, peri-, and neonatal factors and infantile autism. *J. child Psychol. Psychiat.*, **20**, 119–28

Fink, M., Shaw, R., Gross, C. E. & Coleman, F. S. (1958) Comparative study of chlorpromazine and insulin coma in therapy of psychosis. *J. Am. med. Assoc.*, **166**, 1846–50

Fischer, M. (1971) Psychoses in the offspring of schizophrenic monozygotic twins and their normal co-twins. *Brit. J. Psychiat.*, **118**, 43–52

— (1973) Genetic and environmental factors in schizophrenia. *Acta psychiat. scand.*, Supp. 238

Fish, B. (1977) Neurobiological antecedents of schizophrenia in children. *Arch. gen. Psychiat.*, **34**, 1297–1318

— (1979) The recognition of infantile psychoses. In *Modern Perspectives in the Psychiatry of Infancy*, ed. Howells, J. G. New York: Brunner/Mazel

Fish, B. & Ritvo, E. (1979) Childhood psychosis. In *Handbook of Child Psychiatry*, ed. Noshpitz, J., vol. II, pp. 249–304. New York: Basic Books

Fish, B. & Shapiro, T. (1965) A typology of children's psychiatric disorders. *J. Am. Acad. child Psychiat.*, **4**, 32–52

Fish, F. (1967) *Clinical Psychopathology: Signs and Symptoms in Psychiatry.* Bristol: Wright

Fisman, M. (1975) The brain stem in psychosis. *Brit. J. Psychiat.*, **126**, 414–22

Fleiss, J. L., Prien, R. F., Dunner, D. L. & Fieve, R. R. (1978) Actuarial studies of the course of manic depressive illness. *Compr. Psychiatry*, **19**, 355–62

Flood, R. A. & Seager, C. P. (1968) A retrospective examination of

psychiatric case records of patients who subsequently committed suicide. *Brit. J. Psychiat.*, **114**, 443–50

Flor-Henry, P. (1969) Psychosis and temporal lobe epilepsy. A controlled investigation. *Epilepsia*, **10**, 363–95

— (1974) Psychosis, neurosis and epilepsy: developmental and gender-related effects and their aetiological contribution. *Brit. J. Psychiat.*, **124**, 144–50

— (1976) Lateralized temporal-limbic dysfunction and psychopathology. *Ann. N.Y. Acad. Sci.*, **280**, 777–95

Folstein, S. & Rutter, M. (1977) Infantile autism: a genetic study of 21 twin pairs. *J. child Psychol. Psychiat.*, **18**, 297–322

Forrest, A. D. & Ogunremi, O. O. (1974) The prevalence of psychiatric illness in a hospital for the mentally handicapped. *Hlth Bull.*, **32**, 1–4

Forssman, H. & Janssen, B. (1960) Follow-up study of 849 men admitted to the psychiatric ward of a general hospital. *Acta psychiat. scand.*, **35**, 57–72

Foster, F. H. (1962) Maori patients in mental hospitals. Wellington, NZ: Department of Health (Medical Statistics Branch)

Fotherby, K., Ashcroft, G. W., Affleck, J. W. & Forrest, A. D. (1963) Studies on sodium transfer and 5-hydroxyindoles in depressive illness. *J. Neurol. Neurosurg. Psychiat.*, **26**, 71–3

Foulds, G. A. & Bedford, A. (1975) Hierarchy of classes of personal illness. *Psychol. Med.*, **5**, 181–92

Foulds, G. A. & Dixon, P. (1962) The nature of intellectual deficit in schizophrenia. *Brit. J. clin. soc. Psychol.*, **1**, 199

Fox, B. H. (1978) Cancer death risk in hospitalised mental patients. *Science*, **201**, 966

Francis-Williams, J. & Yule, W. (1967) The Bayley infant scales of mental and motor development: an exploratory study with an English sample. *Dev. Med. child Neurol.*, **9**, 391–401

Frankel, F. & Simmons, J. Q. (1976) Self injurious behavior in schizophrenic and retarded children. *Am. J. ment. Defic.*, **80**, 512–22

Freedman, D. A. (1971) Congenital and perinatal sensory deprivation: some studies in early development. *Am. J. Psychiat.*, **127**, 1539–45

Freeman, B. J. (1974) The subjective experience of perceptual and cognitive disturbances in schizophrenia. *Arch. gen. Psychiat.*, **30**, 333–40

— (1976) Evaluating autistic children. *J. paediat. Psychol.*, **1**, 18–21

— (1978) Appraising children for mental retardation: the usefulness and limitations of IQ testing. *Clin. Paediat.*, **17**, 169–73

Fremming, K. H. (1951) The expectation of mental infirmity in a sample of the Danish population. *Occasional Papers on Eugenics*, No. 7. London: Eugenics Society, 104

Freudenberg, R. K. (1967) Theory and practice of the rehabilitation of the psychiatrically disabled. *Psychiat. Quart.*, **41**, 698

Frith, C. D. & Lillie, F. J. (1972) Why does the repertory grid test indicate thought disorder? *Brit. J. soc. clin. Psychol.*, **11**, 73–8

Frith, U. (1970a) Studies in pattern detection in normal and autistic children: I. Immediate recall of auditory sequences. *J. abnorm. Psychol.*, **76**, 413–20

— (1970b) Studies in pattern detection in normal and autistic children: II. Reproduction and production of color sequences. *J. exp. child Psychol.*, **10**, 120–35

— (1971) Spontaneous patterns produced by autistic, normal and subnormal children. In *Infantile Autism: Concepts, Char-*

acteristics and Treatment, ed. Rutter, M., pp. 113–31. London: Churchill Livingstone

— (1972) Cognitive mechanisms in childhood autism. Experiments with colour and tone sequence production. *J. Autism child. schiz.*, **2**, 160–73

Frizel, D., Coppen, A. & Marks, V. (1969) Plasma magnesium and calcium in depression. *Brit. J. Psychiat.*, **111**, 1375–7

Froh, F. (1967) *Clinical Psychopathology*. Bristol: Wright

Fromm-Reichmann, F. (1948) Notes on the development of treatment of schizophrenics by psychoanalytic psychotherapy. *Psychiatry*, **II**, 263–73

Frommer, E. A. (1968) Depressive illness in childhood. In *Recent Developments in Affective Disorders*, ed. Coppen, A. & Walk, A. *Brit. J. Psychiat.* special publication No. 2. Ashford, Kent: Headley

Fuller, R. G. (1935) What happens to mental patients after discharge from hospital. *Psychiat. Q.*, **9**, 95–104

Fulwiler, R. L. & Fouts, R. S. (1976) Acquisition of American sign language by a non-communicating autistic child. *J. Autism child. Schiz.*, **6**, 43–51

Fyffe, C. & Prior, M. (1978) Evidence for language recording in autistic, retarded and normal children. *Brit. J. Psychol.*, **69**, 393–402

Gardos, I., Cole, J. & Orzack, M. H. (1973) The importance of dosage in antipsychotic drug administration – a review of dose-response studies. *Psychopharmacol.*, **29**, 221–30

Gelfand, D. M. & Hartmann, D. P. (1975) *Child Behavior Analysis and Therapy*. New York: Pergamon Press

Gershon, E. S. (1978) The search for genetic markers in affective disorders. In *Psychopharmacology: A Generation of Progress*, ed. Lipton, M. A., DiMascio, A. & Killam, K. F. New York: Raven Press

Gershon, E., Baron, M. & Leckman, J. (1975c) Genetic models of the transmission of affective disorders. *J. psychiat. Res.*, **12**, 301–17

Gershon, E., Bunney, W., Leckman, J., van Eerdewegh, M. & DeBauche, B. (1976) The inheritance of affective disorders: a review of data and of hypotheses. *Behav. Genet.*, **6**, 227–61

Gershon, E., Dunner, D., Stuart, L. & Goodwin, F. (1973) Assortative mating in the affective disorders. *Biol. Psychiat.*, 7(1), 63–74

Gershon, E. & Liebowitz, T. (1975) Sociocultural and demographic correlates of affective disorders in Jerusalem. *J. Psychiat. Res.*, **12**, 37–50

Gershon, E., Mark, A. Cohen, N., Belizon, N., Baron, M. & Knobe, K. (1975b) Transmitted factors in the morbid risk of affective disorders: a controlled study. *J. Psychiat. Res.*, **12**, 283–99

Gershon, E., Mendelwicz, J., Per Bech, M., Goldin, L., Kielholz, P., Rafaelson, O., Vartanian, F. & Bunney, W. (1979) A collaborative study of genetic linkage of bipolar manic-depressive illness and red/green color blindness. Submitted

Gershon, E., Targum, S., Matthysse, S. & Bunney, W. (1979) Color blindness linkage to bipolar illness not supported by new data. *Archiv. gen. Psychiat.*, **36**, 1423–30

Gerver, D. (1967) Linguistic rules and the perception and recall of speech by schizophrenic patients. *Brit. J. soc. clin. Psychol.*, **6**, 204–11

Gibbons, J. L. (1960) Total body sodium and potassium in depressive patients. *Clin. Sci.*, **19**, 133

— (1964) Cortisol secretion rate in depressive illness. *Arch. gen. Psychiat.*, **10**, 572–5

Giel, R., Dijk, S. & Weerden-Dijkstra, J. R. van (1978) Mortality in the long-stay population of all Dutch mental hospitals. *Acta psychiat. scand.*, **57**, 361–8

Gillin, J. C., Kaplan, J., Stillman, R. & Wyatt, R. J. (1976) The psychodelic model of schizophrenia – the case of N,N-dimethyltryptamine. *Am. J. Psychiat.*, **133**, 203–8

Gillin, J. C., Stoff, D. M. & Wyatt, R. J. (1978) Transmethylation hypothesis: a review of progress. In *Psychopharmacology: A Generation of Progress*, ed. Lipton, M. A., DiMascio, A., & Killam, K. F., pp. 1097–112. New York: Raven Press

Gittelman, M. & Birch, H. G. (1967) Childhood schizophrenia: intellect, neurologic status, perinatal risk, prognosis and family pathology. *Arch. gen. Psychiat.*, **17**, 16–25

Gittleson, N. L. (1966a) The effect of obsessions on depressive psychosis. *Brit. J. Psychiat.*, **112**, 253–9

— (1966b) The phenomenology of obsessions in depressive psychosis. *Brit. J. Psychiat.*, **112**, 261–4

— (1967) A phenomenological test of a theory of depersonalization. *Brit. J. Psychiat.*, **113**, 677–8

Glen, A. I. M., Ongley, G. C. & Robinson, K. (1968) Diminished membrane transport in manic depressive psychosis and recurrent depression. *Lancet*, **ii**, 241–3

Glossary of Mental Disorders and Guide to their classification for use in conjunction with the International Classification of Diseases. 8th Revision (1974). (Revised ed., 1978) Geneva: World Health Organization

Goetzl, U., Green, R., Whybrow, P. & Jackson, R. (1974) X-linkage revisited. A further family study of manic-depressive illness. *Arch. gen. Psychiat.*, **31**, 665–72

Goffmann, E. (1961) *Asylums: Essays on the Social Situation of Mental Patients and other Inmates.* New York: Doubleday

— (1961) On the characteristics of total institutions. In *The Prison*, ed. Cressey, D. R. New York: Holt, Rinehart & Winston

Goldberg, E. M. & Morrison, S. L. (1963) Schizophrenia and social class. *Brit. J. Psychiat.*, **109**, 785–802

Goldberg, S. C., Klerman, C. L. & Cole, J. (1965) Changes in schizophrenia psychopathology and ward behaviour as a function of phenothiazine treatment. *Brit. J. Psychiat.*, **111**, 120–33.

Goldberg, S. C., Schooler, N. R., Hogarty, G. E. & Roper, M. (1977) Prediction of relapse in schizophrenic outpatients treated by drug and sociotherapy. *Arch. gen. Psychiat.*, **34**, 171–84

Goldfarb, W. (1961) *Childhood Schizophrenia*. Cambridge, Mass: Harvard University Press

— (1970) Childhood psychosis. In *Carmichael's Manual of Child Psychology*, ed. Massen, P. H., 2nd ed., vol. 2, pp. 765–830. New York: Wiley

— (1974) *Growth and Change of Schizophrenic Children*. New York: Wiley

Goldstein, A. (1967) *The Insanity Defense*. New Haven: Yale University Press

Goldstein, A. S. & Marcus, M. (1977) The McNaughton Rules in the United States. In *Daniel McNaughton: His Trial and the Aftermath*, ed. West, D. J. & Walk, A. Ashford, Kent: Headley Bros.

Goldstein, K. (1939) The significance of special mental tests for diagnosis and prognosis in schizophrenia. *Am. J. Psychiat.*, **96**, 575–87

Goode, D. J., Meltzer, H. Y., Moretti, R., Kupfer, D. J. & McPartland, R. J. (1979) Relationship between wrist-monitored motor activity and serum CPK activity in psychiatric inpatients. *Brit. J. Psychiat.*, **135**, 62–6

Goodwin, F. K. & Bunney, W. E. (1971) Depressions following reserpine: A re-evaluation. *Seminars in Psychiatry*, **3**, 435–48

Goodwin, D. W. & Guze, S. B. (1979) *Psychiatric Diagnosis.* 2nd ed. London: Oxford University Press

Goodwin, D. W., Schulsenger, F., Knop, J., Mednick, S. & Guze, S. B. (1977) Psychopathology in adopted and non-adopted daughters of alcoholics. *Arch. gen. Psychiat.*, **34**, 1005–9

Goodwin, F. K. & Post, R. M. (1973) The use of probenecid in high doses for the estimation of central serotonin turnover in affective illness and addicts on methadone. In *Serotonin and Behavior*, ed. Barchas, J. & Usin, E., p. 469. New York: Academic Press

Gostin, L. (1975) *The Mental Health Act from 1959 to 1975. Observations, Analysis and Proposals for Reform*, Vol. 1. A MIND Special Report. London: National Association for Mental Health

— (1979) The merger of incompetency and certification: the illustration of unauthorised medical contact in the psychiatric context. *Int. J. Law Psychiat.*, **2**, 127–67

Gottesman, I. I. (1974) Developmental genetics and ontogenetic psychology: Overdue détente and propositions from a matchmaker. In *Minnesota Symposium on Child Psychology*, ed. Pick, A., vol. 8. Minneapolis: University of Minnesota Press

Gottesman, I. I. & Shields, J. (1966) Contribution of twin studies to perspectives on schizophrenia. In *Progress in Experimental Personality Research*, ed. Maher, B. A., vol. 3, pp. 1–84. London: Academic Press

— (1967) A polygenic theory of schizophrenia. *Proc. Nat. Acad. Sci., Washington*, **58**, 199–205.

— (1972) *Schizophrenia and Genetics: a Twin Study Vantage Point.* London: Academic Press

— (1976) A critical review of recent adoption, twin and family studies of schizophrenia: behavioral and genetics perspectives. *Schiz. Bull.*, **2**, 360–401 and 447–53

Gould, J. (1976) Assessment: the role of the psychologist. In *An Approach to Teaching Autistic Children*, ed. Everard, M. P., pp. 31–52. Oxford: Pergamon Press

— (1977) The use of the Vineland social maturity scale, the Merrill-Palmer scale of mental tests (non-verbal items) and the Reynell developmental language scales with children in contact with the services for severe mental retardation. *J. men. Def. Res.*, **21**, 213–26

Gour, K. N. & Chaudrey, H. M. (1957) Study of calcium metabolites in electroconvulsive therapy in certain mental diseases. *J. ment. Sci.*, **103**, 275–85

Govaerts, A., Mendelwicz, J. & Verbanck, P. (1977) Manic-depressive illness and HLA. *Tissue Antigens*, **10**, 60–62

Grad, J. & Sainsbury, P. (1968) The effects that patients have on their families in a community care and a control psychiatric service: A two year follow-up. *Brit. J. Psychiat.* **114**, 265–8

Grad de Alarcon, J., Sainsbury, P. & Costain, W. R. (1975) Incidence of referred mental illness in Chichester and Salisbury. *Psychol. Med.*, **5**, 32–54

Graham, L. F. & Rafaelsen, O. J. (1972) Lithium treatment of psychotic children and adolescents. *Acta psychiat. scand.*, **48**, 253–60

Granville-Grossman, K. (1968) The early environment in affective disorder. In *Recent Developments in Affective Disorders*, ed., Coppen, A. & Walk, A. Royal Medico-Psychological Association. Ashford, England: Headley Bros

Greenbaum, J. V. & Lurie, L. A. (1948) Encephalitis as a causative factor in behaviour disorders in children: analysis of 78 cases. *J. Am. Med. Assoc.*, **136**, 923–30

Greenblatt, M. (1977) Efficacy of ECT in affective and schizophrenic illness. *Am. J. Psychiat.*, **134**, 1001–5

Greenblatt, M., Solomon, M., Evans, A. S. & Brooks, C. W. (1965) *Drugs and Social Therapy in Chronic Schizophrenia.* Springfield, Illinois: Charles C. Thomas

Greenhill, L. L., Rieder, R. O. & Wender, P. N. (1973) Lithium carbonate in the treatment of hyperactive children. *Arch. Gen. Psychiat.*, **28**, 636–40

Griffith, J. D., Cavanaugh, J., Held, J. & Oates, J. A. (1972) Dextroamphetamine. Evaluation of psychomimetic properties in man. *Arch. gen. Psychiat.*, **26**, 97–100

Grinker, R. R. (1973) Changing styles in psychiatric syndromes. *Am. J. Psychiat.*, **130**, 151–5

Grinker, R. R. & Werble, B. (1977) *The Borderline Patient.* New York: Aronson

Grinker, R. R., Werble, B. & Drye, R. (1968) *The Borderline Syndrome.* New York: Basic Books

Gruen, P. A., Sachar, E. J., Langer, G., Altman, N., Leifer, M., Franzt, A. & Helpern, F. S. (1978) Prolactin responses to neuroleptics in normal and schizophrenic subjects. *Arch. gen. Psychiat.*, **35**, 108–16

Gruenberg, E. M. (1957) Socially shared psychopathology. In *Explorations in Social Psychiatry*, ed. Leighton, A. H., Clausen, J. A. & Wilson, R. N. New York: Basic Books

Gruer, P. H., Sachar, E. J., Altman, N. & Sassin, J. (1975) Growth hormone responses to hypoglycaemia in postmenopausal depressed women. *Arch. gen. Psychiat.*, **32**, 31–3

Grünfeld, B. & Salveson, C. (1968) Functional psychoses and social status. *Brit. J. Psychiat.*, **114**, 733–8

Gruzelier, J. H. & Venables, P. H. (1972) Skin conductance orienting activity in a heterogeneous sample of schizophrenics. *J. nerv. ment. Dis.*, **155**, 277–87

— (1974) Bimodality and lateral asymmetry of skin conductance activity in schizophrenics. *Biol. Psychiat.*, **11**, 221–30

Gubbay, S. S., Lobascher, M. & Kingerlee, P. (1970) A neurological appraisal of autistic children: results of a Western Australian survey. *Dev. Med. child Neurol.*, **12**, 422–9

Guldberg, H. C., Ashcroft, G. W. & Crawford, T. B. B. (1966) Concentrations of 5-hydroxyindolacetic acid and homovanillic acid in the cerebrospinal fluid of the dog before and during treatment with probenecid. *Life Sci.*, **5**, 1571–5

Gunzburg, H. C. (1974) *The Primary Progress Assessment Chart of Social Development.* Birmingham : SEFA Publications

Gur, R. E. (1978) Left hemisphere dysfunction and left hemisphere overactivation in schizophrenia. *J. abnorm. Psychol.*, **87**, 226–38

Guthrie, R. D. & Wyatt, R. J. (1975) Biochemistry and schizophrenia. III: A review of childhood psychosis. *Schiz. Bull.*, No. 12, 18–32

Guze, S. B. & Perley, M. J. (1963) Observations on the natural history of hysteria. *Am. J. Psychiat.*, **119**, 960–5

Guze, S. B., Woodruff, R. & Clayton, P. (1971) Secondary affective disorder. A study of 95 cases. *Psychol. Med.*, **1**, 426–8

Hackney, M. (1967) Autistic behavior patterns in phenylketonuric children. *Can. Psychiat. Ass. J.*, **12**, 333

Hagnell, O. & Rorsman, B. (1978) Suicide and endogenous depression with somatic symptoms in the Lundby study. *Neuropsychobiol.*, **4**, 180–7

Hajdu-Gaines, L. (1940) Contributions to the aetiology of schizophrenia. *Psychoanal. Rev.*, **27**, 421–38

Haley, J. (1959) The family of the schizophrenic–a model system. *J. nerv. ment. Dis.*, **129**, 357–74

— (1968) Testing parental instructions to schizophrenic and normal children: a pilot study. *J. abnorm. Psychol.*, **73**, 559–65

Hall, K. S., Dunner, D. L., Zeller, G. & Fieve, R. R. (1977) Bipolar illness: a prospective study of life events. *Comprehensive Psychiat.*, **18**, 497–502

Halpern, L. (1938) Some data of the psychic morbidity of Jews and Arabs in Palestine. *Am. J. Psychiat.*, **94**, 1215–22

Hanley, H. G., Stahl, S. M. & Freedman, D. X. (1977) Hyperserotonemia and amine metabolites in autistic and retarded children. *Arch. gen. Psychiat.*, **34**, 521–31

Hanson, D. R. & Gottesman, I. I. (1976) The genetics, if any, of infantile autism and childhood schizophrenia. *J. Autism child. Schiz.*, **6**, 209–34

— (1979) Genetic concepts for psychopathology. In *Handbook of Biological Psychiatry*, vol. I, ed. van Praag, H. M., Lader, M. H., Rafaelsen, O. J. & Sachat, E. J. New York: Dekker

Hanson, D. R., Gottesman, I. I. & Heston, L. L. (1976) Some possible childhood indicators of adult schizophrenia inferred from children of schizophrenics. *Brit. J. Psychiat.*, **129**, 142–54

Haracopos, D. & Kelstrup, A. (1978) Psychotic behaviour in children under the institutions for the mentally retarded in Denmark. *J. Autism child. Schiz.*, **8**, 1–12

Hare, E. H. (1978) Variations in the seasonal distribution of births of psychotic patients in England & Wales. *Brit. J. Psychiat.*, **132**, 155–8

Hare, E. H. & Moran, P. A. P. (1979) Raised parental age in psychiatric patients: evidence for the constitutional hypothesis. *Brit. J. Psychiat.*, **134**, 169–77

Hare, E. H. & Price, J. S. (1970) Birth rank in schizophrenia: with a consideration of the bias due to changes in birth rate. *Brit. J. Psychiat.*, **116**, 409–20

— (1974) Birth order and birth rate bias: findings in a representative sample of the adult population of Great Britain. *J. biosoc. Sci.*, **6**, 139–50

Hare, E. H., Price, J. S. & Slater, E. (1972) Parental social class in psychiatric patients. *Brit. J. Psychiat.*, **121**, 515–24

Hare, E. H. & Shaw, G. K. (1965) *Mental Health on a New Housing Estate: A comparative study of health in two districts in Croydon.* Maudsley Monographs No. 12. London: Oxford University Press

Hare, E. H. & Walter, S. D. (1978) Seasonal variation in admissions of psychiatric patients and its relation to seasonal variation in their births. *J. Epidemiol. Community Health*, **32**, 47–52

Harkey, J., Miles, D. L. & Rushing, W. A. (1976) The relation between social class and functional status: a new look at the drift hypothesis. *J. Hlth soc. Behav.*, **17**, 195–204

Harris, A., Linker, I., Norris, V. & Shepherd, M. (1956) Schizophrenia: a social and prognostic study. *Brit. J. prev. soc. Med.*, **10**, 107–14

Harrow, M. & Quinlan, D. (1977) Is disordered thinking unique to schizophrenia? *Arch. gen. Psychiat.*, **34**, 15–21

Haslam, J. (1809) *Observations on Madness and Melancholy*, pp. 185–206. London: Haydon

Hartmann, E. (1968) Longitudinal studies of sleep and dream patterns in manic-depressive patients. *Arch. gen. Psychiat.*, **19**, 312–29

Hauser, S., DeLong, G. R. & Rosman, N. (1975) Pneumographic findings in the infantile autism syndrome, a correlation with temporal lobe disease. *Brain*, **98**, 667–88

Hawks, D. V. & Robinson, K. N. (1971) Information processing in schizophrenia: The effect of varying the rate of presentation and introducing interference. *Brit. J. soc. clin. Psychol.*, **10**, 30–41

Hays, P. (1976) Etiological factors in manic-depressive psychoses. *Arch. gen. Psychiat.*, **33**, 1187–8

Haywood, H. C. (1977) Alternatives to normative assessment. In *Research to Practice in Mental Retardation. Vol. II. Education and Training*, ed. Mittler, P., pp. 11–19. Baltimore, USA: University Park Press

Hecker, E. (1871) Die Hebephrenie. Ein Beitrag zur klinischen Psychiatrie. *Virchows Arch.*, **52**, 394

Helgason, T. (1964) Epidemiology of mental disorders in Iceland. A psychiatric and demographic investigation of 5395 Icelanders. *Acta psychiat. scand.*, **40**, 173

Helgason, L. (1977) Psychiatric services and mental illness in Iceland. *Acta psychiat. scand.*, Suppl. 268

Heller, T. (1954) Dementia infantilis (translated by W. Hulse). *J. nerv. ment. Dis.*, **119**, 471–7

Helzer, J. & Winokur, G. (1974) A family interview study of male manic-depressives. *Arch. gen. Psychiat.*, **31**, 73–7

Hemsi, L. K. (1967) Psychiatric morbidity of West Indian immigrants. *Soc. Psychiat.*, **2**, 95–100

Hemsley, D. R. (1978) Limitations of operant procedures in the modification of schizophrenic functioning. *Behav. Anal. Modif.*, **2**, 165–73

Hemsley, D. R. & Howlin, P. (1976) Management of behaviour problems. In *An Approach to Teaching Austic Children*, ed. Everard, P. Oxford: Pergamon Press

Hemsley, D. R., Howlin, P., Berger, M., Hersov, L., Holbrook, D., Rutter, M. & Yule, W. (1978) Treating autistic children in family context. In *Autism: A Reappraisal of Concepts and Treatment*, ed. Rutter, M. & Schopler, E. New York: Plenum Press

Hemsley, D. R. & Zawada, S. L. (1976) 'Filtering' and the cognitive deficit in schizophrenia. *Brit. J. Psychiat.*, **128**, 456–61

Henderson, D. K. & Batchelor, I. R. C. (1962) *Textbook of Psychiatry.* pp. 261–2 and 290–295. London: Oxford University Press

Henderson, A. S., Hartigan, J., Davidson, J., Lance, G. N., Duncan-Jones, P., Koller, K. M., Ritchie, K., McAuley, H., Williams, C. L. & Slaghuis, W. (1977) A typology of parasuicide. *Brit. J. Psychiat.*, **131**, 631–41

Henry, G. M., Weingartner, H. & Murphy, D. L. (1971) Idiosyncratic patterns of learning and word association during mania. *Am. J. Psychiat.*, **128**, 564–72

Hermelin, G. (1966) Psychological research. In *Early Childhood Autism*, ed. Wing, L., 1st ed., pp. 159–74. Oxford: Pergamon Press

— (1972) Locating events in space and time: Experiments with autistic, blind and deaf children. *J. Autism child. Schiz.*, **2**, 288–98

— (1976) Coding and the sense modalities. In *Early Childhood*

Autism, ed. Wing, L., 2nd ed, pp. 135–68. Oxford: Pergamond Press

—— (1978) Images and language. In *Autism: A Reappraisal of Concepts and Treatment,* ed. Rutter, M. & Schopler, E. New York: Plenum Press

Hermelin, B. & Frith, U. (1971) Psychological studies of childhood autism. Can autistic children make sense of what they hear? *J. spec. Educ.,* **5,** 1107–17

Hermelin, B. & O'Connor, N. (1968) Measures of the occipital alpha rhythm in normal, subnormal and autistic children. *Brit. J. Psychiat.,* **114,** 603–10

—— (1970) *Psychological Experiments with Autistic Children.* Oxford: Pergamon Press

Hes, J. P. (1960) Manic depressive illness in Israel. *Am. J. Psychiat.,* **116,** 1082–6

Heston, L. L. (1966) Psychiatric disorders in foster home reared children of schizophrenic mothers. *Brit. J. Psychiat.,* **112,** 819–25

Heston, L. L. & Denney, D. (1968) Interactions between early life experiences and biological factors in schizophrenia. In *The Transmission of Schizophrenia,* ed. Rosenthal, D. & Kety, S. S. Oxford: Pergamon Press

Hewett, S. (1979) Somewhere to live. In *Alternative Patterns of Residential Care for Discharged Psychiatric Patients,* ed. Olsen, R. London: BASW

Hewett, S., Ryan, P. & Wing, J. K. (1975) Living without the mental hospitals. *J. soc. Pol.,* **4,** 391–404

Hewitt, M. (1949) The unemployed disabled man. *Lancet,* **ii,** 523–6

Himmelhoch, J. N., Coble, P., Kupfer, D. J. & Ingenito, J. (1976) Agitated psychotic depression associated with severe hypomanic episodes: a rare syndrome. *Am. J. Psychiat.,* **133,** 765–71

Himmelhoch, J M., Mulla, D. & Neil, J. F. (1976) Incidence and significance of mixed affective states in a bipolar population. *Arch. gen. Psychiat.,* **33,** 1062–6

Hirsch, S. R., Gaind, R., Rohde, P. D., Stevens, B. C. & Wing, J. K. (1973) Outpatient maintenance of chronic schizophrenic patients with long-acting fluphenazine: double-blind placebo trial. *Brit. med. J.,* **1,** 633–7

Hirsch, S. R. & Leff, J. P. (1975) *Abnormalities in Parents of Schizophrenics: A review of the literature and an investigation of communication defects and deviances.* Maudsley Monograph No. 22. London: Oxford University Press

Hoch, A. (1910) Die Melancholiefrage. *Zentralbl. Nervenheilk. Psychiat.,* **21,** 193–203

—— (1912) Die Bedeutung der Symptomenkomplexe in der Psychiatrie. *Z. ges. Neurol. Psychiat.,* **12,** 540–51

Hoch, P. & Polatin, P. (1949) Pseudoneurotic forms of schizophrenia. *Psychiat. Quart.,* **23,** 248–76

Hogarty, G. E. (1977) Treatment and the course of schizophrenia. *Schiz. Bull.,* **3,** 587–99

Hogarty, C. E., Goldberg, S., Schooley, N. & Ulrich, R. (1974) Drug and sociotherapy in the aftercare of schizophrenic patients. II. 2 year relapse rates. *Arch. gen. Psychiat.,* **31,** 603–8

Hogarty, C. & Ulrich, R. (1977) Temporal effects of drug and placebo in delaying relapse in schizophrenic outpatients. *Arch. gen. Psychiat.,* **34,** 297–301

Hogarty, C., Ulrich, R., Mussare, F. & Aristigueta, N. (1976) Drug discontinuation among long term, successfully maintained schizophrenic outpatients. *Dis. nerv. Sys.,* **37,** 494–500

Hollister, L. E. (1974) Clinical differences among phenothiazines in schizophrenia. In *Adv. biochem. Psychopharmacol.,* **9,** 667–73, WHO

—— (1978) Antipsychotics. In *Clinical Pharmacology of Psychotherapeutic Drugs,* by Hollister, L., chap. 5. London: Churchill, Livingstone

Holmboe, R., Noreik, K. & Astrup, C. (1968) Follow-up of functional psychoses at two Norwegian mental hospitals. *Acta psychiat. scand.,* **44,** 298–310

Hopkinson, G. & Ley, P. (1969) A genetic study of affective disorder. *Brit. J. Psychiat.,* **115,** 917–22

Howlin, P. (1980) The home treatment of autistic children. In *Language and Language Disorders in Children,* ed. Hersov, L. A., Berger, M. & Nichol, R. Oxford: Pergamon Press

Howlin, P., Marchant, R., Rutter, M., Berger, M., Hersov, L. & Yule, W. (1973) A home-based approach to the treatment of autistic children. *J. Autism child. Schiz.,* **4,** 308–36

Hulse, W. C. (1954) Dementia infantilis. *J. Nerv. ment. Dis.,* **119,** 471–7

Hundley, J. M. (1971) *The Small Outsider.* London: Angus & Robertson

Huntington, E. (1938) *Season of Birth. Its Relation to Human Abilities.* New York: Wiley

Huston, P. E. & Locher, L. M. (1948) Manic depressive psychosis: course when treated and untreated with electric shock. *Arch. Neurol. Psychiat.,* **60,** 37–48

Hutt, S. J., Hutt, C., Lee, D. & Ounsted, C. (1964) Arousal and childhood autism. *Nature,* **204,** 908–9

—— (1965) A behavioural and electro-encephalographic study of autistic children. *J. psychiat. Res.,* **3,** 181–97

Ianzito, B.M., Cadoret, & R. J. Pugh, D. D. (1974) Thought disorder in depression. *Am. J. Psychiat.,* **131,** 703–7

Illingworth, R. S. (1955) Sudden mental deterioration with convulsions in infancy. *Arch. Dis. Child.,* **30,** 529–37

Ingram, T. T. S. (1959) Specific developmental disorders of speech in childhood. *Brain,* **82,** 450–67

International Classification of Disease. (1977) 9th ed. 1975 Revision. Vol. 1. Geneva: WHO

Irvine, D. & Miyashita, H. (1965) Blood groups in relation to depressions and schizophrenia. *Can. med. Ass. J.,* **92,** 551–4

Itard, J. M. G. (1801) *Of the first developments of the young savage of Aveyron.* Reprinted in *Wolf Children and the Wild Boy of Aveyron,* Malson, L. & Itard, J. M. G. (1972) pp. 95–140. London: NLB

—— (1807) *Report on the progress of Victor of Aveyron.* Reprinted in *Wolf Children and the Wild Boy of Aveyron,* Malson, L. & Itard, J. M. G. (1972), pp. 141–79. London: NLB

Iversen, L. L., Iversen, S. D. & Snyder, S. H. (1978) *Handbook of Psychopharmacology.* Vol. 10. *Neuroleptics and Schizophrenia.* New York: Plenum Press

James, N. M. & Chapman, C. J. (1975) A genetic study of bipolar affective disorder. *Brit. J. Psychiat.,* **126,** 449–56

Janssen, P. A. T. & Van Bever, W. F. (1978) Structure-activity relationships of butyrophenones and diphenylbutylpiperidines. In Iversen, L. L., Iversen, S. D. & Snyder, S. H. (1978) *Handbook of Psychopharmacology.* Vol. 10. *Neuroleptics and Schizophrenia.* New York: Plenum Press

Jaspers, K. (1962) *General Psychopathology,* transl. Hoenig, J. & Hamilton, M. W. Manchester: Manchester University Press

Jeffree, D. & McConkey, R. (1976) *Let Me Speak.* London: Souvenir Press

Jeffree, D., McConkey, R. & Hewson, S. (1977) *Let Me Play.* London: Souvenir Press

Jensen, K. (1959) Depressions in patients treated with reserpine for arterial hypertension. *Acta psychiat. scand.*, **34**, 195–204

Jervis, G.A. (1963) The clinical picture. In *Phenylketonuria*, ed. Lyman, F. L., pp. 52–61. Springfield, Illinois: Charles C. Thomas

Johnson, D. A. W. (1976) The expectation of outcome from maintenance therapy in chronic schizophrenic patients. *Brit. J. Psychiat.*, **128**, 246–50

— (1978) The prevalence and treatment of drug-induced extrapyramidal symptoms. *Brit. J. Psychiat.*, **132**, 27–30

Johnson, F. N. (1975) (Ed.) *Lithium Research and Therapy*. London: Academic Press

Johnson, G. & Leeman, M. (1977) Analysis of familial factors in bipolar affective illness. *Arch. gen. Psychiat.*, **24**, 1074–83

Johnstone, E. C., Crow, T. J., Frith, C. D., Carney, M. W. P. & Price, J. S. (1978) The mechanism of the antipsychotic effect in the treatment of acute schizophrenia. *Lancet*, **i**, 848–51

Johnstone, E. C., Crow, T. J., Frith, C. D., Husband, J. & Kreel, L. (1976) Cerebral ventricular size and cognitive impairment in chronic schizophrenia. *Lancet*, **ii**, 924–6

Jones, H. G. (1978) Psychological aspects of treatment of inpatients. In *Schizophrenia: Towards a New Synthesis*, ed. Wing, J. K. London: Academic Press

Jones, I. H. & Frei, D. (1979) Seasonal births in schizophrenia: a southern hemisphere study using matched pairs. *Acta psychiat. scand.*, **59**, 164–72

Jones, K. (1972). *A History of the Mental Health Services*. London: Routledge Kegan Paul

Jones, M. B. & Offord, D. R. (1975) Independent transmission of I.Q. and schizophrenia. *Brit. J. Psychiat.*, **126**, 185–90

Jørgensen, O. S. (1979) Psychopharmacological treatment of psychotic children. *Acta psychiat. scand.*, **59**, 229–38

Joseph, M. H., Baker, H. F., Johnstone, E. C. & Crow, T. J. (1976) Determination of 3-methoxy-4-hydroxyphenylene glycol conjugates in urine. Application to the study of cerebral noradrenaline metabolism in unmedicated chronic schizophrenics. *Psychopharmacol.*, **51**, 47–51

Judd, L. L. & Mandel, A. J. (1968) Chromosome studies in early infantile autism. *Arch. gen. Psychiat.*, **18**, 450–7

Jung, C. G. (1969) (Ed.) *Studies in Word-Association*. London: Routledge & Kegan Paul

Junker, K. S. (1964) *The Child in the Glass Ball* (trans. Gustaf Lannestock). New York: Abingdon Press

Kadrmas, A. & Winokur, G. (1979) Manic-depressive illness and EEG abnormalities. *J. Clin. Psychiat.*, **40**, 306–7

Kahlbaum, K. (1894) *Die Katatonie oder das Spannungsirresein*. Berlin: Hirschwald

Kalinowsky, M. D., Lothar, B. & Hippius, H. (1969) *Pharmacological, Convulsive and other Somatic Treatments in Psychiatry*. New York and London: Grune & Stratton

Kallmann, F. J. (1938) *The Genetics of Schizophrenia*. New York: Augustin

— (1946) The genetic theory of schizophrenia. *Am. J. Psychiat.*, **103**, 309–22

— (1950) The genetics of psychoses: an analysis of 1232 twin index families. *Int. Cong. Psychiat. Rapports, Paris*, 1–27

Kallmann, F. J. & Reisner, D. (1943) Twin studies on genetic variations in resistance to tuberculosis. *J. Hered.*, **34**, 269 and 293

Kallmann, F. J. & Roth, B. (1956) Genetic aspects of pre-adolescent schizophrenia. *Am. J. Psychiat.*, **112**, 599–606

Kanner, L. (1943) Autistic disturbances of affective contact. *Nerv. Child*, **2**, 217–50

— (1946) Irrelevant and metaphorical language in early infantile autism. *Am. J. Psychiat.*, **103**, 242–6

— (1949) Problems of nosology and psychodynamics in early infantile autism. *Am. J. Ortho-psychiat.*, **19**, 416–26

— (1951) The conception of wholes and parts in early infantile autism. *Am. J. Psychiat.*, **108**, 23–6

— (1954) To what extent is early childhood autism determined by constitutional inadequacies? *Proc. Assoc. Res. Nerv. Ment. Dis.*, **33**, 378–85

— (1959) Trends in child psychiatry, *J. ment. Sci.*, **105**, 581–93

— (1968) Early infantile autism revisited. *Psychiat. Dig.*, **29**, 17–28

— (1971) Follow-up study of eleven autistic children originally reported in 1943. *J. Autism child. Schiz.*, **1**, 119–45

— (1973) *Childhood Psychosis: Initial Studies and New Insights*. Washington: Winston

Kanner, L. & Eisenberg, L. (1956) Early infantile autism, 1943–1955. *Am. J. Ortho-psychiat.*, **26**, 55–65

Kanner, L. & Lesser, L. I. (1958) Early infantile autism. *Paed. Clin. North Am.*, **5**, 711–30

Kanner, L., Rodriguez, A. & Ashenden, B. (1972) How far can autistic children go in matters of social adaptation? *J. Autism child. Schiz.*, **2**, 9–33

Kantorowitz, D. & Cohen, B. D. (1977) Referent communication in chronic schizophrenia. *J. abnorm. Psychol.*, **86**, 1–9

Kaplan, J., Mandel, J. R., Stillman, R., Walker, R. W., Vandenheuvel, W. J. A., Gillin, J. C. & Wyatt, R. J. (1974) Blood and urine levels of N,N-dimethyltryptamine following administration of psychoactive doses to human subjects. *Psychopharmacol.*, **38**, 239–45

Karpatkin, S., Khan, Q. & Freedman, M. (1978) Heterogeneity of platelet function. *Am. J. Med.*, **64**, 542–6

Kasanin, J. (1933) The acute schizoaffective psychoses. *Am. J. Psychiat.*, **13**, 97–123

Kay, D. (1959) Observations on the natural history and genetics of old age psychoses. *Proc. R. Soc. Med.*, **52**, 29–32

— (1963) Late paraphrenia and its bearing on the aetiology of schizophrenia. *Acta psychiat. scand.*, **39**, 159–69

— (1978) Assessment of familial risks in the functional psychoses and their application in genetic counselling. *Brit. J. Psychiat.*, **133**, 385–403

Kay, D. W. K. & Roth, M. (1961) Environmental and hereditary factors in the schizophrenias of old age ("late paraphrenia") and their bearing on the general problem of causation in schizophrenia. *J. ment. Sci.*, **107**, 649–86

Keeler, W. R. (1958) Autistic patterns and defective communication in blind children with retrolental fibroplasia. In *Psychopathology of Communication*, ed. Hoch, P. H. & Zubin, J., pp. 64–83. New York: Grune & Stratton

Kelleher, M. J., Copeland, J. R. M. & Smith, A. J. (1974) High first admission rates for schizophrenia in the west of Ireland. *Psychol. Med.*, **4**, 460–62

Kendell, R. E. (1968) *The Classification of Depressive Illnesses*. Maudsley Monograph No. 18. London: Oxford University Press

— (1970) Relationship between aggression and depression. Epidemiological implications of a hypothesis. *Arch. gen. Psychiat.*, **22**, 308–18

— (1974) A new look at hysteria. *Medicine (monthly add-on journal, 1st series)*, **30**, 1780–3

— (1976) The classification of depressions: a review of contemporary confusion. *Brit. J. Psychiat.*, **129**, 15–29

Kendell, R. E. & Discipio, W. J. (1970) Obsessional symptoms and obsessional personality traits in patients with depressive illnesses. *Psychol. Med.*, **1**, 65–72

Kendell, R. E. & Gourlay, J. (1970) The clinical distinction between psychotic and neurotic depression. *Brit. J. Psychiat.*, **117**, 257–60

Kendell, R. E., Wainwright, S., Hailey, A. H. & Shannon, B. (1976) The influence of childbirth on psychiatric morbidity. *Psychol. Med.*, **6**, 297–302

Kendon, A. (1967) Some functions of gaze direction in social interaction. *Acta psychol.*, **26**, 22–63

Kendrick, D. C., Gibson, A. J. Moyes, I. C. A. (1979) The revised Kendrick battery: clinical studies. *Brit. J. soc. clin. Psychol.*, **18**, 329–40

Kenyon, F. E. (1976) Hypochondriacal states. *Brit. J. Psychiat.*, **129**, 1–14

Kessell, A. & Holt, N. F. (1966) Depression–an analysis of a follow-up study. *Brit. J. Psychiat.*, **111**, 1143–53

Kety, S. S. (1978) Schizophrenia: the challenge and the prospects of biologic research. In *Neurochemical and Immunologic Components in Schizophrenia*, ed. Bergsma, D. & Goldstein, A. L. *Birth defects: Original article series*, **14**, 5–15. New York: Alan R. Liss

Kety, S. S., Rosenthal, D., Wender, P. H. & Schulsinger, F. (1968) The types and prevalence of mental illness in the biological and adoptive families of adopted schizophrenics. In *The Transmission of Schizophrenia*, ed. Rosenthal, D. & Kety, S. S., p. 345. Oxford: Pergamon Press

— (1971) The types and prevalence of mental illness in the biological and adoptive families of adopted schizophrenics. In *Genetics, Environment and Psychopathology*, ed. Mednick, S. A., Schulsinger, F., Higgins, J. & Bell, B., p. 159. Amsterdam & Oxford: North-Holland; New York: American Elsevier

Kety, S. S., Rosenthal, D., Wender, P. H., Schulsinger, F. & Jacobsen, B. (1975) Mental illness in the biological and adoptive families of adopted individuals who have become schizophrenic: a preliminary report based on psychiatric interviews. In *Genetic Research in Psychiatry*, ed. Fieve, R. R., Rosenthal, D. & Brill, H., pp. 147–66. Baltimore: Johns Hopkins University Press

Kidd, K. K. & Cavalli-Sforza, L. L. (1973) An analysis of the genetics of schizophrenia. *Soc. Biol., New York*, **20**, 254–65

Kidd, K. K., Reich, T. & Kessler, S. (1973) Sex effect and the single gene. The relevance of sex effect in discriminating between genetic hypotheses. *Genet.*, **73**, 137

Kiev, A. (1976) Cluster analysis profiles of suicide attempters. *Am. J. Psychiat.*, **133**, 150–53

Kiloh, L. G. (1961) Pseudo-dementia. *Acta psychiat. scand.*, **37**, 336–51

— (1977) Commentary on the Report of Inquiry into Psychosurgery. *Med. J. Aust.*, **2**, 296–301

Kiloh, L. G., Andrews, G., Neilson, M. & Bianchi, G. N. (1972) The relationship of the syndromes called endogenous and neurotic depression. *Brit. J. Psychiat.*, **121**, 183–96

Kiloh, L. G., Child, J. P. & Latner, G. (1960) Endogenous depression treated with iproniazid–a follow-up study. *J. ment. Sci.*, **106**, 1425–8

Kiloh, L.G. & Garside, R. F. (1963) The independence of neurotic depression and endogenous depression. *Brit. J. Psychiat.*, **109**, 451–63

King, P. D. (1960) Chlorpromazine and electroconvulsive therapy in the treatment of newly hospitalized schizophrenics. *J. clin. exp. Psychopathol.*, **21**, 101–5

Kinkelin, M. (1954) Verlauf und Prognose des manisch-depressiven Irreseins. *Schweiz. Arch. Neurol. Psychiat.*, **73**, 100–46

Kinney, D. K. & Jacobsen, B. (1978) Environmental factors in schizophrenia: new adoption study evidence. In *The Nature of Schizophrenia*, ed. Wynne, L. C., Cromwell, R. L. & Matthysse, S., pp. 38–51. New York: Wiley

Kirk, S. A., McCarthy, J. & Kirk, W. D. (1968) *Illinois Test of Psycholinguistic Abilities* (revised edition). Urbana: University of Illinois Press

Klein, D. F. (1974) Endogenomorphic depression. *Arch. gen. Psychiat.*, **31**, 447–54

Klein, D. F. & Davis, J. M. (1969) Review of antipsychotic drug literature. In *Diagnosis and Treatment of Psychiatric Disorders*, chap. 5, pp. 51–137. Baltimore: Williams & Wilkins

Kleist, K. (1928) Über zykloide, paranoide und epileptoide Psychosen und über die Frage der Degenerationspsychosen. *Schweiz. Arch. Neurol. Psychiat.*, **23**, 1

— (1953) Die Gliederung der neuropsychischen Erkrankungen. *Mschr. Psychiat. Neurol*, **125**, 526

Klemperer, J. (1933) Zur Belastungsstatistik der Durchschnittsbevölkerung. *Z. ges. Neurol. Psychiat.*, **146**, 277–316

Klerman, G. L. & Cole, J. O. (1965) Clinical pharmacology of imipramine and related antidepressant compounds. *Pharmacol. Rev.*, **17**, 101–41

Kline, N. S. (1954) Use of Rauwolfia serpentinia Benth in neuropsychiatric conditions. *Ann. N.Y. Acad. Sci.*, **59**, 107–32

Knights, A. K., Hirsch, S. R. & Platt, S. D. (1980) Clinical change as a function of brief admission to hospital in a controlled study using the P.S.E. *Brit. J. Psychiat.*, **137**, 170–80

Knights, A. K., Okasha, M. S., Salih, M. A. & Hirsch, S. R. (1979) Depressive and extrapyramidal symptoms and clinical effects: A trial of fluphenazine versus flupenthixol in maintenance of schizophrenic outpatients. *Brit. J. Psychiat.*, **135**, 515–23

Knobloch, H. & Pasamanick, B. (1966) Etiological factors in 'early infantile autism' and 'childhood schizophrenia'. Presented at the 10th Int. Cong. Paediat., Lisbon, 1962

— (1974) Autistic, psychotic and other disturbed behaviour. In *Gesell and Amatruda's Developmental Diagnosis*, ed. Knobloch, H. & Pasamanick, B., 3rd ed., pp. 320–39. New York: Harper & Row

— (1975) Some etiologic and prognostic factors in infantile autism and psychosis. *Pediat.*, **55**, 182—90

Koegel, R. L. & Wilhelm, H. (1973) Selective responding to the components of multiple visual cues by autistic children. *J. exp. child Psychol.*, **15**, 442–53

Koegel, R. L. & Rincover, A. (1974) Treatment of psychotic children in a classroom environment. *J. app. Behav. Anal.*, **7**, 45–9

Koehler, K. (1979) First rank symptoms of schizophrenia: questions concerning clinical boundaries. *Brit. J. Psychiat.*, **134**, 236–48

Koehler, K. & Jacoby, C. (1976) Season of birth & Schneider-oriented diagnosis of affective disorder. *Psychiat. Clin.* (Basel) **9**, 212–19

Koh, S. D., Kayton, L. & Berry, R. (1973) Mnemonic organization in young nonpsychotic schizophrenics. *J. abnorm. Psychol.*, **81**, 299–310

Koh, S. D., Kayton, L. & Schwartz, C. (1974) The structure of word-storage in the permanent memory of nonpsychotic schizophrenics. *J. consult. clin. Psychol.*, **42**, 879–87

Koh, S. D. & Peterson, R. A. (1978) Encoding orientation and the remembering of schizophrenic young adults. *J. abnorm. Psychol.*, **87**, 303–13

Koh, S. D., Szoc, R. & Peterson, R. A. (1977) Short-term memory scanning in schizophrenic young adults. *J. abnorm. Psychol.*, **86**, 451–60

Kohn, M. L. (1973) Social class and schizophrenia: a critical review and reformulation. *Schiz. Bull.*, **7**, 60–79

Kolle, K. (1931a) Paraphrenie und Paranoia. *Fortschr. Neurol. Psychiat.*, **3**, 319–34

— (1931b) *Die primäre Verrücktheit*, p. 19. Leipzig: Thieme

— (1957) *Der Wahnkranke im Lichte alter und neuer Psychopathologie*, pp. 42–43, 8–11. Stuttgart: Thieme

Koluchova, J. (1972) Severe deprivation in twins: A case study. *J. child Psychol. Psychiat.*, **13**, 107–14

— (1976) A report on the further development of twins after severe and prolonged deprivation. In *Early Experience: Myth and Evidence*, ed. Clarke, A. M. & Clarke, A. D. B., pp. 56–66. London: Open Books

Kolvin, I. (1971) Studies in the childhood psychoses: I. Diagnostic criteria and classification. *Brit. J. Psychiat.*, **118**, 381–4

(1972) Infantile autism or infantile psychoses. *Brit. med. J.* **3**, 753–5

Kolvin, I., Garside, R. & Kidd, J. (1971) Studies in the childhood psychoses. IV. Parental personality and attitude and childhood psychosis. *Brit. J. Psychiat.*, **118**, 403–6

Kolvin, I., Humphrey, M. & McNay, A. (1971) Studies in the childhood psychoses. VI. Cognitive factors in childhood psychoses. *Brit. J. Psychiat.*, **118**, 415–20

Kolvin, I., Ounsted, C., Humphrey, M. & McNay, A. (1971) Studies in the childhood psychoses. II. The phenomenology of childhood psychoses. *Brit. J. Psychiat.*, **118**, 385–95

Kolvin, I., Ounsted, C., Richardson, L. & Garside, R. (1971) Studies in the childhood psychoses. III. The family and social background in childhood psychoses. *Brit. J. Psychiat.*, **118**, 396–402

Kolvin, I., Ounsted, C. & Roth, M. (1971) Studies in the childhood psychoses. V. Cerebral dysfunction and childhood psychosis. *Brit. J. Psychiat.*, **118**, 407–14

Korboot, P. J. & Damiani, N. (1976) Auditory processing speed and signal detection in schizophrenia. *J. abnorm. Psychol.*, **85**, 287–95

Korf, J., van Praag, H. M. & Sebens, J. B. (1972) Serum tryptophan decreased, brain tryptophan increased and brain serotonin unchanged after probenecid loading. *Brain Res.*, **42**, 239

Kotin, J. & Goodwin, F. K. (1972) Depression during mania: clinical observations and theoretical implications. *Am. J. Psychiat.*, **129**, 679–86

Kraepelin, E. (1899) *Psychiatrie*. 6th ed. Leipzig: Barth

— (1913) *Lectures on Clinical Psychiatry*. 8th ed. rev. and ed. Johnstone, T. London: Baillière, Tindall & Cox

— (1913) *Psychiatrie*, vol. 8, pt. 2, pp. 967–1022. Leipzig: Barth

— (1920) Die Erscheinungsformen des Irreseins. *Z. ges. Neurol. Psychiat.*, **62**, 1–29

— (1921) *Manic-depressive Insanity and Paranoia*. Trans. Barclay, R. M. Edinburgh: Livingstone

Kramer, M. (1961) Discussion of contribution by J. A. Böök. In *Causes of Mental Disorders: A Review of Epidemiological Knowledge*, 1959. New York: Millbank Memorial Fund

— (1978) Population changes and schizophrenia, 1970–1985. In *The Nature of Schizophrenia*, ed. Wynne, L. C., Cromwell, R. L. & Matthysse, S., pp. 545–71. New York: Wiley

Krauthammer, C. & Klerman, G. L. (1978) Secondary mania. Manic

syndromes associated with antecedent physical illness or drugs. *Arch. gen. Psychiat.*, **35**, 1333–9

Kreitman, N. (1976) The coal gas story: UK suicide rates 1960–1971. *Brit. J. prev. soc. Med.*, **30**, 86

— (1977) *Parasuicide*. London: Wiley

Kreitman, N., Sainsbury, P., Pearce, K. & Costain, W. R. (1965) Hypochondriasis and depression in outpatients at a general hospital. *Brit. J. Psychiat.*, **111**, 607–15

Kretschmer, E. (1925) *Physique and Character*. 2nd ed. (Trans. Sprott, W. J. H., 1936) London: Kegan Paul, Trench & Trubner

— (1966) *Der sensitive Beziehungswahn. Ein Beitrag zur Paranoiafrage und zur psychiatrischen Charakterlehre*. 4th ed. Berlin: Heidelberg & New York: Springer. (English translation: *The Sensitive Delusion of Reference*. Selected sections in *Themes and Variations in European Psychiatry*, ed. Hirsch, S. R. & Shepherd, M. (1974), p. 153. Bristol: Wright)

Kringlen, E. (1967) *Heredity and environment in the functional psychoses. An Epidemiological–Clinical Twin Study*. Oslo: University Press; London: Heinemann

Kulhanek, F., Lunde, O. K. & Meisenberg, G. (1979) Precipitation of insoluble complexes due to interactions between coffee and tea with antipsychotic medication. *Lancet*, **ii**, 1130

Kulhara, P. & Wig, N. N. (1978) The chronicity of schizophrenia in North-West India. *Brit. J. Psychiat.*, **132**, 186–90

Kuriansky, J. B., Gurland, B. J., Spitzer, R. L. & Endicott, J. (1977) Trends in the frequency of schizophrenia by different diagnostic criteria. *Am. J. Psychiat.*, **134**, 631–6

Kysar, J. E. (1968) The two camps in child psychiatry: a report from a psychiatrist-father of an autistic and retarded child. *Am. J. Psychiat.*, **125**, 103–9

Lader, M. (1979) Monitoring plasma concentrations of neuroleptics. *Pharmakopsych.*, **9**, 170–77

Lader, M. H. & Wing, L. (1969) Physiological measures in agitated and retarded depressed patients. *J. psychiat. Res.*, **7**, 89–100

Laing, R. D. (1960) *The Divided Self: a Study of Sanity and Madness*. Chicago: Quadrangle Books

— (1967) The schizophrenic experience. In *The Politics of Experience*. London: Penguin Books

Lancet (1976) Neurological foundations of infantile autism. **ii**, 668–9

Lane, E. A. & Albee, G. W. (1968) On childhood intellectual decline and schizophrenia: a reasssessment of an earlier study. *J. abnorm. Psychol.*, **73**, 774–7

Lane, H. (1977) *The Wild Boy of Aveyron*. London: Allen & Unwin

Lang, P. J. & Buss, A. H. (1965) Psychological deficit in schizophrenia, II. Interference and activation. *J. abnorm. Psychol.* **70**, 77–106

Lang, T. (1931) Zur Frage: Geisteskrankheit und Geburtsmonat. *Arch. Rassen-Biol.*, **25**, 42–57

Langdell, T. (1978) Recognition of faces: an approach to the study of autism. *J. child Psychol. Psychiat.*, **19**, 255–68

Lange, J. (1928) Die endogenen und reaktiven Gemütserkrankungen und die manischdepressive Konstitution. In *Handbuch der Geisteskrankheiten*, ed. Bumke, O. W., vol. 6. Berlin: Springer

Langer, G., Schönbeck, G., Koinig, G., Lesch, O. & Schlüssler, M. (1979) Hyperactivity of hypothalamic pituitary-adrenal axis in endogenous depression. *Lancet*, **ii**, 524

Langfeldt, G. (1937) *The Prognosis in Schizophrenia and the Factors influencing the Course of the Disease*. Copenhagen: Levin & Munksgaard

— (1939) *The Schizophreniform States*. London: Oxford University Press; Copenhagen: Munksgaard

— (1956) The prognosis of schizophrenia. *Acta psychiat. neurol. scand.*, Supp. 13. Copenhagen: Munksgaard

— (1960) Diagnosis and prognosis of schizophrenia. *Proc. R. Soc. Med.*, **53**, 1047–51

Langsley, D. G., Enterline, J. D. & Hickerson, G. (1959) A comparison of chlorpromazine and ECT in treatment of acute schizophrenics and manic reactions. *Arch. Neurol. Psychiat.*, **81**, 384–91

Larsen, S. F. & Fromholt, P. (1976) Mnemonic organization and form recall in schizophrenia. *J. abnorm. Psychol.*, **85**, 61–5

Larson, C. A. & Nyman, G. E. (1973) Differential fertility in schizophrenia. *Acta psychiat. scand.*, **49**, 272–80

Larsson, T. & Sjögren, T. (1954) A methodological, psychiatric, and statistical study of a large Swedish rural population. *Acta psychiat. neurol. scand.*, Supp. 89

Lasèque, C. & Falret, J. (1877) La folie à deux ou folie communiquée. *Ann. méd.-psychol.*, **38**, 321

Laubscher, B. J. F. (1937) *Sex, Custom and Psychopathology*. London: Routledge

Lawson, J. S., McGhie, A. & Chapman, J. (1964) Perception of speech in schizophrenia. *Brit. J. Psychiat.*, **110**, 375–80

Leach, J. & Wing, J. K. (1980) *Helping Destitute Men*. London: Tavistock

Leckman, J., Gershon, E., McGinniss, M., Targum, S. & Dibble, E. (1979) New data do not suggest linkage between the Xg blood group and bipolar illness. *Arch. gen. Psychiat.*, **36**, 1435–41

Lee, T. Seeman, P., Tourtellotte, W. W., Farley. I. J. & Hornykiewicz, O. (1978) Binding of [³H]-neuroleptics and [³H]apomorphine in schizophrenic brains. *Nature, London*, **274**, 897–900

Leff, J. P. (1973) Culture and the differentiation of emotional states. *Brit. J. Psychiat.*, **123**, 299–306.

— (1978) Social and psychological causes of the acute attack. In *Schizophrenia: Towards a New Synthesis*, ed. Wing, J. K. London: Academic Press

Leff, J. P., Fischer, M. & Bertelsen, A. C. (1976) A cross-national epidemiological study of mania. *Brit. J. Psychiat.*, **129**, 428–42

Leff, J., Hirsch, S. R., Rohde, P., Gaind, R. & Stevens, B. C. (1973) Life events and maintenance therapy in schizophrenic relapse. *Brit. J. Psychiat.* **123**, 659–60

Leff, J. & Vaughn, C. (1976) Schizophrenia and family life. *Psychol. To-day*, **2**, 13–18

Leff, J. P. & Wing, J. K. (1971) Trial of maintenance therapy in schizophrenia. *Brit. med. J.*, **3**, 599–604

Lefkowitz, M. M. and Burton, N. (1978) Childhood depression: a critique of the concept. *Psychol. Bull.*, **85**, 716–26

Leighton, A. H., Lambo, T. A., Hughes, C. C., Leighton, D. C., Murphy, J. M. & Macklin, D. B. (1963) *Psychiatric Disorder among the Yoruba*. Ithaca, N.Y.: Cornell University Press

Leiter, R. G. (1952) *Leiter International Performance Scale*. Chicago: Stoelting

Lemert, E. M. (1951) *Social Pathology*, New York: McGraw-Hill

Lennox-Buchthal, M. (1973) Treatment and prevention of febrile convulsions. In *Prevention of Epilepsy and its Consequences*, ed. Parsonage, M. J., pp. 44–50. Proc. Fifth Symp. Epilepsy, London. London: International Bureau for Epilepsy

Leonhard, K. (1959) *Aufteilung der endogenen Psychosen*. Berlin, D. D. R. Akademie Verlag (see also 1979, below)

— (1961) Cycloid psychoses: endogenous psychoses which are neither schizophrenic nor manic-depressive. *J. ment. Sci.*, **107**, 633–48

— (1979) *The Classification of Endogenous Psychoses*, ed. Robins, E., trans. Berman, R., 5th ed. New York: Irvington

Leonhard, K., Korff, I. & Schulz, H. (1962) Die Temperamente in den Familien der Monopolaren und Bipolaren phasischen Psychosen. *Psychiat. Neurol (Basel)*, **143**, 416–34.

Letemendia, F. J. & Harris, A. D. (1967) Chlorpramazine and the untreated chronic schizophrenic. A long term trial. *Brit. J. Psychiat.*, **113**, 950–58

Levy, R. & Maxwell, A. E. (1968) The effect of verbal context on the recall of schizophrenics and other psychiatric patients. *Brit. J. Psychiat.*, **114**, 311–16

Lewine, R. J., Watt, N. F., Prentky, R. A. & Fryer, J. H. (1978) Childhood behaviour in schizophrenia, personality disorder, depression and neurosis. *Brit. J. Psychiat.*, **133**, 347–57

Lewinsohn, P. M., Biglan, A. & Zeiss, A. M. (1976) Behavioral treatment of depression. In *The Behavioral Management of Anxiety, Depression and Pain*, ed. Davidson, P. O. chap. 4, pp. 91–146. New York: Brunner Mazel

Lewis, A. J. (1934) Melancholia: a clinical survey of depressive states. *J. ment. Sci.*, **80**, 277–378

— (1936) Melancholia: prognostic study and case material. *J. ment. Sci.*, **82**, 488–558

— (1955) Psychosis–paranoia and paranoid states. In *British Encyclopaedia of Medical Practice*, 2nd ed. vol. 10, pp. 362–70. London: Butterworths

— (1957) Social Psychiatry. In *Lectures on the Scientific Basis of Medicine*, vol. 6, pp. 116–42. University of London: Athlone Press

— (1962) Ebb and flow in social psychiatry. *Yale J. Biol. Med.*, **35**, 62–83

— (1970) Paranoia and paranoid. *Psychol. Med.*, **1**, 2–12

— (1973) Manfred Bleuler's *The schizophrenic mental disorders*: an exposition and a review. *Psychol. Med.*, **3**, 385–92

Lichstein, K. & Schreibman, L. (1976) Employing electric shock with autistic children: a review of the side-effects. *J. Autism child. Schiz.*, **6**, 163–73

Lidz, T. (1975) *The Origin and Treatment of Schizophrenic Disorders*. London: Hutchinson

— (1978) Egocentric cognitive regression and the family setting of schizophrenic disorders. In *The Nature of Schizophrenia: New Approaches to Research and Treatment*, ed. Wynne, L. C., Cromwell, R. L. & Matthysse, S. New York: Wiley

Lindelius, R. (1970) A study of schizophrenia. *Acta psychiat. scand.*, Supp. 216

Lindelius, R. & Kay, D. W. K. (1973) Some changes in the pattern of mortality in schizophrenia in Sweden. *Acta psychiat. scand.*, **49**, 315–23

Lishman, W. A. (1978) *Organic Psychiatry: The Psychological Consequences of Cerebral Disorder*. Oxford: Blackwell

Littlewood, R. & Lipsedge, M. (1978) Acute psychotic reactions in Africans. *Brit. J. Psychiat.*, **132**, 106–7

Lloyd, K. J., Farley, I. J., Deck, J. H. N. & Hornykiewicz, O. (1974) Serotonin and 5-hydroxyindolacetic acid in discrete areas of the brainstem of suicide victims and control patients. *Adv. Biochem. Psychopharmacol.*, **11**, 387

Lobascher, M. E., Kingerlee, P. E. & Gubbay, S. S. (1970) Childhood autism: an investigation of aetiological factors in twenty-five cases. *Brit. J. Psychiat.*, **117**, 525–9

Lock, A. (Ed.) (1978) *Action, Gesture and Symbol: The Emergence of Language.* London: Academic Press

Lockyer, L. & Rutter, M. (1969) A five to fifteen year follow-up study of infantile psychosis: III. Psychological aspects. *Brit. J. Psychiat.*, **115**, 865–82

Logan, W. P. D. & Cushion, A. A. (1958) *Studies on Medical and Population Subjects. Morbidity Statistics from General Practice.* General Register Office. London: HMSO

Lotter, V. (1966) Epidemiology of autistic conditions in young children, I. Prevalence. *Soc. Psychiat.*, **1**, 124–37

— (1967) Epidemiology of autistic conditions in young children. II. Some characteristics of the parents and children. *Soc. Psychiat.*, **1**, 163–73

— (1974) Factors related to outcome in autistic children. *J. Autism child. Schiz.*, **4**, 263–77

— (1974) Social adjustment and placement of autistic children in Middlesex: a follow-up study. *J. Autism child. Schiz.*, **4**, 11–32

— (1978) Childhood autism in Africa. *J. child Psychol. Psychiat.*, **19**, 231–44

— (1978) Follow-up studies. In *Autism: A Reappraisal of Concepts and Treatment*, ed. Rutter, M. & Schopler, E. New York: Plenum Press

Loudon, J. B., Blackburn, I. M. & Ashworth, C. M. (1977) A study of the symptomatology and course of manic illness using a new scale. *Psychol. Med.*, **7**, 723–9

Lovaas, O. I. (1966) A program for the establishment of speech in psychotic children. In *Early Childhood Autism: Clinical, Educational and Social Aspects*, ed. Wing, J. K. Oxford: Pergamon Press

— (1977) *The Autistic Child: Language Development through Behavior Modification.* New York: Wiley

Lovaas, O. I., Koegel, R., Simmons, J. Q. & Long, J. S. (1973) Some generalisations and follow-up measures on autistic children in behaviour therapy. *J. appl. behav. Anal.*, **6**, 131–65

Lovaas, O. I., Schaeffer, B. & Simmons, J. Q. (1965) Experimental studies in childhood schizophrenia: building social behavior in autistic children by use of electric shock. *J. Exp. Res. Personality*, **1**, 99–109

Lovaas, O. I., Schreibman, L., Koegel, R. & Rehm, R. (1971) Selective responding by autistic children to multiple sensory input. *J. abnorm. Psychol.*, **77**, 211–22

Lovell, A. (1978) *In a Summer Garment*, London: Secker & Warburg

Lowe, M. (1975) Trends in the development of representational play in infants from one to three years, an observational study. *J. child Psychol. Psychiat.*, **16**, 33–47

Lowe, M. & Costello, A. J. (1976) *Manual for the Symbolic Play Test (experimental edition).* Windsor: National Foundation for Educational Research

Lowenthal, M. E. & Haven, C. (1968) Interaction and adaptation: Intimacy as a critical variable. *Amer. sociol. Rev.*, **33**, 20–30

Lundquist, G. (1945) Prognosis and course in manic-depressive psychosis. *Acta psychiat. neurol. scand.*, Supp. 35

Luxenburger, H. (1928) Demographische und psychiatrische Untersuchungen in der engeren biologischen Familie von Paralytiker (Versuch einer Belastung). *Z. ges. Neurol. Psychiat.*, **113**, 331–491

Maas, J. W., Fawcett, J. A. & DeKirmenjian, H. (1972) Catecholamine metabolism, depressive illness and drug response. *Arch. gen. Psychiat.*, **26**, 252–62

Maas, J. W., Hattox, S. E., Greene, N. M. & Landis, D. H. (1979) 3-Methoxy-4-hydroxyphenethyleneglycol production by human brain in vivo. *Science*, **205**, 1025–7

McClelland, H. A. (1976) Discussion on assessment of drug induced extrapyramidal reactions. *Brit. J. clin. Pharmacol.*, supp. **2**, 401–3

McClelland, H. A., Farquharson, R. C., Legburn, P., Furness, J. A. & Schiff, A. A. (1976) Very high dose fluphenazine decanoate. *Arch. gen. Psychiat.*, **33**, 1435–42

MacDonald, J. B. (1918) Prognosis in manic depressive insanity. *J. nerv. ment. Dis.*, **47**, 20–30

McDowall, A. W. T., Brooke, E. M., Freeman-Browne, D. L. & Robin, A. A. (1968) Subsequent suicide in depressed in-patients. *Brit. J. Psychiat.*, **114**, 749–54

MacFarlane, J. W., Allen, L. & Honzik, M. (1962) *A Developmental Study of the Behavior Problems of Normal Children between 21 months and 14 years.* Berkeley: University of California Press

McGeer, P. L. & McGeer, E. G. (1976) Enzymes associated with the metabolisms of catecholamines, acetylcholine and GABA in human controls and patients with Parkinson's disease and Huntington's chorea. *J. Neurochem.*, **26**, 65–76

— (1977) Possible changes in striatal and limbic cholinergic systems in schizophrenia. *Arch. gen. Psychiat.*, **34**, 1319–23

McGhie, A. (1970) Attention and perception in schizophrenia. In *Progress in Experimental Personality Research*, vol. 5, ed. Maher, B. A. New York: Academic Press

McGhie, A. & Chapman, J. (1961) Disorders of attention and perception in early schizophrenia. *Brit. J. med. Psychol.*, **34**, 103–16

McGlashan, T. & Carpenter, W. (1976) Post-psychotic depression in schizophrenia. *Arch. gen. Psychiat.*, **33**, 231–9

McHugh, P. R. & Goodell, H. (1971) Suicidal behaviour: a distinction of patients with sedative poisoning seen in a general hospital. *Arch. gen. Psychiat.*, **25**, 456–64

Mackay, A. V. P., Doble, A., Bird, E. D., Spokes, E. G., Quik, M. & Iversen, L. L. (1978) [³H] Spiperone binding in normal and schizophrenic post-mortem human brain. *Life Sci.*, **23**, 527–32

McKnew, D. H., Cytryn, L., Efron, A. M., Gershon, E. S. & Bunney, W. E., Jr. (1979) Offspring of patients with affective disorders. *Brit. J. Psychiat.*, **134**, 148–52

MacMahon, B. & Pugh, T. F. (1970) *Epidemiology: Principles and Methods.* Boston: Little, Brown

McNeil, T. F. & Kaij, L. (1978) Obstetric factors in the development of schizophrenia: complications in the births of preschizophrenics and in reproduction by schizophrenic parents. In *The Nature of Schizophrenia*, ed. Wynne, W. C., Cromwell, R. L. & Matthysse, S., pp. 401–29. New York: Wiley

MacSweeney, D., Timms, P. & Johnson, A. (1978) Thyro-endocrine pathology, obstetric mortality and schizophrenia: survey of a hundred families with a schizophrenic proband. *Psychol. Med.*, **8**, 151–5

MacVane, J. R., Lange, T. D., Brown, W. A. & Zayat, M. (1978) Psychological functioning of bipolar manic-depressives in remission. *Arch. gen. Psychiat.*, **35**, 1351–4

Magnan, V. (1893) *Leçons Cliniques sur les Maladies Mentales.* Paris: Battaille

Maher, B. A. (1972) The language of schizophrenia: a review and interpretation. *Brit. J. Psychiat.*, **120**, 3–17

Maher, B. A., McKean, K. O. & McLaughlin, B. (1966) Studies in psychotic language. In *The General Inquirer: A Computer Approach to Content Analysis*, ed. Stone, P. J. *et al.* Cambridge, Mass.: MIT Press

Mahler, M. S. (1952) On child psychoses and schizophrenia: autistic and symbiotic infantile psychoses. *Psychoanal. Study Child*, **7**, 286–305

Maisto, C. R., Baumeister, A. A. & Maisto, A. A. (1979) An analysis of variables related to self injurious behavior among institutionalized retarded persons. *J. ment. Defic. Res.*, **22**, 27–36

Malussek, N. (1978) Neuroendokrinologische Untersuchungen bei depressiven Syndromen. *Nervenarzt*, **49**, 569–75

Malzberg, B. (1929) A statistical review of occupational therapy in the New York civil state hospitals. *Psychiat. Q.*, **3**, 413–25

— (1962) The distribution of mental disease according to religious affiliation in New York State 1949–1951. *Ment. Hyg.*, (N.Y.), **46**, 510–22

Mann, S. & Cree, W. (1976) 'New' long-stay psychiatric patients: a national sample survey of fifteen mental hospitals in England and Wales, 1972/3. *Psychol. Med.*, **6**, 603–16

Marchant, R., Howlin, P., Yule, W. & Rutter, M. L. (1974) Graded change in the treatment of the behaviour of autistic children. *J. child Psychol. Psychiat.*, **15**, 221–7

Marsella, A. J. (1978) Thoughts on cross-cultural studies on the epidemiology of depression. *Culture, Med. Psychiat.*, **2**, 343–57

Martin, S., Cadoret, R., Winokur, G. & Ora, E. (1972) Unipolar depression: A family history study. *Biol. Psychiat.*, **4**, 205

Martin, J. R. & Rochester, S. R. (1975) Cohesion and reference in schizophrenic speech. In *The First LACUS Forum*, ed. Makkai, A. & Makkai, V. Columbia, South Carolina: Hornbeam Press

Masters, A. (1967) The distribution of blood groups in psychiatric illness. *Brit. J. Psychiat.*, **113**, 1309–15

Maudsley, H. (1867) *The Physiology and Pathology of the Mind*, 1st ed., pp. 259–93. New York: Appleton

Matthysse, S. & Matthysse, A. G. (1978) Virological and immunological hypotheses of schizophrenia. In *Psychopharmacology: A Generation of Progress*, ed. Lipton, M. A., DiMascio, A. & Killam, K. F., pp. 1125–9. New York: Raven Press

May, A. R. (1972) Suicide – a world health problem. In *Suicide and Attempted Suicide*, ed. Waldenstrom, J., Larsson, T. & Ljungstedt, N. Stockholm: Nordiska Bokhandelns Förlag

May, P. R. A. & Tuma, A. H. (1965) Treatment of schizophrenia. *Brit. J. Psychiat.*, **111**, 503–10

May, P. R. A., Tuma, A. H., Yale, C., Potepan, P. & Dixon, W. (1976) Schizophrenia – a follow-up study of the results of treatment. *Arch. Gen. Psychiat.*, **33**, 481–6

Mayer-Gross, W. (1932) Die Schizophrenie. In *Handbuch der Geisteskrankheiten*, vol. IX, ed. Bumke, O. Berlin: Springer

Mayou, R. (1976) The nature of bodily symptoms. *Brit. J. Psychiat.*, **129**, 55–60

Measel, C. J. & Alfieri, P. A. (1976) Treatment of self injurious behavior by a combination of reinforcement for incompatible behavior and over-correction. *Am. J. ment. Defic.* **81**, 147–53

Medical Research Council (1965) Clinical trial of the treatment of depressive illness. *Brit. med. J.*, **1**, 881–6

Mednick, S. A. (1958) A learning theory approach to research in schizophrenia. *Psychol. Bull.*, **55**, 316–27

Meehl, P. E. (1962) Schizotaxia, schizotypy, schizophrenia. *Am. Psychologist*, **17**, 827–36

— (1964) *Manual for use with Checklist of Schizotypic Signs*. Unpublished manuscript. Psychiatric Research Unit, University of Minnesota Medical Sschool

(1973) Specific genetic etiology, psychodynamics, and therapeutic nihilism. In *Psychodiagnosis: Selected papers*, by Meehl, P. Minneapolis: University of Minnesota Press

— (1977) Specific etiology and other forms of strong influence: Some quantitative meanings. *J. Med. Philos.*, **2**, 33–53

— (1978) Theoretical risks and tabular asterisks: Sir Karl, Sir Ronald, and the slow progress of soft psychology. *J. consult. clin. Psychol.*, **46**, 806–34

Meltzer, H. Y. (1973) Creative phosphokinase activity and clinical symptomatology. *Arch. gen. Psychiat.*, **29**, 589–93

— (1976) Neuromuscular dysfunction in schizophrenia. *Schiz. Bull.*, **2**, 106–35

Mendels, J. (1965) Electroconvulsive therapy and depression. III, A method of prognosis. *Brit. J. Psychiat.*, **111**, 687–90

Mendels, J. & Chernik, D. A. (1975) Sleep changes and affective illness. In *The Nature and Treatment of Depression*, ed. Flach, F. F. & Draghi, S. C., pp. 309–33. New York: Wiley

Mendels, J. & Frazer, A. (1974) Brain biogenic amine depletion and mood. *Arch. gen. Psychiat.*, **30**, 447–51

Mendels, J. & Hawkins, D. R. (1971) Longitudinal sleep study in hypomania. *Arch. gen. Psychiat.*, **25**, 274–7

Mendelson, M. (1974) *Psychoanalytic Concepts of Depression*. 2nd ed. New York: Spectrum Publications

Mendelwicz, J. & Fleiss, J. (1974) Linkage studies with X-chromosome markers in bipolar (manic-depressive) and unipolar (depressive) illness. *Biol. Psychiat.*, **9**, 261–94

Mendelwicz, J., Fleiss, J. & Fieve, R. (1972) Evidence for X-linkage in the transmission of manic-depressive illness. *J. Am. Med. Assoc.*, **222**, 1624–7

Mendelwicz, J., Fleiss, J. & Fieve, R. (1975) Linkage studies in affective disorders. The Xg blood group and manic-depressive illness. In *Genetics and Psychopathology*, ed. Fieve, R., Rosenthal, D. & Brill, H., pp. 220–32. Baltimore: Johns Hopkins Press

Mendelwicz, J. & Linkowski, P. (1978) Linkage between glucose-6-phosphate dehydrogenase deficiency and manic-depressive illness. Paper presented at the Second World Congress of Biological Psychiatry, Barcelona, Spain

Mendelwicz, J., Linkowski, P., Guroff, J. & van Praag, H. (1979) Color blindness linkage to bipolar manic-depressive illness. *Arch. gen. Psychiat.*, **36**, 1442–7

Mendelwicz, J., Massart-Guiot, T. & Wilmotte, J. (1974) Blood groups in manic-depressive illness and schizophrenia. *Dis. nerv. Syst.*, **35**, 39–41

Mendelwicz, J. & Rainer, J. D. (1974) Morbidity risk and genetic transmission in manic-depressive illness. *Am. J. hum. Genet.*, **26**, 692–701

Mendelwicz, J. & Rainer, J. (1977) Adoption study supporting genetic transmission in manic-depressive illness. *Nature*, **268**, 326–9

Mental Disorders: *Glossary and Guide to their Classification in accordance with the Ninth Revision of the International Classification of Diseases*. (1978) Geneva: World Health Organization

Meyers, D. & Goldfarb, W. (1962) Psychiatric appraisals of parents and siblings of schizophrenic children. *Am. J. Psychiat.*, **118**, 902–8

Miles, C. P. (1977) Conditions predisposing to suicide: A review. *J. nerv. ment. Dis.*, **164**, 231–46

Miller, D. H., Clancy, J. & Cumming, E. (1953) A comparison between unidirectional current non-convulsive electrical stimulation given with Reiter's machine, standard alternating current electroshock (Cerletti method) and pentotholin chronic schizophrenia. *Am. J. Psychiat.*, **109**, 617–20

Miller, W. R. (1975) Psychological deficit in depression. *Psychol. Bull.*, **82**, 238–60

Mindham, R. H. S. (1976) Assessment of drug induced extrapyramidal reactions and of drugs given for their control. *Brit. J. clin. Pharmacol.*, Supp. **2**, 395–400

Minkoff, K., Bergman, E. & Beck, A. T. (1973) Hopelessness, depression and attempted suicide. *Am. J. Psychiat.*, **130**, 455–9

Mitsuda, H. (ed.) (1967), *Clinical Genetics in Psychiatry.* Tokyo: Igaku-Shoin

Mittler, P., Gillies, S. & Jukes, E. (1966) Prognosis in psychotic children: report of a follow-up study. *J. ment. Def. Res.*, **10**, 73–83

Modrzewska, K. & Böök, J. A. (1979) Schizophrenia and malignant neoplasms in a North Swedish population. *Lancet*, **i**, 275–6

Moir, A. T. B., Ashcroft, G. W., Crawford, T. B. B., Eccleston, D. & Guldberg, H. C. (1970) Cerebral metabolites in cerebrospinal fluid as a biochemical approach to the brain. *Brain*, **93**, 357–68

Monod, J. (1971) *Chance and Necessity*, pp. 161–2. New York: Alfred A. Knopf

Morel, B. A. (1860) *Traité des Maladies Mentales.* Paris: Masson

Morgan, R. (1979) Conversations with chronic schizophrenic patients. *Brit. J. Psychiat.*, **134**, 187–94

Morris, J. B. & Beck, A. T. (1974) The efficacy of antidepressant drugs. *Arch. gen. Psychiat.*, **30**, 667–74

Morrison, J. R. (1973) Catatonia. *Arch. gen. Psychiat.*, **28**, 39–41

— (1974) Changes in subtype diagnosis of schizophrenia 1920–66. *Am. J. Psychiat.*, **131**, 674–7

— (1975) The family histories of manic-depressive patients with and without alcoholism. *J. nerv. ment. Dis.*, **160**, 227–9

Murillo, L. & Exner, J. E. (1973) The effects of regressive ECT with process schizophrenia. *Am. J. Psychiat.*, **130**, 267–73

Murphy, D. L. & Beigel, A. (1974) Depression, elation and lithium carbonate responses in manic patient subgroups. *Arch. gen. Psychiat.*, **31**, 643–8

Murphy, D. L., Belmaker, R., Carpenter, W. T. & Wyatt, R. J. (1977) Monoamine oxidase in chronic schizophrenia: studies of hormonal and other factors affecting enzyme activity. *Brit. J. Psychiat.*, **130**, 151–8

Murphy, D. L., Brodie, H. K. H., Goodwin, K. K. & Bunney, W. K., Jr. (1971) L-Dopa. Regular induction of hypomania in bipolar manic depressive patients. *Nature*, **229**, 135–6

Murphy, D. L., Wright, C., Buchsbaum, M., Nichols, A., Costa, J. L. & Wyatt, R. J. (1976) Platelet and plasma amine oxidase activity in 680 normals: sex and age differences and stability over time. *Biochem. Med.*, **16**, 254–65

Murphy, G. M., Steele, K., Gilligan, T., Yeow, J. & Spare, D. (1977) Teaching a picture language to a non-speaking retarded boy. *Behav. Res. Ther.*, **15**, 198–201

Murphy, H. B. M. (1968) Cultural factors in the genesis of schizophrenia. In *The Transmission of Schizophrenia*, ed. Rosenthal, D. & Kety, S. S., pp. 137–54. Oxford: Pergamon Press

— (1977) Migration, culture and mental health. *Psychol. Med.*, **7**, 677–84

Murphy, H. B. M. & Raman, A. C. (1971) The chronicity of schizophrenia in indigenous tropical peoples: results of a 12 year follow-up survey. *Brit. J. Psychiat.*, **118**, 489–97

Murray, R. M., Oon, M. C. H., Rodnight, R., Birley, J. L. T. & Smith, A. (1979) Increased excretion of dimethyltryptamine and certain features of psychosis. *Arch. gen. Psychiat.*, **36**, 644–9

Myers, D. H. & Davies, P. (1978) The seasonal incidence of mania and its relation to climatic variables. *Psychol. Med.*, **8**, 433–40

Myrianthopoulos, N. (1976) Congenital malformations in twins. *Acta genet. med. gemell.*, **25**, 331–5

Nachmani, G. & Cohen, B. D. (1969) Recall and recognition free learning in schizophrenics. *J. abnorm. Psychol.*, **74**, 511–16

Nasrallah, H. A., Donnelly, E. F., Bigelow, L. B., Rivera-Calimlim, L., Rogol, A., Potkin, S., Rauscher, F. P., Wyatt, R. J. & Gillin, J. C. (1977) Inhibition of dopamine synthesis in chronic schizophrenia. *Arch. gen. Psychiat.*, **34**, 649–55

National Development Group (1977) *Mentally Handicapped Children: A Plan for Action*, Pamphlet No. 2. London: HMSO

National Schizophrenia Fellowship (1979) *Home Sweet Nothing.* 79 Victoria Road, Surbiton, Surrey KT6 4NS

Naylor, G. J., Dick, D. A. T., Dick, E. G., Le Poidevin, D. & Whyte, S. F. (1973) Erythrocyte membrane cation carrier in depressive illness. *Psychol. Med.*, **3**, 502–8

Naylor, G. J., McNamee, H. B. & Moody, J. P. (1970) Erythrocyte sodium and potassium in depressive illness. *J. psychosom. Res.* **14**, 173–7

— (1971) Changes in erythrocyte sodium and potassium on recovery from a depressive illness. *Brit. J. Psychiat.*, **118**, 219–23

Neale, J. M. (1971) Perceptual span in schizophrenia. *J. abnorm. Psychol.*, **77**, 196–204

Neale, J. M. & Cromwell, R. L. (1970) Attention and schizophrenia. In *Progress in Experimental Personality Research*, ed. Maher, B. A., vol. 5. New York: Academic Press

Neale, J. M. & Oltmanns, T. F. (1980) *Schizophrenia.* New York: Wiley

Nelson J. C. & Bowers, M. B. (1978) Delusional unipolar depression. *Arch. gen. Psychiat.*, **35**, 1321–8

Ney, P. G., Palvesky & A. E. Markeley, J. (1971) Relative effectiveness of operant conditioning and play therapy in childhood schizophrenia. *J. Autism child. Schiz.*, **1**, 337–49

Nordquist, V. M. & Wahler, R. G. (1973) Naturalistic treatment of an autistic child. *J. appl. Behav. Anal.*, **6**, 79–87

Noreik, K. & Ødegård, Ø. (1967) Age of onset of schizophrenia in relation to socio-economic factors. *Brit. J. soc. Psychiat.*, **1**, 243–9

Norris, V. (1959) *Mental Illness in London.* Maudsley Monographs, No. 6. London: Institute of Psychiatry and Chapman & Hall

Noyes, R. & Kletti, R. (1977) Depersonalization in response to life-threatening danger. *Compr. Psychiatry*, **18**, 375–84

Nyhan, W. L., Olivier, W. J. & Lesch, M. (1965) A familial disorder of uric acid metabolism and central nervous system function. *J. Paediat.*, **67**, 257–63

Nyström, S. (1979) Depressions: factors related to 10-year prognosis. *Acta psychiat. scand.*, **60**, 225–38

O'Connor, N. (1973) Psychological studies in subnormality. *Psychol. Med.*, **3**, 137–40

— (1977) Specific and general cognitive deficit. In *Research to Practice in Mental Retardation Education and Training*, ed. Mittler, P., vol. II, IASSMD, pp. 67–75. Baltimore: University Park Press

O'Connor, N. & Hermelin, B. (1967) The selective visual attention of psychotic children. *J. child Psychol. Psychiat.*, **8**, 167–79

— (1971) Cognitive deficits in children. *Brit. med. Bull.*, **27**, 227–31

— (1978) *Seeing and Hearing and Space and Time.* London: Academic Press

Odegård, O. (1932) Emigration and insanity: a study of mental disease among Norwegian-born population in Minnesota. *Acta psychiat. neurol. scand.*, Supp. 4

— (1946) Marriage and mental disease: a study in social psychopathology. *J. ment. Sci.*, **92**, 35–59

— (1946) A statistical investigation of the incidence of mental disorder in Norway. *Psychiat. Q.*, **20**, 381

— (1961) In depression. *Acta psychiat. scand.*, Supp. 162, 37

Office of Population Censuses and Surveys (1974) *Studies on Medical and Population Subjects. Morbidity statistics from general practice*. Second National Study, 1970–71. London: HMSO

Offord, D. R. (1974) School performance of adult schizophrenics, their siblings and age mates. *Brit. J. Psychiat.*, **125**, 12–19

O'Gorman, G. (1970) *The Nature of Childhood Autism*. 2nd ed. London: Butterworths

Oltman, J. E. & Friedman, S. (1962) Life cycles in patients with manic-depressive psychosis. *Am. J. Psychiat.*, **119**, 174–6

Oltmanns, T. F. (1978) Selective attention in schizophrenia and manic psychosis: The effect of distraction on information processing. *J. abnorm. Psychol.*, **87**, 212–25

Oltmanns, T. F. & Neale, J. M. (1975) Schizophrenic performance when distractors are present: Attentional deficit or differential task difficulty? *J. abnorm. Psychol.*, **84**, 205–9

— (1978) Abstraction and schizophrenia: Problems in psychological deficit research. In *Progress in Experimental Personality Research*, ed. Maher, B. A., vol. 8. New York: Academic Press

Oltmanns, T. F., Ohayon, J. & Neale, J. M. (1978) The effect of anti-psychotic medication and diagnostic criteria on distractibility in schizophrenia. *J. psychiat. Res.*, **14**, 81–91

Oltmanns, T. F., Weintraub, S., Stone, A. A. & Neale. J. M. (1978) Cognitive slippage in children vulnerable to schizophrenia. *J. abnorm. child Psychol.*, **6**, 237–45

O'Neal, P. & Robins, L. N. (1958) Childhood patterns predictive of adult schizophrenia: a 30-year follow-up study. *Am. J. Psychiat.*, **115**, 385–91

Oon, M. C. H., Murray, R. M., Rodnight, R., Murphy, M. P. & Birley, J. L.T. (1977) Factors affecting the urinary excretion of endogenously formed dimethyl-tryptamine in normal human subjects. *Psychopharmacol.*, **54**, 171–5

Oppler, W. (1950) Manic psychosis in a case of parasagittal meningioma. *Arch. gen. Psychiat.*, **64**, 417

Orley, J. H. & Wing, J. K. (1979) Psychiatric disorders in two African villages. *Arch. gen. Psychiat.*, **36**, 513–20

Ormrod, R. (1977) The McNaughton case and its predecessors. In *Daniel McNaughton: His Trial and the Aftermath*, ed. West , D. J. & Walk, A. Ashford, Kent: Headley Bros.

Ornitz, E. M. (1970) Vestibular dysfunction in schizophrenia and childhood autism. *Compr. Psychiatry*, **11**, 159–73

— (1974) The modulation of sensory input and motor output in autistic children. *J. Autism child. Schiz.*, **4**, 197–215

Ornitz, E. M. & Forsythe, A. B. (1973) Effect of vestibular and auditory stimulation on the REMs of REM sleep in autistic children. *Arch. Gen. Psychiat.*, **29**, 786–91

Ornitz, E. M. & Ritvo, E. R. (1968a) Perceptual inconstancy in early infantile autism. *Arch. gen. Psychiatr.*, **18**, 76–98

— (1968b) Neurophysiologic mechanisms underlying perceptual inconstancy in autistic and schizophrenic children. *Arch. gen. Psychiat.*, **19**, 22–7

— (1976) Medical assessment. In *Autism: Diagnosis, Current Research and Management*, ed. Ritvo, E. R., pp. 7–23. New York: Spectrum Publications

Ornitz, E. M., Ritvo, E. R., Brown, M. B., La Franchi, S., Paramlee, T. & Walter, R. D. (1969) The EEG and rapid eye movements during REM sleep in normal and autistic children. *Electroenceph. clin. Neurophysiol.*, **26**, 167–75

Ornitz, E. M., Ritvo, E. R., Panman, L. M., Lee, Y. H. & Walter, R. D. (1968) The auditory evoked response in normal and autistic children during sleep. *Electroenceph. clin. Neurophysiol.*, **25**, 221–30

Ornitz, E. M., Ritvo, E. R. & Walter, R. D. (1965a) Dreaming sleep in autistic and schizophrenic children. *Am. J. Psychiat.*, **122**, 419–24

— (1965b) Dreaming sleep in autistic twins. *Arch. gen. Psychiat.*, **12**, 77–9

Ornitz, E. M., Tanguay, P. E., Lee, J. C. M., Ritvo, E. R., Silversten, B. & Wilson, C. (1972) The effect of stimulus interval on the auditory evoked response during sleep in autistic children. *J. Autism child. Schiz.*, **2**, 140–50

Orsulak, P. J., Schildkraut, J. J., Schatzberg, A. F. & Herzog, J. M. (1978) Differences in platelet monoamine oxidase activity in subgroups of schizophrenic and depressive disorders. *Biol. Psychiat.*, **13**, 637–47

Osmond, H. & Smythies, J. R. (1952) Schizophrenia: a new approach. *J. ment. Sci.*, **98**, 309–15

Owen, F., Bourne, R., Crow, T. J., Johnstone, E. C., Bailey, A. R. & Hershon, H. I. (1976) Platelet monoamine oxidase in schizophrenia: an investigation in drug-free hospitalized patients. *Arch. gen. Psychiat.*, **33**, 169–73

Owen, F., Crow, T. J., Poulter, M., Cross, A. J., Longden, A. & Riley, G. J. (1978) Increased dopamine receptor sensitivity in schizophrenia. *Lancet*, **ii**, 223–6

Pallis, D. J. (1977) *The psychiatric assessment of attempted suicide: personality, intent and suicide risk*. Thesis, University of Aberdeen

Pallis, D. J. & Birtchnell, J. (1977) Seriousness of suicide attempt in relation to personality. *Brit. J. Psychiat.*, **130**, 253–9

Pallis, D. J. & Sainsbury, P. (1976) The value of assessing intent in attempted suicide. *Psychol. Med.*, **6**, 487–92

Panse, F. (1924) Untersuchungen über Verlauf und Prognose beim manisch-depressiven Irresein. *Monatsschr. Psychiat. Neurol.*, **56**, 15–32

Paraskevopoulos, J. N. & Kirk, S. A. (1969) *The Development and Psychometric Characteristics of the Revised Illinois Test of Psycholinguistic Abilities*. Urbana: University of Illinois Press

Pare, G. M. B., Young, D. P. H., Price, K. S. & Stacey, R. S. (1969) 5-hydroxytryptamine, noradrenaline and dopamine in brainstem, hypothalamus and caudate nucleus of controls and of patients committing suicide by coal-gas poisoning. *Lancet*, **ii**, 133

Park, C. C. (1967). *The Siege*. New York: Harcourt, Brace/London: Penguin (1972)

— (1978) Book review: Nadia: a case of extraordinary drawing ability in an autistic child, by Lorna Selfe. *J. Autism child. Schiz.*, **8**, 457–72

Park, D. & Youderian, P. (1974) Light and number: ordering principles in the world of an autistic child. *J. Autism child. Schiz.*, **4**, 313–23

Parker, J. B., Theilie, A. & Spielberger, C. (1961) Frequency of blood types in a homogeneous group of manic-depressive patients. *J. ment. Sci.*, **107**, 936–42

Pasamanick, B. & Lilienfeld, A. (1955) Association of maternal and foetal factors with development of mental deficiency. *J. Am. Med. Assoc.*, **159**, 155–60

Passkind, H. (1930) Manic depressive psychosis in private practice. *Arch. Neurol. Psychiat.*, **23**, 789–94

Pauleikhoff, B. & Mester, H. (1972) Abnorme Reaktionen und Entwicklungen. In *Psychiatrie der Gegenwart*, II/I, ed. Kisker, P. K., Meyer, J.-E., Müller, C. & Strömgren, E., pp. 515–16. Berlin: Springer

Paykel, E. S. (1971) Classification of depressed patients: a cluster analysis derived grouping. *Brit. J. Psychiat.*, **118**, 275–88

— (1974) Recent life events and clinical depression. In *Life stress and illness*, ed. Gunderson, E. K. & Rahe, R. H., chap. 9, pp. 134–63. Springfield: Illinois, Charles C. Thomas

— (1977) Depression and appetite. *J. psychosom. Res.*, **21**, 401–7

— (1978) Contribution of life events to causation of psychiatric illness. *Psychol. Med.*, **8**, 245–53

— (1979) Predictors of treatment response. In *Psychopharmacology of Affective Disorders*, ed. Paykel, E. S. & Coppen, A., pp. 193–220, Oxford: Oxford University Press

(1982) Life events and early environment. In *Handbook of Affective Disorders*, ed. Paykel, E. S. Edinburgh: Churchill Livingstone

Paykel, E. S. & Coppen, A. (1979) (Eds.) *Psychopharmacology of Affective Disorders*. Oxford: Oxford University Press

Paykel, E. S., Fleminger, R. & Watson, J. P. (1982) Psychiatric side effects of antihypertensive drugs other than reserpine. In *P. clin. Psychopharm.* (In press)

Paykel, E. S., Klerman, G. L. & Prusoff, B. A. (1974) Prognosis of depression and the endogenous-neurotic distinction. *Psychol. Med.*, **4**, 57–64

Paykel, E. S., Myers, J. K., Dienelt, M. N., Klerman, G. L., Lindenthal, J. J. & Pepper, M. P. (1969) Life events and depression: a controlled study. *Arch. gen. Psychiat.*, **21**, 753–60

Paykel, E. S. & Rowan, P. (1979) Recent advances in research on affective disorders. In *Recent Advances in Clinical Psychiatry*. Edinburgh: Churchill Livingstone

Paykel, E. S. & Tanner, J. (1976) Life events, depressive relapse and maintenance treatment. *Psychol. Med.*, **6**, 481–5

Paykel, E. S., Weissman, M. M., Prusoff, B. A. & Tonks, C. M. (1971) Dimensions of social adjustment in depressed women. *J. nerv. ment. Dis.*, **152**, 158–72

Payne, R. W., Matussek, P. & George, E. I. (1959) An experimental study of schizophrenic thought disorder. *J. ment. Sci.*, **103**, 627–652

Pearlin, L. I. & Johnson, J. S. (1977) Marital status, life-strains and depression. *Am. sociol. Rev.*, **42**, 704–715

Pearlin, L. I. & Schooler, C. (1978) The structure of coping. *J. Health & soc. Behav.*, **19**, 2–21

Peet, M. & Coppen, A. (1979) The pharmacokinetics of antidepressant drugs: relevance to their therapeutic effect. In *Psychopharmacology of Affective Disorders*, ed. Paykel, E. S. & Coppen, A., pp. 91–107. Oxford: Oxofrd University Press

Perris, C. (1966) A study of bipolar (manic-depressives) and unipolar recurrent affective psychoses. *Acta psychiat. scand.*, **42**, Suppl. 194

— (1968) The course of depressive psychoses. *Acta psychiat. scand.* **44**, 238–48

— (1974) A study of cycloid psychoses. *Acta psychiat. scand.*, supp. 253

— (1976) Frequency and hereditary aspects of depression. In *Depression: Behavioral, Biochemical, Diagnostic and Treatment Concepts*, ed. Gallant, D. & Simpson, G. New York: Spectrum Press

Perris, C., Strandman, E. & Wåhlby, L. (1979) HLA antigens and the responses to prophylactic lithium. *Neuropsychobiol.*, **5**, 114–18

Perry, T. L., Kish, S. J., Buchanan, J. & Hansen, S. (1979) γ-Aminobutyric acid deficiency in brain of schizophrenic patients. *Lancet*, **i**, 237–9

Petersen, W. F. (1935) *The Patient and the Weather*. Michigan: Edwards

Piaget, J. (1951) *Play, Dreams and Imitation in Childhood*. London: Routledge & Kegan Paul

(1972) *Play, Dreams and Imitation in Childhood*. London: Routledge & Kegan Paul

Pierce, S. & Bartolucci, G. (1977) A syntactic investigation of verbal autistic, mentally retarded and normal children. *J. Autism child. Schiz.*, **7**, 121–33

Pitfield, M. & Oppenheim, A. N. (1964) Child rearing attitudes of mothers of psychotic children. *J. child Psychol. Psychiat.*, **5**, 51–7

Pogue-Geile, M. F. & Oltmanns, T. F. (1980) Sentence perception and distractibility in schizophrenic, manic, and depressed patients. *J. abnorm. Psychol.*, **89**, 115–24

Pokorney, A. D. (1964) Suicide rates in various psychiatric disorders. *J. nerv. ment. Dis.*, **139**, 499–506

Pollin, W., Stabenau, J. R., Mosher, L. & Tupin, J. (1966) Life history differences in identical twins discordant for schizophrenia. *Am. J. Orthopsychiat.* **36**, 492

Pollitt, J. (1972) The relationship between genetic and precipitating factors in depressive illness. *Brit. J. Psychiat.*, **121**, 67–70

Pollock, H. M. (1931) Recurrence of attacks in manic depressive psychosis. *Am. J. Psychiat.*, **88**, 567–73

Pond, D. (1963) The EEG in paediatrics. In *Electroencephalography*, ed. Hill, D. & Parr, G., pp. 207–31. London: MacDonald

— (1974) Prognosis of severe childhood epilepsy. In *Total Care in Severe Epilepsy*, ed. Parsonage, M. J., pp. 43–4. Proc. Sixth Int. Symp. Epilepsy, Belgium. London: International Bureau for Epilepsy

Poort, R. (1945) Catamnestic investigations on manic-depressive psychosis with special reference to the prognosis. *Acta psychiat. neurol. scand.*, **20**, 59–74

Pope, H. G. & Lipinski, J. F. (1978) Diagnosis in schizophrenia and manic-depressive illness. *Arch. gen. Psychiat.*, **35**, 811–28

Post, F. (1962) *The Significance of Affective Symptoms in Old Age*. Maudsley Monograph No. 10. London: Oxford University Press

— (1966) *Persistent Persecutory States of the Elderly*. Oxford: Pergamon Press

— (1966) Somatic and psychic factors in the treatment of elderly psychiatric patients. *J. psychosom. Res.*, **10**, 13–18

— (1976) Diagnosis of depression in geriatric patients and treatment modalities appropriate for the population. In *Depression: Behavioral, Biochemical, Diagnostic and Treatment Concepts*, ed. Gallant, D. M. & Simpson, G. M., pp. 205–31. New York: Spectrum Publications

— (1978) The functional psychoses. In *Studies in Geriatric Psychiatry*, ed. Isaacs, A. D. & Post, F., pp. 77–98. Chichester: Wiley

— (1980) Paranoid, schizophrenia-like and schizophrenic states in the aged. In *Handbook of Mental Aging*, ed. Birren, J. E. & Sloane, R. B. Englewood Cliffs: Prentice-Hall

Post, R. M., Fink, E., Carpenter, T., Jr. & Goodwin, F. K. (1975) Cerebrospinal fluid amine metabolites in acute schizophrenia. *Arch. gen. Psychiat.*, **32**, 1063–9

Potkin, S. G., Cannon, H. E., Murphy, D. L. & Wyatt, R. J. (1978) Are paranoid schizophrenics different from other schizophrenics? *New Eng. J. Med.*, **298**, 61–6

Prange, A. J., Wilson, I. C., Lara, P. P., Alltop, L. B. & Breese, G. R. (1972) Thyrotrophin releasing hormone in depression. *Lancet*, **ii**, 999–1002

Prange, A. J., Wilson, I. C., Rabon, A. M. & Lipton, M. A. (1969) Enhancement of imipramine antidepressant activity by thyroid hormone. *Am. J. Psychiat.*, **126**, 457–69

Price, J. (1968) The genetics of depressive behaviour. In *Recent Developments in Affective Disorders*, ed. Coppen, A. & Walk, A. Royal Medico-Psychological Association. Ashford, England: Headley

Prien, R. F. (1979) Lithium in the treatment of schizophrenia and schizoaffective disorders. *Arch. gen. Psychiat.*, **36**, 852–3

Prien, R. F. & Cole, J. (1968) High dose chlorpromazine therapy in chronic schizophrenia. *Arch. gen. Psychiat.*, **18**, 482–95

Prien, R. F., Gillis, R. D. & Caffey, E. M. (1973) Intermittent pharmacotherapy in chronic schizophrenia. *Hosp. comm. Psychiat.*, **24**, 317–22

Prien, R. F. & Klett, C. C. (1972) An appraisal of the long term use of tranquillizing medication with hospitalized chronic schizophrenics. *Schiz. Bull.*, **5**, 64–73

Priestley, D. (1979) *Tied Together with String*. Surbiton, Surrey: National Schizophrenia Fellowship

Prior, M. & Chen, C. S. (1976) Short-term and serial memory in autistic retarded and normal children. *J. Autism child. Schiz.*, **6**, 121–31

Prior, M., Perry, D. & Gajzago, C. (1975) Kanner's syndrome or early onset psychosis: taxonomic analysis of 142 cases. *J. Autism child. Schiz.*, **5**, 71–80

Procci, W. R. (1976) Schizoaffective psychosis. Fact or fiction? *Arch. gen. Psychiat.*, **33**, 1167–78

Protheroe, C. (1969) Puerperal psychoses: a long term study 1927–1961. *Brit. J. Psychiat.*, **115**, 9–30

Prusoff, B., Williams, D. M., Weissman, M. & Astrachan, B. (1979) Treatment of secondary depression in schizophrenia. *Arch. gen. Psychiat.*, **36**, 569–75

Puig-Antich, J., Blau, S., Mark, N., Greenhill, L. L. & Chambers, W. (1977) Prepubertal major depressive disorder: A pilot study. Paper presented at the Annual Meeting of the American Academy of Child Psychiatry, Houston, Texas

Quitkin, F., Rifkin, A., Cockfeld, L. & Klein, D. (1977) Tardive dyskinesia: are first signs reversible? *Amer. J. Psychiat.*, **134**, 84–7

Quitkin, F., Rifkin, A., Kane, J., Ramor-Lorenzi, J. & Klein, D. (1978). Long acting oral vs injectable antipsychotic drugs in schizophrenics. *Arch. gen. Psychiat.*, **35**, 889–92

Quitkin, F., Rifkin, A. & Klein, D. E. (1975) Very high dosage vs standard dosage fluphenazine in schizophrenia. *Arch. gen. Psychiat.*, **32**, 1276–81

Rainer, J. D. & Kallmann, F. J. (1959) Genetic and demographic aspects of disordered behavior patterns in a deaf population. In *Epidemiology of Mental Disorders*, ed. Pasamanick, B., pp. 229–39. Washington: American Association for the Advancement of Science

Ramsey, P. (1970) *The Patient as Person*. New Haven: Yale University Press

Rank, B. (1949) Adaptation of the psycho-analytical technique for the treatment of young children with atypical development. *Am. J. Ortho-psychiat.*, **19**, 130–9

Ratcliff, R. A. W. (1962) The open door. Ten years' experience in Dingleton. *Lancet*, **ii**, 188–90

Rawnsley, K. (1968) Epidemiology of affective disorders. In *Recent Developments in Affective Disorders*, ed. Coppen, A. & Walk, A. *Brit. J. Psychiat.*, Special Publication No.2. London: Royal Medico-Psychological Association

Reed, G. F. (1963) Elective mutism in children: a reappraisal. *J. child Psychol. Psychiat.*, **4**, 99–107

Rees, S. C. & Taylor, A. (1975) Prognostic antecedents and outcome in a follow-up study of children with a diagnosis of childhood psychosis. *J. Autism child Schiz.*, **5**, 309–22

Registrar General (1960) *Statistical Review of England & Wales, 1954–56*. Supplement on Mental Health. London: HMSO

— (1964) *Statistical Review of England & Wales, 1960*. Supplement on Mental Health. London: HMSO

Reich, T., Clayton, P. & Winokur, G. (1969) Family history studies: V. The genetics of mania. *Am. J. Psychiat.*, **125**, 1358–69

Reich, T., Cloninger, C. R. & Guze, S. B. (1975). The multifactorial model of disease transmission: I. Description of the model and its use in psychiatry. *Brit. J. Psychiat.*, **127**, 1–10

Reich, T., James, S. W. & Morris, C. A. (1972) The use of multiple thresholds in determining the mode of transmission of semi-continuous traits. *Ann. hum. Genet., London*, **36**, 163–84

Reich, T., Rice, J., Cloninger, C. R., Wette, R. & James, J. (1979) The use of multiple thresholds and segregation analysis in analyzing the phenotypic heterogeneity of multifactorial traits. *Ann. hum. Genet., London*, **42**, 371–90

Rennie, T. A. C. (1942) Prognosis in manic depressive psychosis. *Am. J. Psychiat.*, **98**, 801–14

Retterstöl, N. (1966) *Paranoid and Paranoiac Psychoses*. Oslo: Universitets-forlaget

— (1968) Paranoid psychoses. *Brit. J. Psychiat.*, **114**, 553–62

— (1970) *Prognosis in Paranoid Psychoses*. Springfield, Illinois: Charles C. Thomas

Revitch, E. (1954) The problem of conjugal paranoia. *Dis. nerv. Syst.*, **15**, 271–7

Reynell, J. (1977) *Reynell Developmental Language Scales – revised*. Windsor: National Foundation for Educational Research

Reynolds, B. S., Newsom, C. D. & Lovaas, O. I. (1974) Auditory over-selectivity in autistic children. *J. Abnorm. child Psychol.*, **2**, 252–63

Rice, J., Cloninger, C. R. & Reich, T. (1978) Multifactorial inheritance with cultural transmission and assortative mating. I. Description and basic properties of the unitary models. *Am. J. hum. Genet.*, **30**, 618–43

Ricks, D. M. (1975) Vocal communication in pre-verbal normal and autistic children. In *Language, Cognitive Deficits and Retardation*, ed. O'Connor, N. London: Butterworths

— (1972) *The Beginning of Vocal Communication in Infants and Autistic Children*. M.D. Thesis, University of London

Ricks, D. M. & Wing, L. (1975) Language, communication and the use of symbols in normal and autistic children. *J. Autism child. Schiz.*, **5**, 191–221

— (1976) Language, communication and the use of symbols in normal and autistic children. In *Early Childhood Autism*, ed. Wing, L., 2nd ed. Oxford: Pergamon Press.

Riding, J. & Munro, A. (1975) Pimozide in the treatment of mono-symptomatic hypochondriacal psychosis. *Acta psychiat. scand.*, **52**, 23–30

Rieder, R. O., Broman, S. H. & Rosenthal, D. (1977) The offspring of schizophrenics: II. Perinatal factors and IQ. *Arch. gen. Psychiat.*, **34**, 789–801

Rieder, R. O. & Gershon, E. S. (1978) Genetic strategies in biological psychiatry. *Amer. J. Psychiat.*, **35**, 866–73

Rifkin, A., Quitkin, F. & Klein, D. (1975) Akinesia: a poorly recognized drug induced extrapyramidal disorder. *Arch. gen. Psychiat.*, **32**, 672–4

Rifkin, A. Quitkin, F., Rabiner, L. & Klein, D. (1977) Fluphenazine decanoate, fluphenazine hydrochloride given orally and placebo in remitted schizophrenics. *Arch. gen. Psychiat.*, **34**, 43–7

Rimland, B. (1965) *Infantile Autism*, pp. 187–217. London: Methuen

Rimmer, J. & Jacobsen, B. (1976) Differential fertility of adopted schizophrenics and their half-siblings. *Acta psychiat. scand.*, **54**, 161–66

Rimon, R., Halonen, P., Anttinen, E. & Evoler, K. (1971) Complement fixing antibody to herpes simplex virus in patients with psychotic depression. *Dis. nerv. Syst.*, **32**, 822–4

Rincover, A. & Koegel, R. L. (1975) Setting generality and stimulus control in autistic children. *J. applied Behav. Anal.*, **8**, 235–46

Ringuette, E. & Kennedy, T. (1966) An experimental study of the double-bind hypothesis. *J. abnorm. Psychol.*, **71**, 136–141

Ritvo, E. R. (1977) Biochemical studies of children with the syndromes of autism, childhood schizophrenia, and related developmental disabilities: a review. *J. child Psychol. Psychiat.*, **18**, 373–9

Ritvo, E. R., Cantwell, D., Johnson, E., Clements, M., Benbrook, F., Slagle, S., Kelly, P. & Ritz, M. (1971) Social class factors in autism. *J. Autism child. Schiz.*, **1**, 297–310

Ritvo, E. R., Ornitz, E. M., Walter, R. D. & Hanley, J. (1970) Correlation of psychiatric diagnoses and EEG findings. A double-blind study of 184 hospitalized children. *Am. J. Psychiat.*, **126**, 988–96

Ritvo, E. R., Rabin, K., Yuwiler, A., Freeman, B. J. & Geller, E. (1978) Biochemical and hematologic studies: A critical review. In *Autism: A Reappraisal of Concepts and Treatment*, ed. Rutter, M. & Schopler, E., pp. 163–83. New York: Plenum Press

Roberts, J. A. F. & Pembrey, M. E. (1978) *An Introduction to Medical Genetics.* 7th ed. London: Oxford University Press

Robin, A. A., Brooke, E. M. & Freeman-Browne, D. L. (1968) Some aspects of suicide in psychiatric patients in Southend. *Brit. J. Psychiat.*, **114**, 739–47

Robins, E. & Guze, S. B. (1970) Establishment of diagnostic validity in psychiatric illness: its application to schizophrenia. *Am. J. Psychiat.*, **126**, 983–7

— (1972) Classification of affective disorders: the primary–secondary, the endogenous–reactive, and the neurotic–psychotic concepts. In *Recent Advances in the Psychology of Depressive Illness*. Publication HSM 70-9053. U.S. Department of Health, Education and Welfare

Robins, E., Murphy, G. E., Wilkinson, R. H., Gassner, S. & Kayes, J. (1959) Some clinical considerations in the prevention of suicide based on a study of 134 successful suicides. *Am. J. pub. Health*, **49**, 888–98

Robins, L. N. (1970) Follow-up studies investigating childhood disorders. In *Psychiatric Epidemiology*, ed. Hare, E. H. & Wing, J. K. London: Oxford University Press

Rochester, S. R. (1973) The role of information processing in the sentence decoding of schizophrenic listeners. *J. nerv. ment. Dis.*, **157**, 217–23

— (1978) Are language disorders in acute schizophrenia actually information processing problems? *J. psychiat. Res.*, **14**, 275–83

Rochester, S. R., Harris, J. & Seeman, M. V. (1973) Sentence processing in schizophrenic listeners. *J. abnorm. Psychol.*, **82**, 350–56

Rochester, S. R., Martin, J. R. & Thurston, S. (1977) Thought-process disorder on schizophrenia: the listener's task. *Brain and Language*, **4**, 95–114

Rochester, S. R., Thurston, S. & Rupp, J. (1977) Hesitations as clues to failures in coherence: a study of the thought-disordered speaker. In *Sentence Production: Developments in Theory and Research*, ed. Rosenberg, S. New York: Erlbaum

Rodnick, E. H. & Garmezy, N. (1957) An experimental approach to the study of motivation in schizophrenia. In *Nebraska Symposium on Motivation*, ed. Jones, M. R., vol. 5. Lincoln, USA: University of Nebraska Press

Rodnick, E. H. & Shakow, D. (1940) Set in the schizophrenic, as measured by a composite reaction time index. *Am. J. Psychiat.*, **97**, 214–25

Rodnight, R. (1975) The significance of some biochemical abnormalities in schizophrenia. *Acta neurol.*, **30**, 84–101

— (1980) Biochemical perspectives in psychiatric research. In *Priorities in Psychiatric Research*, ed. Lader, M. H. Chichester, UK: Wiley

Rodnight, R., Murray, R. M., Oon, M. C. H., Brockington, R. F., Nicholls, P. & Birley, J. L. T. (1976) Urinary dimethyltryptamine and psychiatric symptomatology and classification. *Psychol. Med.*, **6**, 649–57

Roe, D. (1973) *A Plague of Corn: A Social History of Pellagra.* Ithaca, N.Y.: Cornell University Press

Roisin, L. (1972) Histopathologic observations in schizophrenia (including effects of somatic and biochemical therapies). In *Pathology of the Nervous System*, ed. Winkler, W., Vol. 3, pp. 2670–77. New York: McGraw Hill

Roos, B. E. & Sjöström, R. (1969) 5-Hydroxyindolacetic acid and homovanillic acid levels in the cerebrospinal fluid after probenecid application in patients with manic depressive psychosis. *Pharmac. Clin.*, **1**, 153

Rosanoff, A. J., Hardy, L. M. & Plesset, R. (1935) The etiology of manic-depressive syndromes with special reference to their occurrence in twins. *Am. J. Psychiat.*, **91**, 725–62

Rosen, D. H. (1970) The serious suicide attempt: epidemiological and follow-up study of 886 patients. *Am. J. Psychiat.*, **127**, 764–70

Rosenthal, D. (1960) Confusion of identity and the frequency of schizophrenia in twins. *Arch. gen. Psychiat.*, **3**, 297–304

— (1972) Three adoption studies of heredity in the schizophrenic disorders. *Int. J. ment. Hlth.*, **1**, 63–75

Rosenthal, D., Goldberg, I., Jacobsen, B., Wender, P. I., Kety, S. S., Schulsinger, F. & Eldred, C. A. (1974) Migration, heredity and schizophrenia. *Psychiat.*, **37**, 321–39

Rosenthal, D. & Kety, S. S. (1968) (Eds.) *The Transmission of Schizophrenia*. Oxford: Pergamon Press

Rosenthal, D., Wender, P. H., Kety, S. S., Schulsinger, F., Welner, J. & Østergaard, L. (1968) Schizophrenics' offspring reared in adoptive homes. In *The Transmission of Schizophrenia*, ed. Rosenthal, D. & Kety, S. S., pp. 377–92. Oxford: Pergamon Press

Rosenthal, S. H. (1968) The involutional depressive syndrome. *Am. J. Psychiat.*, **124**, Supp. 21–35

Rosenthal, S. H. & Klerman, G. L. (1966) Content and consistency in the endogenous depressive pattern. *Brit. J. Psychiat.*, **112**, 471–84

Ross, E. M. & Mesulam, M. M. (1979) Dominant language functions of the right hemisphere? Prosody and emotional gesturing. *Arch. Neurol.*, **36**, 144

Ross, E. M., Peckham, C. S., West, B. B. & Butler, N. R. (1980) Epilepsy in childhood: findings from the National Child Development Study. *Brit. med. J.*, **1**, 207–10

Roth, M. (1955) The natural history of mental disorder in old age. *J. Ment. Sci.*, **101**, 281–301

— (1960) The phobic anxiety-depersonalisation syndrome and some general aetiological problems in psychiatry. *J. Neuropsychiat.*, **1**, 292–306

Royal College of Psychiatrists (1977) Memorandum on the Use of Electroconvulsive Therapy. *Brit. J. Psychiat.*, **131**, 261–72

— (1981) *Psychiatric Rehabilitation in the 1980s.* London: Royal College of Psychiatrists

Rowitz, L. & Levy, L. (1968) Ecological analysis of treated mental disorders in Chicago. *Arch. gen. Psychiat.*, **19**, 571–9

Rümke, H. C. (1958) Die klinische Differenzierung innerhalb der Gruppe der Schizophrenien. *Nervenarz*, **29**, 49

Russell, P. N. & Beekhuis, M. E. (1976) Organization in memory: a comparison of psychotics and normals. *J. abnorm. Psychol.*, **85**, 527–34

Russell, P. N. & Knight, R. G. (1977) Performance of process schizophrenics on tasks involving visual search. *J. abnorm. Psychol.*, **86**, 16–26

Rutschmann, J., Cornblatt, B. & Erlenmeyer-Kimling, L. (1977) Sustained attention in children at risk for schizophrenia. *Arch. gen. Psychiat.*, **34**, 571–5

Rutter, M. L. (1965) The influence of organic and emotional factors on the origins, nature and outcome of childhood psychosis. *Dev. med. child Neurol.*, **7**, 518–28

— (1966) *Children of Sick Parents.* London: Oxford University Press

— (1966) Behavioural and cognitive characteristics. In *Early Childhood Autism*, ed. Wing, J. K., 1st ed., pp. 51–82. Oxford: Pergamon Press

— (1967) Psychotic disorders in early childhood. In *Recent Developments in Schizophrenia*, ed. Coppen, A. J. & Walk, A., pp. 133–51. Ashford, England: Headley

— (1968) Concepts of autism: a review of research. *J. child Psychol. Psychiat.*, **9**, 1–25

— (1970) Autistic children: infancy to adulthood. *Seminars in Psychiatry*, **2**, 435–50

— (1972a) Childhood schizophrenia reconsidered. *J. Autism child. Schiz.*, **2**, 315–37

— (1972b) *Maternal Deprivation Reassessed.* Harmondsworth: Penguin Books

— (1974) The development of infantile autism. *Psychol. med.*, **4**, 147–63

— (1977) Infantile autism and other child psychoses. In *Child Psychiatry: Modern Approaches*, ed. Rutter, M. & Hersov, L. Oxford: Blackwell Scientific Publications

— (1978a) Communication deviances and diagnostic differ-

ences. In *The Nature of Schizophrenia: New Approaches to Research and Treatment*, ed. Wynne, L. C., Cromwell, R. L. and Matthysse, S., pp. 512–16. New York: Wiley

— (1978b) Diagnosis and definition. In *Autism: A Reappraisal of Concepts and Treatment*, ed. Rutter, M. & Schopler, E., pp. 1–26. New York: Plenum Press

— (1978c) Language disorder and infantile autism. In: *Autism: A Reappraisal of Concepts and Treatment*, ed. Rutter, M. & Schopler, E. New York: Plenum Press

— (1979) Language, cognition and autism. In *Congenital and Acquired Cognitive Disorders*, ed. Katzman, R. New York: Raven Press

— (1980) Language training with autistic children. How does it work and what does it achieve? In *Language and Language Disorders in Children*, ed. Hersov, L. A., Berger, M. & Nichol, R. Oxford: Pergamon Press.

Rutter, M. & Bartak, L. (1973) Special educational treatment of autistic children: a comparative study: II. Follow-up findings and implications for services. *J. child Psychol. Psychiat.*, **14**, 241–70

Rutter, M. L., Bartak, L. & Newman, S. (1971) Autism – a central disorder of cognition and language? In *Infantile Autism: Concepts, Characteristics and Treatment*, ed. Rutter, M., pp. 148–71. New York: Longman

Rutter, M. & Brown, G. W. (1966) The reliability and validity of measures of family life and relationships in families containing a psychiatric patient. *Soc. Psychiat.*, **1**, 38–53

Rutter, M. L., Greenfeld, D. & Lockyer, L. (1967) A five to fifteen year follow-up study of infantile psychosis. II. Social and behavioural outcome. *Brit. J. Psychiat.*, **113**, 1183–99

Rutter, M., Lebovici, S., Eisenberg, L., Sneznevskij, A. V., Sadoun, R., Brooke, E. & Tsung-Yi Lin (1969) A tri-axial classification of mental disorders in childhood: an international study. *J. child Psychol. and Psychiat.*, **10**, 41–61

Rutter, M. & Lockyer, L. (1967) A five to fifteen year follow-up study of infantile psychosis: I. Description of the sample. *Brit. J. Psychiat.*, **113**, 1169–82

Rutter, M., Shaffer, D. & Sturge, C. (1975) *A Guide to a Multi-Axial Classification Scheme for Psychiatric Disorders in Childhood and Adolescence.* London: Institute of Psychiatry

Rutter, M. L. & Sussenwein, F. (1971) A development and behavioural approach to the treatment of preschool autistic children. *J. Autism child. Schiz.*, **1**, 376–97

Rwegellera, G. G. C. (1977) Psychiatric morbidity in West Africans and West Indians in London. *Psychol. med.*, **7**, 317–30

Ryan, P. (1979) New forms of residential care for the mentally ill. In *Community Care for the Mentally Disabled*, ed. Wing, J. K. & Olsen, R. London: Oxford University Press

Ryan, P. & Wing, J. K. (1979) Patterns of residential care. In *Alternative Patterns of Residential Care for Discharged Psychiatric Patients*, ed. Olsen, R. London: BASW

Sachar, E. J., Finkelstein, J. & Hellman, L. (1971) Growth hormone responses in depressive illness. 1. Responses to insulin tolerance test. *Arch. gen. Psychiat.*, **25**, 263–9

Sachar, E. J., Frantz, A. B., Altman, N. & Sassin, J. (1973a) Growth hormone and prolactin in unipolar and bipolar depressed-patients. Responses to hypoglycaemia and L-dopa. *Am. J. Psychiat.*, **130**, 1362–7

Sachar, E. J., Hellman, L., Roffwarg, H. P., Halpern, F. S., Fukushima, D. K. & Gallagher, T. F. (1973b) Disrupted 24-hour patterns of cortisol secretion in psychotic depression. *Arch. gen. Psychiat.*, **28**, 19–24

Sackeim, H. A. & Gur, R. C. (1978) Lateral asymmetry in intensity of emotional expression. *Neuropsychologie*, **16**, 473–81

Sainsbury, P. (1973) Suicide: opinions and facts. *Proc. R. Soc. Med.*, **66**, 579–87

— (1975) Suicide and attempted suicide. In *Psychiatrie der Gegenwart*, ed. Kisker, K. P. *et al.* Berlin: Springer

Sainsbury, P., Baert, A. & Jenkins, J. (1978) *Suicide Trends in Europe: a study of the decline in suicide in England and Wales and of the increase elsewhere.* A report to the World Health Organisation Regional Office for Europe, Copenhagen

Sainsbury, P. & Barraclough, B. M. (1968) Differences between suicide rates. *Nature* (Lond.), **220**, 1252

Sands D. E. (1956) The psychoses of adolescence. *J. ment. Sci.*, **102**, 308–18

Sass, J. K., Itabashi, H. H. & Dexter, R. H. (1965) Juvenile gout with brain involvement. *Arch. Neurol.*, **13**, 639–55

Sattler, J. M. (1974) *Assessment of Children's Intelligence.* London: W. B. Saunders

Saugstad, L. F. & Ødegård, Ø. (1979) Mortality in psychiatric hospitals in Norway 1950–74. *Acta psychiat. scand.*, **59**, 431–47

Sauvage Nolting, W. J. J. de (1955) Considerations regarding a possible relation between the vitamin C content of the blood of pregnant women and schizophrenia, debilitas mentis and psychopathia. *Folia psychiat. neerl.*, **58**, 285–95

Sayers, A. C., Burki, H. R., Rueh, W. & Asper, H. (1975) Neuroleptic induced hypersensitivity of striatal dopamine receptors in the rat as a model of tardive dyskinesia. *Psychopharmacol.* (Berlin) **41**, 97–104

Schaffer, H. R. (1974) Early social behaviour and the study of reciprocity. *Bull. Brit. Psychol. Soc.*, **27**, 209–16

Schain, R. J. & Yannet, H. (1960) Infantile Autism. *J. Pediat.*, **57**, 560–76

Scheff, T. J. (1964) The societal reaction to deviance; ascriptive elements in the psychiatric screening of mental patients in a Midwestern State. *Soc. Problems*, **2**, 401–13

— (1966) *Being Mentally Ill.* Chicago: Aldine

Schildkraut, J. J. (1978) Current status of the catecholamine hypothesis of affective disorders. In *Psychopharmacology: A Generation of Progress*, ed. Lipton, M.A., Di Mascio, A. & Killam, K. F. New York: Raven Press

Schildkraut, J. J., Keeler, B. A., Papousek, M. & Hartmann, E. (1973) MHPG excretion in depressive disorders: relation to clinical subtypes and desynchronized sleep. *Science*, **181**, 762–4

Schlesser, M. A., Winokur, G. & Sherman, B. M. (1979). Genetic subtypes of unipolar primary depressive illness distinguished by hypothalamic-pituitary-adrenal axis activity. *Lancet*, **i**, 739–741

Schmale, A. H. (1973) Adaptive role of depression in health and disease. In *Separation and Depression: clinical and research aspects*, ed. Scott, J. P. & Senay, E. C. Washington DC: American Association for the Advancement of Science

Schmidt, E. H., O'Neal, P. & Robins, E. (1954) Evaluation of suicide attempts as a guide to therapy: clinical and follow-up study of 109 patients. *J. Am. Med. Assoc.*, **155**, 549–57

Schneider, K. (1959) *Clinical Psychopathology.* Translated by Hamilton, M. W. New York: Grune & Stratton

— (1971) *Klinische Psychopathologie.* 9th ed. Stuttgart: Thieme

— (1976) *Klinische Psychopathologie.* 11th ed. Stuttgart: Thieme. (English translation 1959: *Clinical Psychopathology.* New York: Grune & Stratton)

Schneider, W. & Shiffrin, R. M. (1977) Controlled and automatic human information processing: I. Detection, search, and attention. *Psychol. Rev.*, **81**, 1–66.

Schopler, E., Andrews, C. E. & Strupp, K. (1979) Do autistic children come from upper middle class parents? *J. Autism Dev. Dis.*, **9**, 139–52

Schopler, E., Brehm, S. S., Kinsbourne, M. & Reichler, R. J. (1971) Effects of treatment structure on development in autistic children. *Arch. gen. Psychiat.*, **24**, 415–21

Schopler, E. & Loftin, J. (1969a) Thought disorders in parents of psychotic children. A function of test anxiety. *Arch. gen. Psychiat.*, **20**, 174–81

— (1969b) Thinking disorders in parents of young psychotic children. *J. abnorm. Psychol.*, **74**, 281–7.

Schopler, E. & Reichler, R. J. (1971) Parents as co-therapists in the treatment of psychotic children. *J. Autism child. Schiz.*, **1**, 87–102

Schopler, E., Reichler, R. J. & Lansing, M. (1979a) *Individualized Assessment and Treatment for Autistic and Developmentally Disabled Children.* Vol. 1. *Psychoeducational Profile.* Baltimore: University Park Press.

Schopler, E., Reichler, R. J. & Lansing, M. (1979b) *Individualized Assessment and Treatment for Autistic and Developmentally Disabled Children.* Vol. 2. *Teaching Strategies for Parents and Professionals.* Baltimore: University Park Press

Schroeder, S. R., Schroeder, C. S., Smith, B. & Dalldorf, J. (1978) Prevalence of self-injurious behaviors in a large state facility for the retarded. A 3-year follow-up. *J. Autism child. Schiz.*, **8**, 261–9

Schulsinger, H. (1976) A 10-year follow-up of children of schizophrenic mothers: clinical assessment. *Acta psychiat. scand.*, **53**, 371–86

Schulz, B. & Leonhard, K. (1940) Erbbiologischklinische Untersuchungen an insgesamt 99 im Sinne Leonhards typischen bzw. atypischen Schizophrenen. *Z. ges. Neurol. Psychiat.*, **168**, 587

Schwab, J. J. & Schwab, M. E. (1978) *Sociocultural Roots of Mental Illness: An Epidemiologic Survey.* New York: Plenum Medical Book Co

Sedman, G. (1966) Depersonalization in a group of normal subjects. *Brit. J. Psychiat.*, **112**, 907–12

— (1970) Theories of depersonalization: a reappraisal. *Brit. J. Psychiat.*, **117**, 1–14

Sedman, G. & Kenna, J. C. (1963) Depersonalization and mood changes in schizophrenia. *Brit. J. Psychiat.*, **109**, 669–73

Sedman, G. & Reed, G. F. (1963) Depersonalization phenomena in obsessional personalities and in depression. *Brit. J. Psychiat.*, **109**, 376–9

Seegmiller, J. E. (1972) Lesch-Nyhan syndrome and the X-linked uric acidurias. *Hosp. Practice*, April, 79–90

Selfe, L. (1977) *Nadia: a Case of Extraordinary Drawing Ability in an Autistic Child.* London: Academic Press

Seligman, M. E. P. (1975) *Helplessness.* San Francisco: Freeman

Schaffer, D. (1977a) Brain injury. In *Child Psychiatry*, ed. Rutter, M. & Hersov, L. Oxford: Blackwell

— (1977b) Drug treatment. In *Child Psychiatry*, ed. Rutter, M. & Hersov, L. Oxford: Blackwell

Shaffer, D. & Greenhill, L. (1979) A critical note on the predictive validity of 'The Hyperkinetic Syndrome'. *J. child Psychol. Psychiat.*, **20**, 61–72

Shakespeare, R. (1970) Severely subnormal children. In *The Psychological Assessment of Mental and Physical Handicaps*, ed. Mittler, P., pp. 519–41. London: Methuen

Shapiro, R., Bock, E., Rafaelsen, O., Ryder, L. & Svejgaard, A. (1976) Histocompatibility antigens and manic-depressive disorders. *Arch. gen. Psychiat.*, **33**, 823–5

Shapiro, R., Rafaelsen, O., Ryder, L., Svejgaard, A. & Sorensen, H. (1977) ABO blood groups in unipolar and bipolar manic-depressive patients. *Am. J. Psychiat.*, **134**, 197–200

Shapiro, T. & Huebner, H. F. (1976) Speech patterns of five psychotic children now in adolescence. *J. child Psychiat.*, **15**, 278–93

Sharan, S. N. (1966) Family interaction with schizophrenics and their siblings. *J. abnorm. Psychol.*, **71**, 345–53

Shaw, D. M. (1977) The practical management of affective disorders. *Brit. J. Psychiat.*, **130**, 432–51

Shaw, D. M., Camps, F. E. & Eccleston, E. G. (1967) 5-Hydroxytryptamine in the hind brain of depressive suicides. *Brit. J. Psychiat.*, **113**, 1407

Shaw, D. M. & Coppen, A. (1966) Potassium and water distribution in depression. *Brit. J. Psychiat.*, **112**, 269–76

Shaw, D. M., Frizel, D., Camps, F. E. & White, S. (1969) Brain electrolytes in depressive and alcoholic suicides. *Brit. J. Psychiat.*, **115**, 69–77

Sheldrick, C., Jablensky, A., Sartorius, N. & Shepherd, M. (1977) Schizophrenia succeeded by affective illness: catamnestic study and statistical enquiry. *Psychol. Med.*, **7**, 619–24

Shepherd, M. (1957) *A Study of the Major Psychoses in an English county.* Maudsley Monographs, No. 3. London: Chapman & Hall

— (1961) Morbid jealousy: some clinical and social aspects of a psychiatric symptom. *J. ment. Sci.*, **107**, 687–753

Shepherd, M., Cooper, B., Brown, A. C. & Kalton, G. W. (1966) *Psychiatric Illness in General Practice.* London: Oxford University Press

Shepherd, M., Lader, M. & Rodnight, R. (1968) *Clinical Psychopharmacology.* London: English Universities Press Ltd

Sheridan, M. D. (1969) Playthings in the development of language. *Hlth Trends*, **1**, 7–10

Shields, J. (1976) Personal communication to L. & J. Wing

— (1978) In *Schizophrenia: Towards a New Synthesis*, ed. Wing, J. K., p. 56. London: Academic Press

Shields, J. & Gottesman, I. I. (1977) Obstetric complications and twin studies in schizophrenia: clarifications and affirmations. *Schiz. Bull.*, **3**, 351–4

Shobe, F. O. & Brion, P. (1971) Long-term prognosis in manic-depressive illness. *Arch. gen. Psychiat.*, **24**, 334–7

Shorvon, H. J. (1946) The depersonalisation syndrome. *Proc. R. Soc. Med.*, **39**, 779–92

Siever, L. J. & Gunderson, J. G. (1979) Genetic determinants of borderline conditions. *Schiz. Bull.*, **5**, 59–86

Sigel, I. E. (1963) How intelligence tests limit understanding of intelligence. *Merrill-Palmer Quart.*, **9**, 39–56

Silver, M. A., Bohnert, M., Beck, A. T. & Marcus, D. (1971) Relation of depression to attempted suicide and seriousness of intent. *Arch. gen. Psychiat.*, **25**, 573–6

Silverman, C. (1968) *The Epidemiology of Depression.* Baltimore: Johns Hopkins Press

Simon W. & Wirt, R. (1961) Prognostic factors in schizophrenia. *Am. J. Psychiat.*, **117**, 887

Sims, A., Salmons, P. & Humphreys, P. (1977) Folie à quatre. *Brit. J. Psychiat.*, **130**, 134–6

Singer, M. T., Wynne, L. C. & Toohey, M. L. (1978) Communication disorders and the families of schizophrenics. In *The Nature of Schizophrenia: New Approaches to Research and Treatment*, ed. Wynne, L. C., Cromwell, R. L. & Matthysse, S. New York: Wiley

Sjöström, R. & Roos, B. E. (1972) 5-Hydroxyindolacetic acid and homovanillic acid in cerebrospinal fluid in manic depressive psychosis. *Eur. J. Pharmacol.* **4**, 170–76

Slater, E. (1938) Zur Erbpathologie des manisch-depressiven Irreseins. Die Eltern und Kinder von Manisch-Depressiven. *Z. ges. Neurol. Psychiat.*, **163**, 1–147

— (1935) The incidence of mental disorder. *Ann. Eugen.*, **6**, 172

— (1938) Zur Periodik des manisch-depressiven Irreseins. *Z. ges. Neurol. Psychiat.*, **162**, 794–801

— (1953) *Psychotic and Neurotic Illness in Twins.* Special Reports Service, Medical Research Council, No. 278. London: HMSO

Slater, E., Beard, A. W. & Glithero, E. (1963) The schizophrenic-like psychoses of epilepsy. *Brit. J. Psychiat.*, **109**, 95–150

Slater, E. & Cowie, V. (1971) *Genetics of Mental Disorders*, chap. 2. London: Oxford University Press

Slater, E. & Roth M. (1969) *Clinical Psychiatry.* 3rd ed. New York: Williams & Wilkins

Sloan, W. (1955) The Lincoln-Oseretsky Motor Development Scale. *Genet. Psychol. Monog.*, **51**, 183–252

Sloane, H. N. MacAulay, B. D. (1968) *Operant procedures in remedial speech and language training.* Boston: Houghton Mifflin

Small, J. G. (1968) Epileptiform electro encephalographic abnormalities in mentally ill children. *J. nerv. ment. Dis.*, **147**, 341–8

— (1971) Sensory evoked responses of autistic children. In: *Infantile Autism*, ed. Alpern, G. D. & DeMyer, M. K., pp. 224–42. Springfield, Illinois: Charles C. Thomas

— (1975) EEG and neurophysiological Studies of early infantile autism. *Biol. Psychiat.*, **10**, 385–97

Small, J. G., DeMyer, M. K. & Kendall, J. K. (1969) Experiences with response averaging in autistic children. *Electroenceph. clin. Neurophysiol.*, **26**, 112–3

Small, J. G. & Small, I. (1972) Clinical results: Indoklan versus ECT. *Seminars in Psychiatry*, **4**, 13–26

Small, J. G., Small, I. F., Milstein, V. & Moore, D. F. (1975) Familial associations with EEG variants in manic-depressive disease. *Arch. gen. Psychiat.*, **32**, 43–8

Smeraldi, E., Kidd, K. K., Negri, F., Heimbuch, R. & Melica, A. M. (1979) Genetic studies of affective disorders. In *Biological Psychiatry Today*, ed. Obiols, J., Ballús, E., González Monclús, E., & Pujol, J., pp. 60–65. New York: Elsevier/North-Holland

Smeraldi, E., Negri, F. & Melica, A. M. (1977) A genetic study of affective disorders. *Acta psychiat. scand.*, **56**, 382–98

Smeraldi, E., Negri, F., Melica, A. & Scorza-Smeraldi, R. (1978) HLA system and affective disorders: A sibship genetic study. *Tissue Antigens*, **12**, 270–74

Smeraldi, E., Negri, F., Melica, A., Scorza-Smeraldi, R., Fabio, G., Bonara, P., Bellodi, L., Sacchetti, E., Sabbadini-Villa, M., Cazzullo, C. & Zanussi, C. (1978) HLA typing and affective disorders: A study in the Italian population. *Neuropsychobiol.*, **4**, 344–52

Smith, K., Surphlis, W., Gynther, M. & Shimkunas, A. (1967) ECT-chlorpromazine and chlorpromazine compared in the treatment of schizophrenia. *J. nerv. ment. Dis.*, **144**, 284–90

Snyder, S. H. (1974) *Madness and the brain.* New York: McGraw-Hill

Sommer, R. (1969) *Personal Space: the Behavioural Basis of Design.* New Jersey: Prentice-Hall

Soni, S. D. (1976) Serum creatine phosphokinase in acute psychosis. *Brit. J. Psychiat.*, **128**, 181–3

Spence, M. A., Elston, R. C., Namboodiri, K. K. & Rainer, J. D. (1976) A genetic study of schizophrenia pedigrees. I. Demographic studies: sample distribution, age of onset ascertainment and classification. *Neuropsychobiol., Basel*, **2**, 328–40

Spitzer, R. L. & Endicott, J. (1979) *Schedule for Affective Disorders and Schizophrenia*. 3rd ed. Biometrics Research, New York State Department of Mental Hygiene. New York (Instrument)

Spitzer, R. L., Endicott, J. & Robins, E. (1978) *Research Diagnostic Criteria (RDC) for a Selected Group of Functional Disorders.* 3rd ed. New York: New York State Psychiatric Institute

— (1978) Research diagnostic criteria: Rationale and reliability. *Arch. gen. Psychiat.*, **35**, 773–82

Spokes, E. G. S. (1979) An analysis of factors influencing measurements of dopamine, noradrenaline, glutamate decarboxylase and choline acetylase in human post-mortem brain tissue. *Brain*, **102**, 333–46

Squire, L. R. & Chace, P. M. (1975) Memory functions six to nine months after electroconvulsive therapy. *Arch. gen. Psychiat.*, **32**, 1557–64

Steadman, H. J. (1979) Attempting to protect patients' rights under a medical model. *Int. J. Law Psychiat.*, **2**, 185–97

Steen, R. R. (1933) Prognosis in manic depressive psychosis. *Psychiat. Q.*, **7**, 419–29

Steffy, R. A. & Galbraith, K. (1974) A comparison of segmental set and inhibitory deficit explanations of the crossover pattern in process schizophrenic reaction time. *J. abnorm. Psychol.*, **83**, 227–33

Steinberg, D., Hirsch, S. R., Marston, S. D., Reynolds, K. & Sutton, R. N. P. (1972) Influenza infection causing manic psychosis. *Brit. J. Psychiat.*, **120**, 531–5

Stember, R. & Fieve, R. (1976) Histocompatibility complex in affective disorders. *Scientific proceedings of the 129th Annual Meeting of the American Psychiatric Association*

Stengel, E. (1950) A follow-up investigation of 330 cases treated by prefrontal leucotomy. *J. ment. Sci.*, **96**, 633–62

— (1960) Discussion of paper by G. Langfeldt. *Proc. R. Soc. Med.*, **53**, 1052

— (1972) A survey of follow-up examinations of attempted suicides. *Skandia International Symposia: Suicide and attempted suicide*. Stockholm: Nordiska Bockhandelns Forlag

Stengel, E. & Cook, N. (1958) *Attempted Suicide: Its Social Significance and Effects.* Maudsley Monographs, No. 4. London: Chapman and Hall

Stenstedt, A. (1952) A study in manic depressive psychosis. *Acta psychiat. neurol. scand.*, Supp. 79

— (1959) Involutional melancholia. *Acta psychiat scand.*, **34**, Supp. 127

— (1966) Genetics of neurotic depression. *Acta psychiat. scand.*, **42**, 392–409

Stephens, J. H. (1970) Long-term course and prognosis in schizophrenia. *Seminars in Psychiatry*, **2**, 464–85

Stephens, J. H., Astrup, C. & Mangrum, J. S. (1966) Prognostic factors in recovered and deteriorated schizophrenics. *Am. J. Psychiat.*, **122**, 1116

Stern, K. & Dancey, T. (1942) Glioma of the diencephalon in a manic patient. *Am. J. Psychiat.*, **98**, 716

Sternberg, D. E. & Jarvik, M. E. (1976) Memory functions in depression: Improvement with antidepressant medication. *Arch. gen. Psychiat.*, **33**, 219–24

Stevens, B. (1969) *Marriage and Fertility of Women suffering from Schizophrenia or Affective Disorders.* Maudsley Monographs No. 19. London: Oxford University Press

— (1973) Role of fluphenazine decanoate in lessening the burden of chronic schizophrenics in the community. *Psychol. Med.*, **3**, 141–58

Stevens, J. R. (1973) An anatomy of schizophrenia? *Arch. gen. Psychiat.*, **29**, 177–89

Stevens, J. R. & Milstein, V. (1970) Severe psychiatric disorders of childhood. *Am. J. Dis. Children*, **120**, 182–92

Stone, A. A. & Eldred, S. H. (1959) Delusional formation during the activation of chronic schizophrenic patients. *Arch. gen. Psychiat.*, **1**, 177–9

Stonehill, E., Crisp, A. H. & Koval, J. (1976) The relationship of reported sleep characteristics to psychiatric diagnosis and mood. *Brit. J. med. Psychol.*, **49**, 381–91

Strömgren, E. (1965) Schizophreniform psychoses. *Acta psychiat. scand.*, **41**, 483

— (1974) Psychogenic psychoses. In *Themes and Variations in European Psychiatry*, ed. Hirsch, S. R. & Shepherd, M., p. 97. Bristol: Wright

Strömgren, L. S. (1977) The influence of depression on memory. *Acta psychiat. scand.*, **56**, 109–28

Stubns, E. G. (1978) Autistic symptoms in a child with congenital cytomegalo-virus infection. *J. Autism child. Schiz.*, **8**, 37–43

Student, M. & Sohmer, N. (1978) Evidence from auditory nerve and brainstem evoked responses for an organic brain lesion in children with autistic traits. *J. Autism child. Schiz.*, **8**, 13–20

Stutsman, R. (1931) *Mental Measurement of Pre-school Children.* New York: World Book Company

Sundby, P. & Nyhus, P. (1963) Major and minor psychiatric disorders in males in Oslo. *Acta psychiat. scand.*, **39**, 519–47

Swift, H. M. (1907) The prognosis of insanity of the recurrent type. *Am. J. Insanity*, **64**, 311–26

Symonds, R. L. & Williams, P. (1976) Seasonal variations in the incidence of mania. *Brit. J. Psychiat.*, **129**, 45–8

Szurek, S. A. (1956) Psychotic episodes and psychotic maldevelopment. *Am. J. Ortho-psychiat.*, **26**, 519–43

Taft, L. T. & Cohen, H. J. (1971) Hypsarrhythmia and infantile autism: a clinical report. *J. Autism child. Schiz.*, **1**, 327–36

Tanna, V. & Winokur, G. (1968) A study of association and linkage of ABO blood types and primary affective disorder. *Brit. J. Psychiat.*, **114**, 1175–81

Tanna, V., Go, R., Winokur, G. & Elston, R. (1977) Possible linkage between group-specific component (Gc protein) and pure depressive disease. *Acta psychiat. scand.*, **55**, 111–15

— (1979) Possible linkage between α-Haptoglobin (Hp) and depression spectrum disease. *Neuropsychobiol.*, **5**, 102–13

Tanna, V., Winokur, G., Elston, R. & Go, R. (1976a) A linkage study of depression spectrum disease: The use of the sib-pair method. *Neuropsychobiol.*, **2**, 52–62

— (1976b) A linkage study of pure depressive disease: The use of the sib-pair method. *Biol. Psychiat.*, **11**, 767–71

— (1977b) A genetic linkage study in support of the concept of depression spectrum disease. *Alcoholism: clin. exper. Res.*, **1**, 119–23

Targum, S., Gershon, E., van Eerdewegh, M. & Rogentine, N. (1979) Human leukocyte antigen system not closely linked to or associated with bipolar manic-depressive illness. *Biol. Psychiat.*, **14**, 615–36

Tarrier, N., Vaughn, C., Lader, M. H. & Leff, J. P. (1978) Bodily reactions to people and events in schizophrenics. *Arch. gen. Psychiat.*, **36,** 311–15

Taschev, T. (1965) Statistisches über die Melancholie. *Fortschr. Neurol. Psychiat.*, **33,** 25–36

— (1974) The course and prognosis of depression on the basis of 652 patients deceased. In *Classification and Prediction of Outcome of Depression*, ed. Angst, J. Stuttgart: Schattauer

Taylor, F. K. (1979) *Psychopathology: Its Causes and Symptoms.* 2nd ed. Sunbury-on-Thames: Quartermaine House

Taylor, J. (1976) Language problems and a method of assessment and teaching. In *An Approach to Teaching Autistic Children,* ed. Everard, M. P., pp. 99–119. Oxford: Pergamon Press

Taylor, M. A. T. & Abrams, R. (1973) The phenomenology of mania. *Arch. gen. Psych.*, **29,** 520–2

— (1973) Manic states: a genetic study of early and late onset affective disorders. *Arch. gen. Psychiat.*, **28,** 656–8

Taylor, Lord & Chave, S. (1964) *Mental Health and Environment.* London: Longmans Green

Temoche, A., Pugh, T. & MacMahon, B. (1964) Suicide rates among current and former mental institution patients. *J. nerv. ment. Dis.*, **138,** 124–30

Tennant, C. & Bebbington, P. (1978) The social causation of depression: a critique of the work of Brown and his colleagues. *Psychol. Med.*, **8,** 565–75

Tennant, C., Bebbington, P. & Hurry, J. (1980a) Parental death in childhood and risk of adult depressive disorders: a review. *Psychol. Med.*, **10,** 289–99

Tennant, C., Hurry, J. & Bebbington, P. (1980b) Parent-child separations during childhood. In *Epidemiological Research as a Basis for the Organization of Extramural Psychiatry*, ed. Strömgren, E., Dupont, A. & Nielsen, J. A. Copenhagen: Munksgaard

Terris, M. (1964) (Ed.) *Goldberger on Pellagra.* Baton Rouge: Louisiana State University Press

Tewfik, G. I. (1958) Psychoses in Africa. In *Mental Disorders and Mental Health in Africa South of the Sahara.* Geneva: WHO

Thompson, I. E. (1976) Implications of medical ethics for ethics in general. *J. med. Ethics*, **2,** 74–82

Thomson, K. C. & Hendrie, H. C. (1972) Environmental stress in primary depressive illness. *Arch. gen. Psychiat.*, **26,** 130–32

Tienari, P. (1963) Psychiatric illness in identical twins. *Acta psychiat. neurol. scand.*, Supp. 171

Tilton, J. R. & Ottinger, D. R. (1964) Comparison of toy-play behaviour of autistic, retarded, and normal children. *Psychol. Reports*, **15,** 967–75

Tooth, G. (1950) *Studies in Mental Illness in the Gold Coast.* London: HMSO

Torrey, E. F. (1973a) Is schizophrenia universal? An open question. *Schiz. Bull.*, **7,** 53–9

— (1973b) Slow and latent viruses in schizophrenia. *Lancet*, **ii,** 22–4

Torrey, E. F. & Peterson, M. R. (1974) Schizophrenia and the limbic system. *Lancet*, **ii,** 942–6

— (1976) The viral hypothesis of schizophrenia. *Schiz. Bull.*, **2,** 136–46

Torrey, E. F., Torrey, B. B. & Burton-Bradley, B. G. (1974) The epidemiology of schizophrenia in Papua, New Guinea. *Am. J. Psychiat.*, **131,** 567–73

Torrey, E. F., Torrey, B. B. & Peterson, M. R. (1977) Seasonality of schizophrenic births in the United States. *Arch. gen. Psychiat.*, **34,** 1065–70

Traupman, K. L. (1975) Effects of categorization and imagery on

recognition and recall by process and reactive schizophrenics. *J. abnorm. Psychol.*, **84,** 307–14

Traupman, K. L., Berzofsky, M. & Kesselman, M. (1976) Encoding of taxonomic word categories by schizophrenics. *J. abnorm. Psychol.*, **85,** 350–5

Treffert, D. A. (1970) Epidemiology of infantile autism. *Arch. gen. Psychiat.*, **22,** 431–8

Trevarthen, C. (1974) Conversations with a two-month old. *New Scientist*, **62,** 230–5

Trostorff, S. v. (1968a) Über die hereditäre Belastung bei den zykloiden Psychosen, den unsystematischen und systematischen Schizophrenien. *Psychiat. Neurol. med. Psychol.* (Lpz.), **20,** 98

— (1968b) Über die hereditäre Belastung bei den bipolaren und monopolaren phasischen Psychosen. *Schweiz. Arch. Neurol. Neurochir. Psychiat.*, **102,** 235

Tsuang, M. T. (1978) Suicide in schizophrenics, manics, depressives and surgical controls. *Arch. gen. Psychiat.*, **35,** 153–5

— (1979) Schizoaffective disorder. *Arch. gen. Psychiat.*, **35,** 633–4

Tsuang, M. T. (1978) Familial sub-typing of schizophrenia and affective disorders. In *Critical Issues in Psychiatric Diagnosis,* ed. Spitzer, R. L. & Klein, D. F., pp. 203–11. New York: Raven Press

Tsuang, M. T. & Woolson, R. F. (1978) Excess mortality in schizophrenia and affective disorders. *Arch. gen. Psychiat.*, **35,** 1181–5

Tsuang, M. T., Woolson, R. F. & Fleming, J. A. (1980) Causes of death in schizophrenia and manic-depression. *Brit. J. Psychiat.*, **136,** 239–42

Tubbs, V. K. (1966) Types of linguistic ability in psychotic children. *J. ment. Defic. Res.*, **10,** 230–40

Tuomisto, J. & Tukiainen, E. (1976) Decreased uptake of 5-hydroxytryptoamine in blood platelets from depressed patients. *Nature*, **262,** 596–9

Turek, I. S. (1973) Combined use of ECT and psychotropic drugs – antidepressants and antipsychotics. *Compr. Psychiatry*, **14,** 495–504

Turek, I. S. & Hanlon, T. E. (1977) The effectiveness and safety of electroconvulsive therapy (ECT). *J. nerv. ment. dis.*, **164,** 419–31

Turner, R. J. & Wagenfeld, M. O. (1967) Occupational morbidity in schizophrenia: an assessment of the social causation and social selection hypotheses. *Am. sociol. Rev.*, **32,** 104–13

Tymchuk, A. J., Simmons, J. Q. & Neafsey, S. (1977) Intellectual characteristics of adolescent childhood psychotics with high verbal ability. *J. ment. def. Res.*, **21,** 133–8

Tyrer, P. (1976) Towards rational therapy with monoamine oxidase inhibitors. *Brit. J. Psychiat.*, **128,** 354–60

— (1979) Anxiety states. In *Recent Advances in Clinical Psychiatry,* ed. Granville-Grossman, K., vol. 3, pp. 161–83. Edinburgh: Churchill Livingstone

Tyrell, D. A. J., Crow, T. J., Parry, R. P., Johnstone, E. & Ferrier, I. N. (1979) Possible virus in schizophrenia and some neurological disorders. *Lancet*, **i,** 839–41

Ueno, Y., Aoki, N., Yaluki, T. & Kuraishi, F. (1963) Electrolyte metabolism in blood and cerebrospinal fluid in psychoses. *Folia psychiat. neurol. jap.* **15,** 304–26

Uhlenhuth, E. H., Lipmann, R. S., Balter, M. B. & Stern, M. (1974) Symptom intensity and life stress in the city. *Arch. gen. Psychiat.*, **31,** 759–64

Urstein, M. (1909) *Die Dementia praecox und ihre Stellung zum man-*

isch-depressiven Irresein. Berlin & Wien: Urban & Schwarzenberg

U.S. National Commission for the Protection of Human Subjects of Biomedical and Behavioral Research. (1977) *Report and Recommendations on Psychosurgery*. Department of Health, Education and Welfare Publication No. (OS) 77-0001 Washington, D.C.

Vaillant, G. E. (1962a) The prediction of recovery in schizophrenia. *J. nerv. ment. Dis.*, **135**, 534

— (1962b) Historical notes: John Haslam on early infantile autism. *Am. J. Psychiat.*, **119**, 376

— (1964) An historical review of the remitting schizophrenias. *J. nerv. mental. Dis.*, **138**,48

van Eerdewegh, M., Gershon, E. & van Eerdewegh, P. (1980) X-chromosome threshold models of bipolar manic-depressive illness. *J. psychiat. Res.*, **15**, 215–38

Vanggaard, T. (1979) *Borderlands of Sanity. Neuroses. Schizophrenic Borderline States. Atypical Endogenous Depression*. Copenhagen: Munksgaard

van Krevelen, D. A. (1971) Early infantile autism and autistic psychopathy. *J. Autism child. Schiz.*, **1**, 82–6

van Praag, H. M. (1973) Monoamine metabolism in depression: clinical application of the probenecid test. In *Serotonin and Behaviour*, ed. Barchas, J. & Usdin, E., p. 457. New York: Academic Press

van Praag, H. M. & Korf, J. (1971) Retarded depressions and dopamine metabolism. *Psychopharmacol.*, **19**, 199

van Praag, H. M., Korf, J. & Dols, L. C.W. (1976) Clozapine versus perphanazine: the value of the biochemical mode of action of neuroleptics in predicting their therapeutic activity. *Brit. J. Psychiat.*, **129**, 547–55

van Praag, H. M. & Puite, J. (1970) 5-Hydroxyindolacetic acid levels in the cerebrospinal fluid of depressive patients treated with probenecid. *Nature*, London, **225**, 1259

Vaugn, C. E. & Leff, J. P. (1976) The influence of family and social factors on the course of psychiatric illness: a comparison of schizophrenic and depressed neurotic patients. *Brit. J. Psychiat.*, **129**, 125–37

Venables, P. H. (1964) Input dysfunction in schizophrenia. In *Progress in Experimental Personality Research*, ed. Maher, B., vol. 1. New York: Academic Press

— (1977) The electrodermal physiology of schizophrenia and children at risk for schizophrenia: controversies and developments. *Schiz. Bull.*, **3**, 28–48

— (1978) Cognitive disorder. In *Schizophrenia: Towards a New Synthesis*, ed. Wing, J. K. London: Academic Press

Venables, P. H. & Wing, J. K. (1962) Level of arousal and the subclassification of schizophrenia. *Arch. gen. Psychiat.*, **7**, 114–19

Videbech, T., Weeke, A. & Dupont, A. (1974) Endogenous psychoses and season of birth. *Acta psychiat. scand.*, **50**, 202–18

Wadsworth, M., Butterfield, W. J. H. & Blaney, R. (1971) *Health and Sickness: the Choice of Treatment*. London: Tavistock Publications

Wakabayashi, S. (1979) A case of infantile autism associated with Down's syndrome. *J. Autism Develop. Dis.*, **9**, 31–6

Wålinder, J., Skott, A., Nagy, A., Carlsson, A. & Roos, B. E. (1975) Potentiation of antidepressant action of clomipramine by tryptophan. *Lancet*, **i**, 984

Walk, D. (1967) Suicide and Community Care. *Brit. J. Psychiat.*, **113**, 1381–91

Walker, R. W., Mandel, L. R., Kleinman, J. E., Gillin, J. C., Wyatt,

R. J. & Vandenheuvel, W. J. A. (1979) Improved selective ion monitoring mass-spectrometry assay for the determination of N,N-dimethyltryptamine in human blood utilising capillary column gas chromatography. *J. Chromatog.*, **162**, 539–46

Wansbrough, N. & Cooper, P. (1980) *Open Employment after Mental Illness*. London: Tavistock Publications

Warheit, G. J., Holzer, C. E. & Schwab, J. J. (1973) An analysis of social class and racial differences in depressive symptomatology: a community study. *J. Hlth. soc. Behav.*, **14**, 291–5

Waring, M. & Ricks, D. M. (1965) Family patterns of children who became adult schizophrenics. *J. nerv. ment. Dis.*, **140**, 351–64

Warneke, L. (1975) A case of manic-depressive illness in childhood. *Can. Psychiat. Ass. J.*, **20**, 195–200

Warren, S. A. (1977) Using tests to assess intellectual functioning. In *Research to Practice in Mental Retardation*, ed. Mittler, P. Vol. II. *Education and Training*, pp. 3–11, Baltimore, U.S.A.: University Park Press.

Warren, W. (1965) A study of adolescent psychiatric in-patients and the outcome six or more years later. *J. child Psychol. Psychiat.* **6**, 1–17

Watt, N. F. & Lubensky, A. W. (1976) Childhood roots of schizophrenia. *J. consult. clin. Psychol.*, **44**, 363–75

Watts, C. A. H. (1966) *Depressive Disorders in the Community*. Bristol: John Wright

Watts, C. A. H., Cawte, E. C. & Kuenssberg, E. V. (1964) Survey of mental illness in general practice. *Brit. Med. J.*, **2**, 1351–9

Watzlawick, P., Beavin, J. H. & Jackson, D. (1968) *Pragmatics of Human Communications*. London: Faber

Wechsler, D. (1949) *Wechsler Intelligence Scale for Children*. New York: The Psychological Corporation

— (1955) *The Manual for the Wechsler Adult Intelligence Scale*. New York: The Psychological Corporation

— (1967) *The Manual for the Wechsler Pre-school* and *Primary Scale of Intelligence*. New York: The Psychological Corporation

— (1974) *The Manual for the Wechsler Intelligence Scale for Children-Revised*. New York: The Psychological Corporation

Weckers, W. & Meyer, J.-E. (1977) Zur Schlafstörung in der Manie. *Nervenarzt*, **48**, 557–9

Weckowicz, T. E. & Blewett, D. E. (1959) Size constancy and abstract thinking in schizophrenic patients. *J. ment. Sci.*, **105**, 909–34

Weinberg, S. K. (1965) Cultural aspects of manic-depression in West Africa. *J. Hlth. hum. Behav.*, **6**, 246–53

Weinberger, D. R., Torrey, E. F., Neophytides, A. N. & Wyatt, R. J. (1979a) Lateral ventricle enlargement in chronic schizophrenia. *Arch. gen. Psychiat.*, **36**, 735–9

— (1979b) Structural abnormalities in the cerebral cortex of chronic schizophrenic patients. *Arch. gen. Psychiat.*, **36**, 935–9

Weiner, B. P. & Marvit, R. C. (1977) Schizophrenia in Hawaii: analysis of cohort mortality risk in a multi-ethnic population. *Brit. J. Psychiat.*, **131**, 497–503

Weinstein, M. R. & Fisher, A. (1971) Combined treatment with ECT and antipsychotic drugs in schizophrenia. *Disord. ner. Syst.*, **32**, 801–8

Weiss, J. M. A., Nunez, N. & Schaie, K. W. (1961) Quantification of certain trends in attempted suicide. In *Proc. Third World Congress of Psychiatry*, Montreal, 1236–40

Weissman, M. M. (1972) Casework and pharmacotherapy in treatment of depression. *Soc. Casework*, January 1972, 38–44

Weissman, M. M. & Klerman, G. L. (1977) The chronic depressive in the community: unrecognised and poorly treated. *Compr. Psychiatry*, **18**, 523–32

— (1977) Sex differences and the epidemiology of depression. *Arch. gen. Psychiat.*, **34**, 98–111

Weissman, M. M. & Myers, J. K. (1978) Affective disorders in a U.S. Urban community. *Arch. gen. Psychiat.*, **35**, 1304–11

Weissman, M. M. & Paykel, E. S. (1974) *The Depressed Woman. A Study of Social Relationships.* Chicago: University of Chicago

Weissman, M., Pottenger, M., Kleber, H., Ruben, H. L., Williams, D. & Thompson, W. D. (1977) Symptom patterns in primary and secondary depression. *Arch. gen. Psychiat.*, **34**, 854–62

Wells, C. A. (1973) Electroconvulsive treatment for schizophrenia, a ten year survey. *Compr. Psychiatry*, **14**, 291–8

Welner, A., Welner, Z. & Fishman, R. (1979) The group of schizoaffective and related psychoses. IV. A family study. *Compr. Psychiatry*, **20**, 21–6

Welner, A., Welner, Z. & Leonard, M. A. (1977) Bipolar manic depressive disorder: a reassessment of course and outcome. *Compr. Psychiatry*, **18**, 327–32

Welner, J. & Strömgren, E. (1958) Clinical and genetic studies on benign schizophreniform psychoses based on follow-up. *Acta psychiat. neurol. scand.*, **33**, 377

Welner, Z. (1978) Childhood depression: an overview. *J. nerv. ment. Dis.*, **166**, 588–93

Welner, Z., Welner, A., McCrary, M. A. & Leonard, M. A. (1977) Psychopathology in children of inpatients with depression: a controlled study. *J. nerv. ment. Dis.*, **164**, 408–13

Wender, P. H., Rosenthal, D., Kety, S. S., Schulsinger, F. & Welner, J. (1973) Social class and psychopathy in adoptees. *Arch. gen. Psychiat.*, **28**, 318–25

— (1974) Cross-fostering: a research strategy for clarifying the role of genetic and experiential factors in the etiology of schizophrenia. *Arch. gen. Psychiat.*, **30**, 121–8

Wender, P. H., Rosenthal, D., Rainer, J. D., Greenhill, L. & Sarlin, M. B. (1977) Schizophrenics' adopting parents: psychiatric status. *Arch. gen. Psychiat.*, **34**, 777–84

Wertham, F. I. (1929) A group of benign chronic psychoses: prolonged manic excitements. *Am. J. Psychiat.*, **86**, 17–78

White, P. T., DeMyer, W. & DeMyer, M. (1964) EEG abnormalities in early childhood schizophrenia: a double-blind study of psychiatrically disturbed and normal children during promazine sedation. *Am. J. Psychiat.*, **120**, 950–8

White, J. H. & O'Shanick, G. (1977) Juvenile manic-depressive illness. *Am. J. Psychiat.*, **134**, 1035–6

Whitlock, F. A. (1978) Suicide, cancer and depression. *Brit. J. Psychiat.*, **132**, 269–74

WHO. See World Health Organization

Wijsenbeek, H., Steiner, M. & Goldberg, S. C. (1974) Trifluoperazine: a comparison between regular and high doses. *Psychopharmacol.*, **36**, 147–50

Wing, J. K. (1961) A simple and reliable sub-classification of chronic schizophrenia. *J. ment. Sci.*, **107**, 862

— (1962) Institutionalism in mental hospitals. *Brit. J. soc. clin. Psychol.*, **1**, 38

— (1966) Diagnosis, epidemiology, aetiology. In *Early Childhood Autism*, ed. Wing, J. K. 1st ed. Oxford: Pergamon Press

— (1975) (Ed.) *Schizophrenia from Within*. London: National Schizophrenia Fellowship

— (1977) The management of schizophrenia in the community. In *Psychiatric Medicine*, ed. Usdin, G. New York: Brunner Mazel

— (1978a) Clinical concepts of schizophrenia. In *Schizophrenia: Towards a New Synthesis*, ed. Wing, J. K., pp. 1–30. London: Academic Press

— (1978b) (Ed.) *Schizophrenia: Towards a New Synthesis*. London: Academic Press

— (1978c) *Reasoning about Madness*. London and New York: Oxford University Press

Wing, J. K., Bennett, D. H. & Denham, J. (1964) *The Industrial Rehabilitation of Long-stay Schizophrenic Patients*. Med. Res. Council Memorandum No. 42. London: HMSO

Wing, J. K. & Brown, G. W. (1970) *Institutionalism and Schizophrenia*. London: Cambridge University Press

Wing, J. K., Cooper, J. E. & Sartorius, N. (1974) *Description and Classification of Psychiatric Symptoms*. London: Cambridge University Press

Wing, J. K. & Freudenberg, R. K. (1961) The response of severely ill chronic schizophrenic patients to social stimulation. *Amer. J. Psychiat.*, **118**, 311

Wing, J. K. & Fryers, T. (1976) *Psychiatric Services in Camberwell and Salford: Statistics from the Camberwell and Salford Registers, 1964–74*. MRC Social Psychiatry Unit, Institute of Psychiatry, London

Wing, J. K., Leff, J. & Hirsch, S. H. (1973) Preventive treatment of schizophrenia: some theoretical and methodological issues. In *Psychopathology and Psychopharmacology*, ed. Cole, J. O., Freedman, A. M. & Friedhoff, A. J. Baltimore: Johns Hopkins University Press

Wing, J. K., Mann, S. A., Leff, J. P. & Nixon, J. N. (1978) The concept of a 'case' in psychiatric population surveys. *Psychol. Med.*, **8**, 203–17

Wing, J. K. & Morris, B. (Eds.) (1981) *Handbook of Psychiatric Rehabilitation Pracice*. London: Oxford University Press.

Wing, J. K. & Nixon, J. (1975) Discriminating symptoms in schizophrenia. A report from the international pilot study of schizophrenia. *Arch. gen. Psychiat.*, **32**, 853–9

Wing, J. K. & Olsen, R. (Eds.) (1979) *Social Care for the Mentally Disabled*. London: Oxford University Press

Wing, L. (1966) The diagnosis of early childhood autism. *A.E.P. News Letter*, July 1966, Illustrated Supplement

— (1969) The handicaps of autistic children – a comparative study. *J. child Psychol. Psychiat.*, **10**, 1–40

— (1970) Observations on the psychiatric section of the International Classification of Diseases and the British Glossary of Mental Disorders. *Psychol. Med.*, **1**, 79–85

— (1971) Perceptual and language development in autistic children: A comparative study. In *Infantile Autism: Concepts, Characteristics and Treatment*, ed. Rutter, M. London: Churchill

— (1976) *Children Apart*. London: National Association for Mental Health

— (1976) (Ed.) *Early Childhood Autism*. 2nd ed. Oxford: Pergamon Press

— (1976) Diagnosis, clinical description and prognosis. In *Early Childhood Autism*, ed. Wing, L., 2nd ed., pp. 15–64. Oxford: Pergamon Press

— (1978) Social, behavioural and cognitive characteristics: an epidemiological approach. In *Autism: A Reappraisal of Concepts and Treatment*, ed. Rutter M. & Schopler, E. New York: Plenum Press

— (1979a) Differentiation of retardation and autism from specific communication disorders. *Child: Care, Health and Development*, 5, 57–68

— (1979b) Mentally retarded children in Camberwell (London). In *Estimating Needs for Mental Health Care*, ed. Häfner, H., pp. 107–12. Heidelberg: Springer

— (1980a) *Autistic children: A Guide for Parents*. 2nd ed. London: Constable

— (1980b) Childhood autism and social class: a question of selection? *Brit. J. Psychiat.* 137, 410–17

— (1981a) Language, social and cognitive impairments in autism and severe mental retardation. *J. Autism dev. Disord.* 11, 31–44

— (1981b) Asperger's Syndrome *Psychol. Med.*, 11, 115–29

— (1981c) Sex ratios in early childhood autism and related conditions. *Psychiat. Res.*, 5, 129–37

Wing, L. & Gould, J. (1978) Systematic recording of behaviour and skills of retarded and psychotic children. *J. Autism child. Schiz.*, 8, 79–97

— (1979) Severe impairments of social interaction and associated abnormalities in children: epidemiology and classification. *J. Autism dev. Disord.*, 9, 11–29

Wing, L., Gould, J., Yeates, S. R. & Brierley, L. M. (1977) Symbolic play in severely mentally retarded and in autistic children. *J. child Psychol. Psychiat.*, 18, 167–78

Wing, L. & Wing, J. K. (1971) Multiple impairments in early childhood autism. *J. Autism child. Schiz.* 1, 256–66

Wing, L., Wing, J. K., Griffith, D. & Stevens, B. (1972) An epidemiological and experimental evaluation of industrial rehabilitation of chronic psychotic patients in the community. In *Evaluating a Community Psychiatric Service*, ed. Wing, J. K. & Hailey, A. M. London: Oxford University Press

Wing, L., Yeates, S. R., Brierley, L. M. & Gould, J. (1976) The prevalence of early childhood autism: comparison of administrative and epidemiological studies. *Psychol. med.*, 6, 89–100

Winokur, G. (1973) The types of affective disorders. *J. nerv. ment. Dis.*, 156, 82–96

— (1974) Genetic and clinical factors associated with course in depression. *Pharmakopsychiat. Neuropharmakol.*, 7, 122–6

— (1975) The Iowa 500: Heterogeneity and course in manic-depressive illness (bipolar). *Compr. Psychiatry*, 16, 125–31

— (1976) Duration of illness prior to hospitalisation (onset) in the affective disorders. *Neuropsychobiol.*, 2, 87–93

— (1977) Delusional disorder (paranoia). *Compr. Psychiat.*, 18, 511–21

— (1977) Genetic patterns as they affect psychiatric diagnosis. In *Psychiatric Diagnoses*, ed. Rakoff, V. M., Stancer, H. C. & Kedward, H. B. New York: Brunner/Mazel

— (1978) A survey of the genetics of affective disorders. In *Mood Disorders: The World's Major Public Health Problem*, ed. Ayd, F. J., Jr., chap. 2, pp. 9–21. Baltimore: Ayd Medical Communications

— (1979) Familial (genetic) subtypes of pure depressive disease. *Am. J. Psychiat.*, 136, 911–13

— (1979) Unipolar depression: is it divisible into autonomous subtypes? *Arch. gen. Psychiat.*, 36, 47–52

Winokur, G., Behar, D., vanValkenberg, C. & Lowry, M. (1978) Is a familial definition of depression both feasible and valid? *J. nerv. ment. Dis.*, 166, 764–8

Winokur, G., Cadoret, R., Baker, M. & Dorzab, J. (1975) Depression spectrum disease versus pure depressive disease: some further data. *Brit. J. Psychiat.*, 127, 75–7

Winokur, G., Cadoret, R., Dorzab, J. & Baker, M. (1971). Depressive disease: a genetic study. *Arch. gen. Psychiat.*, 24, 135–44

Winokur, G. & Clayton, P. (1967) Family history studies. I. Two types of affective disorders separated according to genetic and clinical factors. *Rec. Adv. Biol. Psychiatry*, 9, 35–50

Winokur, G., Clayton, P. J. & Reich, T. (1969) *Manic-Depressive Illness*. St. Louis: Mosby

Winokur, G. & Morrison, J. (1973) The Iowa 500: follow-up of 225 depressives. *Brit. J. Psychiat.*, 123, 543–8

Winokur, G. & Pitts, F. N. (1964) Affective disorder: I. Is reactive depression an entity? *J. nerv. ment. Dis.*, 138, 541–7

Winokur, G. & Tanna, V. (1969) Possible role of X-linked dominant factors in manic-depressive disease. *Dis. nerv. Syst.*, 30, 89

Winter, W. D. & Ferreira, A. J. (1967) Interaction process analysis of family decision making, *Family Process*, 6, 155–72

Winter, H., Herschel, M., Propping, P., Friedl, W. & Vogel, F. (1978) A twin study of three enzymes (DβH, COMT, MAO) of catecholamine metabolism. *Psychopharmacol.*, 57, 63–9

Wise, C. D., Baden, M. M. & Stein, L. (1974) Post mortem measurements of enzymes in human brain: evidence of a central noradrenergic deficit in schizophrenia. *J. psychiat. Res.*, 11, 185–98

Wolff, S. & Barlow, A. (1979) Schizoid personality in childhood: a comparative study of schizoid, autistic and normal children. *J. child Psychol. Psychiat.*, 20, 29–46

Wolraich, M., Bzostek, B., Neu, R. L. & Gardner, L. (1970) Lack of chromosome aberrations in autism. *New Eng. J. Med.*, 283, 1231

Woodruff, R. A., Guze, S. B. & Clayton, P. J. (1971) Unipolar and bipolar primary affective disorder. *Brit. J. Psychiat.*, 119, 33–8

Woodruff, R., Pitts, F. N. & Winokur, G. (1964) Affective disorder: II. A comparison of patients with endogenous depressions with and without family history of affective disorder. *J. nerv. ment. Dis.*, 139, 49–52

World Health Organization (1968) *World Health Statistics Report*, 21, No. 6. Geneva: WHO

— (1973) *World Health Statistics Report*, 26, No. 3. Geneva: WHO

— (1973) *Schizophrenia: Report of an International Pilot Study*, vol. 1. Geneva: WHO

— (1975) *Schizophrenia: A Multi-national Study*. Geneva: WHO

— (1976) *World Health Statistics Report*, 29, No. 7. Geneva: WHO

— (1978) *Mental Disorders: Glossary and Guide to their Classification in accordance with ICD9*. Geneva: WHO

— (1979) *Schizophrenia: An International Follow-up Study*. New York: Wiley

Wurst, E. (1976) *Autismus*. Bern: Huber

Wyatt, R. J., Murphy, D. L., Belmaker, R., Cohen, S., Donnelly, C. H. & Pollin, W. (1973) Reduced monoamine oxidase activity in platelets: a possible genetic marker for vulnerability to schizophrenia. *Science*, 179, 916–18

Wyatt, R. J., Potkin, S. G., Gillin, J. C. & Murphy, D. L. (1978) Enzymes involved in phenylethylamine and catecholamine metabolism in schizophrenics and controls. In *Psychopharmacology: A Generation of Progress*, ed. Lipton, M. A., DiMascio, A. & Gillam, K. F., pp. 1083–95. New York: Raven Press

Wyatt, R. J., Potkin, S. G. & Murphy, D. L. (1979) Platelet monoamine oxidase activity in schizophrenia: a review of the data. *Am. J. Psychiat.*, **136**, 377–85

Wykes, T. (1982) A hostel-ward for 'new' long-stay patients: an evaluative study of a 'ward in a house'. In *Long-term Community Care: Experience in a London borough*, ed. Wing, J. K. *Psychol. Med.*, Supp. No. 2

Wynne, L. C., Cromwell, R. L. & Matthysse, S. (1978) (Eds.) *The Nature of Schizophrenia: New Approaches to Research and Treatment*. New York: Wiley

Wynne, L. C., Singer, M. T. & Bartko, J. (1977) Recent research on parental communication. In *Developments in Psychiatric Research*, ed. Tanner, J. M. London: Hodder & Stoughton

Yates, A. J. (1966) Data-processing levels and thought disorder in schizophrenia. *Aust. J. Psychol.*, **18**, 103–17

Yolles, S. F. & Kramer, M. (1969) Vital statistics. In *The Schizophrenic Syndrome*, ed. Bellak, L. & Loeb, L., chap. 3. New York: Grune & Stratton

Young, J. G., Belendiuk, K., Freedman, D. X., Sternstein, G. & Cohen, D. J. (1982a) Hypersertornemia in infantile autism: Clinical studies and biochemical correlates of platelet concentrations of sertonin. Submitted for publication

Young, J. G., Caparulo, B. K., Shaywitz, B. A., Johnson, W. T. & Cohen, D. J. (1977) Childhood autism: cerebrospinal fluid examination and immunoglobulin levels. *J. Am. Acad. child Psychiat.*, **16**, 174–9

Young, J. G. & Cohen, D. J. (1979) The molecular biology of development. In *Basic Handbook of Child Psychiatry*, ed. Ioshpitz, J., pp. 22–62. New York: Basic Books

Young, J. G., Cohen, D. J., Anderson, G. M. & Shaywitz, B. A. (19820b) Neurotransmitter ontogeny as a perspective for studies of child development and pathology. In *The Psychobiology of Childhood: A Profile of Current Issues*, ed. Shopsin, B. & Greenhill, L. New York: Spectrum Publications.

Young, J. G., Cohen, D. J., Brown, S.-L. & Caparulo, B. K. (1978) Decreased urinary free catecholamines in childhood autism. *J. Am. Acad. child Psychiat.*, **17**, 671–8

Young, J. G., Cohen, D. J., Caparulo, B. K., Brown, S.-L. & Maas,

J. W. (1979) Decreased 24-hour urinary MHPG in childhood autism. *Am. J. Psychiat.*, **136**, 1055–7

Young, J. G., Cohen, D. J., Waldo, M. C., Feiz, R. & Roth, J. A. (1980a) Platelet monoamine oxidase activity in children and adolescents with psychiatric disorders. *Schiz. Bull.* **6**, 324–33

Young, J. G., Holliday, J., Lowe, T. L. & Cohen, D. J. (1982c) Developmental changes in thyroxine indices in children and adolescents with autism and other developmental disorders. Submitted for publication.

Young, J. G., Kyprie, R. M., Ross, N. T. & Cohen, D. J. (1980b) Serum dopamine-beta-hydroxylase activity: Clinical applications in child psychiatry. *J. Autism devel. Disord.* **10**, 1–14

Youngerman J. & Canino I. A. (1978) Lithium carbonate use in children and adolescents. *Arch. gen. Psychiat.*, **35**, 216–27

Yule, W., Berger, M., Butler, S., Newham, V. & Tizard, J. (1969) The W.P.P.S.I.: an empirical evaluation with a British sample. *Brit. J. educ. Psychol.*, **39**, 1–13

Yule, W. & Carr, J. (eds.) (1979) *Behaviour Modification with the Mentally Retarded*. London: Croom-Hall

Zahn, T. P. (1964) Autonomic reactivity and behavior in schizophrenia. *Psychiat. Res. Reports*, **1**, 156–73

Zahn, T. P., Rosenthal, D. & Lawlor, W. G. (1968) Electrodermal and heart rate orienting reactions in chronic schizophrenia. *J. psychiat. Res.* **6**, 117–34

Zerbin-Rudin, E. (1967) *Endogene Psychosen in human Genetik*, Thieme ein kurzes Handbuch, vol. 2, ed. Becker, P. E. Stuttgart:

— (1979) Genetics of affective psychoses. In *Origin, Prevention and Treatment of Affective Disorders*, ed. Schon, M. & Strömgren E. London: Academic Press

Zis, A. P. & Goodwin, F. K. (1979) Major affective disorder as a recurrent illness. A critical review. *Arch. gen. Psychiat.*, **36**, 835–9

Zubin, J. (1978) Introduction to Section XII, Onset and Course. In *The Nature of Schizophrenia*, ed. Wynne, L. C., Cromwell, R. L. & Matthysse, S. New York: Wiley

Zubin, J. & Spring, B. (1977) Vulnerability—a new view of schizophrenia. *J. abnorm. Psychol.*, **86**, 103-26

Zubin, J., Sutton, S., Salzinger, K. *et al.* (1961) A biometric approach to prognosis in schizophrenia. In *Epidemiology in the Mental Disorders*, ed. Hoch, P. H. & Zubin, J. New York: Grune & Stratton

Cross-references to other volumes in the series

KEY TO VOLUMES AND CHAPTERS
(e.g. 1.4 indicates vol 1, chapter 4)

CROSS-REFERENCES

In addition to specific references given below, the reader is referred to volumes 1 and 5 for a discussion of the concepts, descriptive and developmental phenomena, principles of classification, diagnosis, assessment and treatment, forensic aspects, and the scientific foundations of psychiatry; to volume 2 for the relationship between mental disorder and somatic illness, and to volume 4 for a review of the neuroses and personality disorders.

(See also the key to volumes and chapters.)

Author index

Subject index

DATE DUE